Fundamentals of
Pharmacology for Paramedics

T0287263

To all those health professionals who have put themselves in harm's way to care for patients in the front lines of the COVID-19 pandemic.

Fundamentals of
Pharmacology
for Paramedics

Edited by

IAN PEATE, OBE, FRCN

Senior Lecturer
University of Roehampton
London, UK

SUZANNE EVANS, PhD

Associate Professor
University of Newcastle Australia
Callaghan, Australia

LISA CLEGG, PhD, MHLTHSC, BHLTHSC

Senior Lecturer
Charles Sturt University
Australia

WILEY Blackwell

This edition first published 2022
© 2022 John Wiley & Sons Ltd

All rights reserved. No part of this publication may be reproduced, stored in a retrieval system or transmitted, in any form or by any means, electronic, mechanical, photocopying, recording or otherwise, except as permitted by law. Advice on how to obtain permission to reuse material from this title is available at http://www.wiley.com/go/permissions.

The right of Ian Peate, Suzanne Evans and Lisa Clegg to be identified as the authors of the editorial material in this work has been asserted in accordance with law.

Registered Offices
John Wiley & Sons, Inc., 111 River Street, Hoboken, NJ 07030, USA
John Wiley & Sons Ltd, The Atrium, Southern Gate, Chichester, West Sussex, PO19 8SQ, UK

Editorial Office
9600 Garsington Road, Oxford, OX4 2DQ, UK

For details of our global editorial offices, customer services and more information about Wiley products, visit us at www.wiley.com.

Wiley also publishes its books in a variety of electronic formats and by print-on-demand. Some content that appears in standard print versions of this book may not be available in other formats.

Limit of Liability/Disclaimer of Warranty
The contents of this work are intended to further general scientific research, understanding and discussion only and are not intended and should not be relied upon as recommending or promoting scientific method, diagnosis or treatment by physicians for any particular patient. In view of ongoing research, equipment modifications, changes in governmental regulations and the constant flow of information relating to the use of medicines, equipment and devices, the reader is urged to review and evaluate the information provided in the package insert or instructions for each medicine, equipment or device for, among other things, any changes in the instructions or indication of usage and for added warnings and precautions. While the publisher and authors have used their best efforts in preparing this work, they make no representations or warranties with respect to the accuracy or completeness of the contents of this work and specifically disclaim all warranties, including without limitation any implied warranties of merchantability or fitness for a particular purpose. No warranty may be created or extended by sales representatives, written sales materials or promotional statements for this work. The fact that an organization, website or product is referred to in this work as a citation and/or potential source of further information does not mean that the publisher and authors endorse the information or services the organization, website or product may provide or recommendations it may make. This work is sold with the understanding that the publisher is not engaged in rendering professional services. The advice and strategies contained herein may not be suitable for your situation. You should consult with a specialist where appropriate. Further, readers should be aware that websites listed in this work may have changed or disappeared between when this work was written and when it is read. Neither the publisher nor authors shall be liable for any loss of profit or any other commercial damages, including but not limited to special, incidental, consequential or other damages.

Library of Congress Cataloging-in-Publication Data

Names: Peate, Ian, editor. | Evans, Suzanne, editor. | Clegg, Lisa, editor.
Title: Fundamentals of pharmacology for paramedics / edited by Ian Peate,
    Suzanne Evans, Lisa Clegg.
Description: Hoboken, NJ : Wiley-Blackwell, 2022. | Includes
    bibliographical references and index.
Identifiers: LCCN 2022000521 (print) | LCCN 2022000522 (ebook) | ISBN
    9781119724285 (paperback) | ISBN 9781119724315 (Adobe PDF) | ISBN
    9781119724322 (epub)
Subjects: MESH: Pharmacology–methods | Emergency Medical Technicians
Classification: LCC RM300 (print) | LCC RM300 (ebook) | NLM QV 704 | DDC
    615.1–dc23/eng/20220119
LC record available at https://lccn.loc.gov/2022000521
LC ebook record available at https://lccn.loc.gov/2022000522

Cover Design: Wiley
Cover Image: © sturti/Getty Images

Set in 9/11pt Myriad by Straive, Pondicherry, India

Printed and bound by CPI Group (UK) Ltd, Croydon CR0 4YY

C9781119724285_010222

Contents

Contributors

Dawn Ball
PGCert ROM, Dip IMC (RCSEd), MCPara. Senior Lecturer University of Cumbria, Enhanced Care Paramedic (Bank) North East Ambulance Service.

Dawn started her medical career in the Royal Army Medical Corps in 1997 where she trained as a combat medical technician. Deploying across the globe in both operational and humanitarian roles, she gained invaluable experience in both trauma and primary care. In 2014 Dawn qualified as a paramedic at the University of Cumbria and has since used her knowledge and experience to help train others in combat casualty care and prehospital emergency care. Dawn has a keen interest in trauma and paediatrics and regularly instructs on several Resuscitation Council UK courses.

Emma Beadle
BSc(Hons), PGCert, MCPara. Advanced Paramedic Practitioner (Urgent Care).

Emma has 20 years' experience with the London Ambulance Service. She started as a qualified ambulance technician and became a paramedic in 2007. In 2011 she joined the Clinical Education department as a training officer with an IHDC instructor qualification. Emma graduated with a degree in paramedic science with emergency care practice in 2012 from the University of Hertfordshire. In 2016 she gained a postgraduate certificate in healthcare education from Anglia Ruskin University. Currently Emma is an advanced paramedic practitioner in urgent care and is studying for a master's in advanced clinical practice at St George's University London.

George Bell-Starr
FdSc, MCPara. Trainee Advanced Clinical Practitioner.

George began his career in paramedicine studying at the University of Worcester before starting with South Western Ambulance Foundation Trust as a newly qualified paramedic in 2017. He has continued to study, focusing particularly on clinical reasoning. His key areas of interest include mentoring, developing paramedic practice and frailty. In late 2020 he began training as an advanced practitioner in primary care within the Mid-Dorset Primary Care Network.

Geoffrey Bench
PGCert Medical Healthcare Education, Dip HE (Emergency Care), CAVA. Clinical Tutor/Driving Instructor, L4CERADI Motorcycle Response Unit/Cycle Response Unit, Paramedic.

Geoff began his ambulance career as an emergency medical technician (EMT) with the London Ambulance Service (LAS) 27 years ago, progressing to paramedic and then emergency care practitioner. Geoff has a passion for motorcycles which culminated in him joining the Motorcycle Response Unit with the LAS. Geoff moved into the education department 7 years ago and still works clinical shifts to maintain the high standards he sets himself.

Lisa Clegg
PhD, MHlthSc, BHlthSc. Senior Lecturer.

Dr Lisa Clegg has worked in healthcare delivery since 1980. After qualifying as a registered nurse, Lisa worked in several different areas within the hospital and aged care settings. From 1998 to 2009 she was employed with Ambulance Tasmania in the roles of paramedic, intensive care paramedic and paramedic educator. Whilst employed as a paramedic educator, Lisa worked with University of Tasmania academics to develop and deliver the Associate Degree in Paramedicine. In 2009 Lisa was appointed senior lecturer in paramedicine at the University of Tasmania where she was part of a team that developed and delivered the Bachelor of Paramedic Practice (BPP). Lisa was course coordinator for the BPP for 2 years. In 2016, Lisa was appointed as a senior lecturer in paramedicine at the University of the Sunshine Coast (USC). Lisa has completed a PhD researching mental healthcare in out-of-hospital practice. In 2021, Lisa commenced employment as a senior lecturer in paramedicine at Charles Sturt University (CSU).

Nigel Conway
MSc, BA (Hons). Cert Ed, RODP, Principal Lecturer, Programme Leader.

Nigel qualified in 1988 as an operating department practitioner initially working in a number of anaesthetic and surgical specialties in Oxford. He went on to develop his clinical career in the Midlands, London and the south coast of the UK. Alongside this Nigel continued to study, leading to roles in clinical practice education, lecturer practitioner and full-time academic employment in higher education, working his way up to principal lecturer. He has a wealth of experience, having lead and taught on a number of undergraduate and postgraduate healthcare programmes including paramedic science, non-medical prescribing, leadership and management and community nurse upskilling projects in the UK and internationally. He has also been involved with professional and regulatory projects and published a number of professional healthcare-focused articles and textbooks as well as undertaking a number of external examiner and clinical advisory roles.

Hayley Croft
BPharm, GCert Diabetes, PhD (Pharmacy), AACP, MPS. Pharmacist – Accredited Consultant.

Hayley began her pharmacy career in Newcastle, New South Wales, Australia, becoming a pharmacist and then accredited consultant pharmacist practising in the primary health sector. She later undertook a postgraduate certificate in diabetes education and management and a PhD in pharmacy which has led to her developing role as a clinician scientist in multimorbidity care with a focus on effective and safe utilisation of pharmacotherapies for complex, chronic patients. She has been delivering clinical pharmacy services to patients living in the community since 2000 and has worked in pharmacy education and research since 2007. Her key areas of interest are cardiometabolic health, disability care and pharmacy practice and education. Hayley has published in international peer-reviewed journals.

Dan Davern
MSc, GDip, BSc, Dip NQEMT-AP, MCPara.

Dan began his career completing a diploma in emergency medical technology – paramedic at the Royal College of Surgeons in Ireland and working as a firefighter/paramedic with a statutory fire, rescue and ambulance service. He later undertook a graduate diploma and master of science in emergency medical science. He is currently a PhD candidate in the field of emergency medicine. Dan currently practises as an advanced paramedic and is registered in both the UK and Ireland. He has worked in education since 2010 and is currently Head of Institution at DX2 in Dublin. His key areas of interest are prehospital airway management and clinical practice guideline development. Dan sits on the NAEMT European Education Committee and Pre-Hospital Emergency Care Council's education and standards committee.

Sarah Dineen-Griffin
PhD, MPharm, GradCertPharmPrac, BBSci, AACPA, AdvPP(II), MPS. Lecturer.

Sarah is a lecturer in health management and leadership at Charles Sturt University, Australia. She has been a research investigator on national and international pharmacy projects and has published in international journals. At an international level, she is an editorial board member for *Pharmacy Practice and Research in Social and Administrative Pharmacy*. Sarah is an executive committee member of the Community Pharmacy Section of the International Pharmaceutical Federation. At a national level, she is Vice President of the Pharmaceutical Society of Australia's New South Wales Branch, and appointed to the Expert Advisory Committee leading the Review of the Australian National Medicines Policy. Sarah was named Early Career Pharmacist of the Year in 2021.

Matt Dixon
MSc, PGCert, BSc (Hons), FdSc, MCPara. Advanced Clinical Practitioner/Bank Specialist Paramedic (Urgent and Emergency Care).

Matt began his career in 2007 as a community first responder, graduating as a paramedic in 2011. He initially worked on ambulances in Wiltshire, UK, providing the normal range of paramedic care, before taking on additional responsibility as a mentor and educator working with new students and developing colleagues. He moved into urgent care in 2016, completing an MSc and working in a senior admission avoidance role within the ambulance service. In 2018 he left to work in general practice in a surgery in Bristol, going on to be one of the first paramedic prescribers in the UK. He has a small portfolio of publications and recently has written on the topic of prescribing for paramedics and pharmacology.

Jennifer Dod
BSc (Hons), FdSc, Paramedic. Lecturer – Paramedic Practice.

Jenny graduated from the University of Sussex in 2006 with a first class honours degree in chemistry. She then worked for 5 years as a research scientist for an Oxfordshire pharmaceutical company. She worked in early-stage drug design and discovery on a variety of clinical projects, including those targeting Alzheimer disease and neuropathic pain via sodium ion channels. In 2011 she joined South Central Ambulance Service as an emergency care assistant. She qualified as an ambulance technician in 2014 and gained a foundation degree in paramedic sciences from Oxford Brookes in 2015. After gaining her paramedic registration, she worked at Kidlington Ambulance Station as a paramedic and clinical mentor. In 2018 she returned to Oxford Brookes to join the paramedic sciences teaching team as a lecturer specialising in pharmacology. She is also a qualified prehospital trauma life support instructor and is currently studying part time for a master's in pharmacology.

Paul Doherty
Paramedic Science (FdSc), Paramedic Science (PGCert), Medical and Healthcare Education (PGCert). Clinical Education Tutor.

Paul has worked for the NHS since 2012 and began his ambulance career with the London Ambulance Service in 2013. After graduating from Teesside University, Paul undertook a PGCert in paramedic science at Hertfordshire University. He has always been passionate about education and enjoyed mentoring paramedic students before deciding to join the clinical education department at the LAS in 2019 in a formal teaching role.

Alastair Dolan
Biomedical Science (BSc), Medical and Heathcare Education (PGCert), Clinical Education Tutor.

Alastair graduated from the University of Sheffield in 2007. He has worked for the London Ambulance Service since 2009, starting as student paramedic and qualifying as a paramedic in 2012. Alastair undertook a PGCert at Anglia Ruskin University in 2019, when he joined the London Ambulance Services Clinical Education Team.

Suzanne Evans
Physiology (BSc), Neuropharmacology (PhD), Associate Professor, Biomedical Sciences.

Suzanne gained her PhD in neuroscience at the University of Wales in 1989 and has been researching and teaching in universities in the UK, USA, the Caribbean, New Zealand and Australia ever since, receiving numerous teaching awards along the way. She has taught human physiology, pathophysiology and pharmacology at undergraduate and postgraduate level for many years and her special interest is teaching and assessing these subjects in health professional degrees.

Michael Fanner
RN(Adult), SCPHN(HV), FHEA, PhD, PGDip, PGCert, BSc (Hons). Senior Lecturer.

Michael graduated in adult nursing (2012) and specialist community public health nursing/health visiting (2013) at King's College London and was awarded a PhD in social policy at the University of Greenwich in 2020. Michael was a main architect of the UK's first MSc in paramedic science (pre-registration) and subsequent module leader for a range of paramedic theory modules. Michael is currently a senior lecturer in specialist community public health nursing at the University of Hertfordshire and is an external examiner for the BSc (Hons) paramedic science programmes at the University of Huddersfield. Michael has research interests in ethically complex social issues in clinical practice and is an associate editor for *Child Abuse Review*.

Deborah Flynn

Doctor of Nursing, MA Medical Education, PGC Academic Practice, BSc (Hons) Health and Social Care, DipHE General Nursing, Registered Nurse (RN), Registered Teacher (NMC), Fellow (FHEA), Senior Lecturer Adult Nursing, Northumbria University.

Deborah became a student nurse in 1986 at BG Alexander Nursing College and Johannesburg General Hospital (now Charlotte Maxeke Johannesburg Academic Hospital) in Johannesburg, South Africa, completing her studies as a registered nurse (general, community health and psychiatry) and midwife in 1990. Deborah worked across the South African public and private sector in general surgical and neuro medical wards. From 1993 to 2002, she worked as a staff nurse. rising to a charge nurse, in Germany and Switzerland in a variety of disciplines. In 2002, she returned to Britain to work as a staff nurse on an acute stroke unit. Entering the educational sector in 2005, Deborah progressed from practice educator to senior lecturer and has taught on both under-graduate and postgraduate programmes. In 2018, she completed her doctorate exploring student nurses' experience of humour use in the clinical setting. Her key interests are clinical skills, humour in clinical care, stroke care, pharmacology and practice supervisor/assessor preparation.

Annette Hand

Prof. Doc (Health), MA, PGDip (CR), Dip HE, RGN. Nurse Consultant/Associate Professor/Clinical Lead – Nursing.

Annette has a clinical academic position and divides her time between three roles. She has worked within the Parkinson's Northumbria Team in the UK for over 23 years, starting as the research associate before obtaining a nurse specialist post. For the past 16 years she has worked as a nurse consultant in Parkinson's. Her main role is to co-ordinate the Parkinson's service, support patients and their families and manage a team of Parkinson's specialist nurses. As an autonomous practitioner she is responsible for diagnosis and management of all stages of Parkinson's. She has worked on and been involved with multiple research studies at a local, national and international level, including non-motor symptoms, sexual dysfunction, information prescriptions and care needs in Parkinson's. Her doctorate focused on understanding carer strain and its relationship to care home placement for people with Parkinson's. Annette was appointed to an associate professor post with Northumbria University in recognition of her research work within the field of Parkinson's. She also has the UK national role of clinical lead for nursing within the Parkinson's UK Excellence Network, as part of the clinical leadership team. This role was developed to support service improvements through education, knowledge exchange and evidence-based practice and support the role of the Parkinson's nurse across the UK.

Ashley Ingram

BSc (Hons), MCPara. Frailty Practitioner.

Ashley began his career with South Western Ambulance Foundation Trust as an ambulance care assistant. Over the space of 7 years he worked his way up to a registered paramedic, training whilst working full time. He worked as an ambulance paramedic for 3 years, during which time he took a keen interest in palliative and end-of-life care. He has recently embarked on a primary care role as a frailty practitioner. Working within a multidisciplinary team, they focus on admission avoidance, with patients who reside in care homes in Dorset, UK. He looks forward to developing this role in the future.

Anthony Kitchener

MSc, PGCert. Paramedic Educationalist.

As a leader within the health and social care network, Ant has held senior management and educationalist positions within the public, voluntary and academic sector. He holds a number of publications, consultancies and award nominations. He is a Master of Science (Education) and a Master of Arts (Educational Leadership) with various other clinical and professional qualifications.

Ricky Lawrence
Clinical Education Tutor.

Ricky has been working in the Clinical Education Standards for the past 2 years. He joined the London Ambulance Service in 1982 after leaving the army, as a qualified ambulance technician working in London, qualifying as a NHSTD registered paramedic in 1990. Since then he has had various roles within the London Ambulance Service and a secondment to the Department of Health Equality and Human Rights Group, as lead adviser on EQIA. He returned in 2007 as Equality and Inclusion Officer until 2016 when due to organisational restructuring, he had a number of short roles in safeguarding and infection prevention control before joining the CES department full time.

Claire Leader
RN, RM, PGCAP, MA, BSc (Hons), FHEA. Senior Lecturer.

Claire qualified as a registered nurse from York University in 1998 after which she moved to Leeds, working in cardiothoracic surgery and emergency nursing. In 2003 she commenced her midwifery education at Huddersfield University where she was awarded a first class BSc (Hons). Working initially at Sheffield Teaching Hospitals, she later moved to the North East where she commenced her role as a staff midwife before moving into the area of research as a research nurse and midwife. She was awarded a distinction for her MA in sociology and social research at Newcastle University in 2012. Claire moved to Northumbria University in 2018 and is now a senior lecturer and programme lead for pre-registration nursing programmes, while also studying for her PhD in the area of nurse and midwife wellbeing.

Tom Mallinson
BSc (Hons), MBChB, PGCHE, MRCGP(2020), MCPara, MCoROM, FAWM, FHEA, FRGS. Prehospital Doctor, Rural Generalist, Responder Support Clinician.

Tom began his career in London, undertaking the IHCD ambulance aid and paramedic qualifications alongside a Bachelor's degree in paramedic science at the University of Hertfordshire. After working as a paramedic for the London Ambulance Service NHS Trust, he attended Warwick Medical School to qualify as a medical practitioner. He continued his studies with postgraduate qualifications in healthcare education, wilderness medicine and primary care. Tom has published a variety of primary research and educational resources and is a member of the editorial board for the *Journal of Paramedic Practice*.

Jason McKenna
BSc, GDip, DipNQEMT AP. Advanced Paramedic Supervisor.

Jason began his prehospital career as an emergency medical technician within the private ambulance services in Ireland. In 2011 he joined the National Ambulance Service as a student paramedic, graduating from University College Dublin (UCD) with a diploma in emergency medical technology. In 2015 he continued his education as part of the Bachelor degree programme in paramedic studies at the University of Limerick. He subsequently joined the advanced paramedic programme, graduating from UCD in 2018 with a graduate diploma in emergency medical science. He is also a graduate of the University of South Wales where he studied Acute Medicine. He is a registered assistant tutor with PHECC and is involved with training and education of all levels of prehospital care from community first responder to paramedic. His interests lie in prehospital education and research.

Ian Peate
OBE, FRCN. Visiting Professor of Nursing, St George's University of London and Kingston University London; Visiting Professor, Northumbria University; Visiting Senior Clinical Fellow, University of Hertfordshire, and Editor-in-Chief of the British Journal of Nursing. Senior Lecturer University of Roehampton.

Ian began his nursing career at Central Middlesex Hospital, becoming an enrolled nurse practising in an intensive care unit. He later undertook 3 years' student nurse training at Central Middlesex and Northwick Park Hospitals, becoming a staff nurse and then a charge nurse. He has worked in nurse education since 1989. His key areas of interest are nursing practice and theory. Ian has published widely. He is editor in chief of the *British Journal of Nursing*, founding consultant editor of the *Journal* of *Paramedic Practice* and editorial board member of the *British Journal of Healthcare Assistants*. Ian was awarded an OBE in the Queen's 90th Birthday Honours List for his services to nursing and nurse education and was granted a fellowship from the Royal College of Nursing in 2017.

Liam Rooney
BSc (Hons), GDip, DipNQEMT-AP. Assistant Tutor.

Liam has worked as a firefighter/paramedic with Dublin Fire Brigade since 2007, where he completed his diploma in emergency medical technology – paramedic with the Royal College of Surgeons, Ireland. In 2016 he completed a BSc (Hons) in paramedic studies at the University of Limerick, winning the Graduate Entry Medical School Award for overall performance. In 2017, he undertook a graduate diploma in emergency medical science through University College Dublin. Liam currently practises as an advanced paramedic in Ireland. In 2017, he joined the faculty of DX2, where he delivers multiple courses in prehospital education. He has a keen interest in geriatric medicine and pain management in dementia patients.

Fraser D. Russell
BSc (Deakin), PhD (Univ. Melb.). Associate Professor, University of the Sunshine Coast, Queensland, Australia.

Fraser's PhD investigating the regulation of cardiac beta-adrenoceptors was awarded by the University of Melbourne in 1994. A series of successful postdoctoral appointments followed at the University of Cambridge, UK (1995–1998), University of Otago, NZ (1998–2000) and University of Queensland, Australia (2000–2004). Fraser's research interests have focused on providing a better understanding of the intracellular trafficking and cardiovascular function of endothelin-1, urotensin II and glial cell line-derived neurotrophic factor. Since taking a faculty position at the University of the Sunshine Coast (2005–), Fraser has developed a research programme in natural product therapies, with a focus on providing new ideas for the management of patients with abdominal aortic aneurysm and aberrant wound healing responses, where there are limited pharmacological treatment options.

Emma Senior
MSc Academic and Professional Learning, BSc (Hons) Promoting Practice Effectiveness (Public Health/Health Visiting), DipHE Nursing Studies (Adult), Registered Nurse (RN), Registered Specialist Community Public Health Nurse (SCPHN), Registered Teacher (NMC), Fellow (FHEA). Senior Lecturer, Northumbria University.

Emma is an NMC registered teacher, nurse and health visitor with over 10 years of experience in the NHS and 10 years teaching experience with Northumbria University. She began her nurse career in theatres specialising in women's and children's health before qualifying as a health visitor in 2006. She then went on to work as a sexual health advisor across North Yorkshire where she was able to work collaboratively with a range of services and organisations which included the military, primary care and secondary education. Emma joined higher education in 2009, taking her first post as a senior lecturer/practitioner implementing a workforce development initiative called Northumbria Integrated Sexual Health Education (NISHE) for postqualified nurses across County Durham and Darlington and then project managed delivery across the south west of England with the University of West England. This involved the development and delivery of e-learning educational materials along with supporting academic staff and students in their practice setting. In 2012, Emma joined the pre-registration nurse team where she has been able to introduce, develop and co-ordinate e-learning packages on the programme. Along with teaching pre-registration healthcare, Emma has maintained her postregistration nurse teaching within sexual health, safeguarding and public health within the Specialist Community Public Health Nurse programme. During her time at Northumbria University, Emma was part of the workforce development team working in collaboration with external partners to create education packages to develop the workforce. In 2015, Emma became involved with and is programme lead for Northumbria University's innovative programme for professional non-surgical aesthetic practice which has been a trailblazer nationally. Emma's key areas of interest are public health, sexual health, military families and technology-enhanced learning. She has published widely in journals and is a fellow of the Higher Education Academy.

Lena Solanki
DipHe Paramedic Practice. Paramedic Clinical Tutor.

Lena's career began in 1998 with the Lancashire Ambulance Service as a call taker. After a brief spell adjusting to life as a new mum, she started training with the London Ambulance Service in 2010 as a student paramedic. She joined the clinical education and standards department in 2018 and trained as a clinical tutor, achieving her teaching qualification in 2020. Lena has enjoyed her career with the London Ambulance Service and finds it immensely rewarding. Lena likes to help others especially during their times of need and supports them in achieving their goals.

Tanya Somani
MSc. Registered Paramedic.

Tanya began her career in paramedicine in 2008 practising in metropolitan and regional NSW Australia. Tanya completed a Bachelor Paramedicine (University of Tasmania) and undertook volunteer work in Papua New Guinea. She developed an interest in infection control, attaining a graduate certificate in clinical redesign (University of Tasmania), with a focus on environmental cleaning of ambulances, and an infection prevention and control qualification from the Australian College of Infection Prevention and Control. Tanya worked as part of the Sydney Metropolitan Ambulance Infrastructure program as program manager for the Make Ready Model and as station officer. Tanya has been the recipient of the Safety Thinker Award 2021 for NSW Ambulance, International Woman of the Year award 2021 from Council Ambulance Authorities and received a Commissioner Citation in 2021. Currently she is health relationship manager for NSW Ambulance. Tanya is passionate about patient and paramedic safety with a focus on systems improvement and project management.

Olivia Thornton
BEnvSc, Dip Pre-hospital Care, MPharm (Dist), AACPa, MSHPA. Pharmacist – Accredited Consultant.

Olivia began her career as a paramedic with the New South Wales Ambulance Service. During her 10 years of service as a paramedic, she worked at multiple sites in NSW, including metropolitan and regional areas. Olivia undertook a master's in pharmacy through the University of Newcastle, graduating with distinction. Her pharmacy career has included working in community pharmacy, hospital pharmacy, consultancy work and as a clinical associate lecturer for an undergraduate pharmacy program. She has an interest in improving medication safety for people with complex chronic health conditions throughout their medical journey, including during hospital admissions, aged care/disability care or at home. Her clinical interest areas are pre- and postsurgical admission, diabetes, Parkinson disease and mental health pharmacology.

Charlotte White
BSc (Hons) Paramedic Science and PGCert Medical Healthcare Education. Education Centre Manager.

Charlotte has worked in paramedicine since 2012. Previously, she worked within a learning disability and dementia setting, then moved into clinical settings in numerous hospitals. Charlotte has enjoyed mentoring students during her operational duties, which sparked her passion to move into a formal education working environment, where she is currently undertaking a secondment. Charlotte enjoys the dynamic and challenging work education can bring, always striving for continuous developmental practice.

Dean Whiting
RN, BN (Hons), BSc (Hons), PgCAP, PgDip(ACP), MSc, FHEA. Principal Lecturer in Advanced Clinical Practice, University of Hertfordshire. Advanced Clinical Practitioner, Berryfields Medical Centre, Buckinghamshire. Advanced Clinical Practitioner, London Scottish RFC.

Dean began his career in the British Army as a combat medical technician and then studied at the Royal Centre for Defence Medicine and the University of Portsmouth to become a registered nurse. During his time in the military, he mainly specialised in trauma and critical care nursing and was fortunate enough to work all over the UK and around the world. Since 2012, Dean has worked in higher education and pursued a clinical career in general practice and sports nursing. He now leads the MSc in Advanced Clinical Practice at the University of Hertfordshire.

Carol Wills

MSc Multidisciplinary Professional Development and Education, PGDip Advanced Practice, Bsc (Hons) Specialist Community Public Health Nursing (SCPHN) (Health Visiting), DipHE Adult Nursing, Registered Nurse (RN), Enrolled Nurse (EN), Registered Health Visitor (HV), Community Practitioner Prescriber (NP), Registered Lecturer/Practice Educator (RLP), Senior Fellow (SFHEA), Subject and Programme Leader Non-Medical Prescribing at Northumbria University.

Carol began her career undertaking enrolled nurse training in 1983 at Hexham Hospital in Northumberland. She then worked within neurotrauma at Newcastle General Hospital and then for several years in coronary care and intensive care at Hexham Hospital. This experience and additional training to complete registered nurse qualification then stimulated her to focus on primary care and prevention of ill health. Carol worked as a practice nurse and nurse practitioner in Newcastle city centre and as a staff nurse within Northumberland community nursing teams before going on to complete a health visiting degree and working in Newcastle as a health visitor for several years. During this time, she undertook several leadership and teaching roles including immunisation training co-ordinator, community practice teacher and trust lead mentor. Carol has been a senior lecturer at Northumbria University since 2002 and has led several postgraduate professional programmes including MSc Education in Professional Practice (NMC Teacher programme), PGDip SCPHN and the Non-Medical Prescribing programme. She has also undertaken national roles including Policy Advice Committee member and Treasurer for the UK Standing Conference SCPHN Education and subject expert for several quality approval panels and external examiner roles. Her key areas of interest and research are around developing learning and teaching and advanced level practice.

Barbara C. Wimmer

BPharm (Hons), MSc (Clin Pharm), PhD. Lecturer.

Barbara brings together experience in community and hospital pharmacy and clinical research in Europe and in Australia. She worked in community pharmacies as pharmacist in charge and is an approved hospital pharmacist. Barbara has experience teaching pharmacology to nursing students and oversaw quality assurance in a hospital setting in Austria. Following on from her master of clinical pharmacy at the University of Strathclyde, Scotland, she returned to Steyr Hospital in Austria to lead the service for drugs information and clinical pharmacy. Barbara's PhD studies at Monash University in Melbourne focused on factors associated with medication regimen complexity. She joined the University of Tasmania in 2016 and teaches clinical pharmacokinetics to undergraduate students.

Paul Younger

MClinRes, PGCert (Medical Ultrasound), PGCE, BSc(Hons), BA(Hons), DipPUC, FCPara. Advanced Paramedic Practitioner. North East Ambulance Service.

Paul joined the North East Ambulance Service in 2002, completing his paramedic training in 2005. He has a master's in clinical research from Newcastle University, a PGCE, and a postgraduate qualification in medical ultrasound. He studied non-medical prescribing at Northumbria University, becoming one of the first paramedics in the UK to complete their training. He works clinically as an advanced practitioner for the North East Ambulance Service. A member of the College of Paramedics council and board since 2010, he has held various posts including regional and alternative regional representative for the North East, vice and deputy chair before being appointed as vice president in 2021. For his work with the profession and the college, Paul was made a fellow of the College of Paramedics in 2016. He has presented on paramedic practice at conferences around the world, including the UK, USA, Canada, Australia, Finland and The Netherlands.

Preface

The key aim of *Fundamentals of Pharmacology for Paramedics* is to provide the reader with an understanding of the essentials associated with pharmacology and paramedic practice so as to enhance patient safety and patient outcomes. This book can help readers improve and expand their expertise and self-confidence within the field of paramedicine and enable them to recognise and respond appropriately to the needs of those they offer care and support to, wherever this may be. The contributors to the text are all experienced clinicians and academics who have expertise in their sphere of practice.

Pharmacology is the study of how drugs, medicines and substances work together with the body when they are being used for the management of illness, disease, pain relief and other conditions. This can be everything from drugs that are used in respiratory care to the action of medications used as a vaccine.

The paramedic scope of practice at the point of registration continues to be developed within pre-registration programmes of study around the world, ensuring that the newly qualified paramedic has the required knowledge and skills to provide best practice healthcare to patients. In many countries, this also includes ensuring that pre-registration paramedic students are 'prescriber ready' once they have successfully completed their undergraduate programme of study.

If undergraduate paramedic students are to offer care that is safe and effective, then they must be prepared in such a way that they become accountable practitioners who are able to carry out their role in a meaningful manner that adheres to professional standards and aligns with the law. *Fundamentals of Pharmacology for Paramedics* will help paramedics add to their repertoire of skills as they gain appropriate pharmacological knowledge. Whilst there is a need to ensure that emphasis is placed on the principles of safe drug administration in undergraduate curricula, there is also a need to ensure that students are provided with the pharmacological foundations associated with the bigger issues related to medicines management. Knowing how to study this subject effectively is about developing an effective workable learning strategy. *Fundamentals of Pharmacology for Paramedics* provides the reader with an overview of the key issues that can support them as they begin to understand and apply the complexities associated with pharmacology as well as the exciting challenges that are ahead of them.

The text integrates comprehensive knowledge of pharmacology enabling the reader to formulate a plan of care that can improve the overall health and wellbeing of the patient. When advising on and dispensing or administering medicines, this must be done within the limits of the individual's education, training and competence, professional body guidance and other relevant policies and regulations. It is essential to ensure that you keep to the laws of the country in which you are practising.

The paramedic must know the names, mechanism of action, indications, contraindications, complications, routes of administration, side-effects, interactions, dose and any specific administration considerations for a range of medications. They have to understand relevant pharmacology as well as the administration of therapeutic medications.

The chapters in this book offer a range of teaching and learning resources that can help you come to terms with the often complex area of pharmacology and paramedicine. The book can be used in a number of ways; for example, you may choose to read Chapters 1–7 first and then dip in and out of the remaining chapters as you need them. Trying to learn everything at once has the potential to cause confusion which can eventually result in a loss of confidence, affecting your ability to learn and assimilate. Avoid trying to learn large volumes of information and copious amounts of detail all at once; focus instead on only those details that can help you achieve your aims.

Often pharmacology modules, as part of the wider curriculum, will require the student to safely administer the appropriate medication, correctly monitor medicated patients in accordance with established protocols/policy, understand the drug's mechanism of action, indication for use, routes of administration, how the drug is absorbed, distributed, metabolised and eliminated, contraindications, drug interactions and a lot more. Recognising each drug you use and learning the differences and similarities between drugs is key to understanding the fundamentals of pharmacology. Pharmacology is an important subject and it is vital that you effectively learn the various drugs, their categories, mechanisms of action, pharmacodynamics and pharmacokinetics. The 17 chapters in this book will help you come to terms with what is often seen as a complex and sometimes terrifying subject.

The paramedic scope of practice at the point of registration continues to be developed within pre-registration programmes of study, ensuring that the newly qualified paramedic is fit for practice. The scope of practice for specialist, advanced and consultant paramedics is being defined and refined around the world. A sound understanding of the fundamentals of pharmacology related to paramedicine will help you attain the goals that you set today.

We hope you enjoy using this book as you develop personally and professionally. Having a detailed understanding of how drugs work and why they are given has the potential to help you become a great paramedic.

Ian Peate, London, UK
Suzanne Evans, Newcastle, New South Wales, Australia
Lisa Clegg, New South Wales, Australia

Acknowledgements

Ian wishes to thank his partner Jussi Lahtinen for his unfailing encouragement and Mrs Frances Cohen for her ongoing support.

Suzanne would like to thank everyone who has contributed to the writing of this text at such a difficult time for health professionals.

Lisa wishes to thank her wife Jennie for her ongoing love and support.

Prefixes, suffixes and abbreviations

Prefix: A prefix is positioned at the beginning of a word to modify or change its meaning. Pre means 'before'. Prefixes may also indicate a location, number, or time.

Suffix: The ending part of a word that changes the meaning of the word.

Prefix or suffix	Meaning	Example(s)
a-, an-	not, without	analgesic, apathy
ab-	from; away from	abduction
abdomin(o)-	of or relating to the abdomen	abdomen
acous(io)-	of or relating to hearing	acoumeter, acoustician
acr(o)-	extremity, topmost	acrocrany, acromegaly, acroosteolysis, acroposthia
ad-	at, increase, on, toward	adduction
aden(o)-, aden(i)-	of or relating to a gland	adenocarcinoma, adenology, adenotome, adenotyphus
adip(o)-	of or relating to fat or fatty tissue	adipocyte
adren(o)-	of or relating to adrenal glands	adrenal artery
-aemia	blood condition	anaemia
aer(o)-	air, gas	aerosinusitis
-aesthesi(o)-	sensation	anaesthesia
alb-	denoting a white or pale colour	albino
-alge(si)-	pain	analgesic
-algia, -alg(i)o-	pain	myalgia
all(o-)	denoting something as different, or as an addition	alloantigen, allopathy
ambi-	denoting something as positioned on both sides	ambidextrous
amni-	pertaining to the membranous fetal sac (amnion)	amniocentesis
ana-	back, again, up	anaplasia
andr(o)-	pertaining to a man	android, andrology
angi(o)-	blood vessel	angiogram
ankyl(o)-, ancyl(o)-	denoting something as crooked or bent	ankylosis
ante-	describing something as positioned in front of another thing	antepartum
anti-	describing something as 'against' or 'opposed to' another	antibody, antipsychotic
arteri(o)-	of or pertaining to an artery	arteriole, arterial

Prefix or suffix	Meaning	Example(s)
arthr(o)-	of or pertaining to the joints, limbs	arthritis
articul(o)-	joint	articulation
-ase	enzyme	lactase
-asthenia	weakness	myasthenia gravis
ather(o)-	fatty deposit, soft gruel-like deposit	atherosclerosis
atri(o)-	an atrium (especially heart atrium)	atrioventricular
aur(i)-	of or pertaining to the ear	aural
aut(o)-	self	autoimmune
axill-	of or pertaining to the armpit (uncommon as a prefix)	axilla
bi-	twice, double	binary
bio-	life	biology
blephar(o)-	of or pertaining to the eyelid	blepharoplast
brachi(o)-	of or relating to the arm	brachium of inferior colliculus
brady-	'slow'	bradycardia
bronch(i)-	bronchus	bronchiolitis obliterans
bucc(o)-	of or pertaining to the cheek	buccolabial
burs(o)-	bursa (fluid sac between the bones)	bursitis
carcin(o)-	cancer	carcinoma
cardi(o)-	of or pertaining to the heart	cardiology
carp(o)-	of or pertaining to the wrist	carpal tunnel
-cele	pouching, hernia	hydrocele, varicocele
-centesis	surgical puncture for aspiration	amniocentesis
cephal(o)-	of or pertaining to the head (as a whole)	cephalalgy
cerebell(o)-	of or pertaining to the cerebellum	cerebellum
cerebr(o)-	of or pertaining to the brain	cerebrology
chem(o)-	chemistry, drug	chemotherapy
cholecyst(o)-	of or pertaining to the gallbladder	cholecystectomy
chondr(i)o-	cartilage, gristle, granule, granular	chondrocalcinosis
chrom(ato)-	colour	haemochromatosis
-cidal, -cide	killing, destroying	bacteriocidal
cili-	of or pertaining to the cilia, the eyelashes	ciliary
circum-	denoting something as 'around' another	circumcision
col(o)-, colono-	colon	colonoscopy
colp(o)-	of or pertaining to the vagina	colposcopy
contra-	against	contraindicate
coron(o)-	crown	coronary
cost(o)-	of or pertaining to the ribs	costochondral
crani(o)-	belonging or relating to the cranium	craniology

Prefix or suffix	Meaning	Example(s)
-crine, -crin(o)-	to secrete	endocrine
cry(o)-	cold	cryoablation
cutane-	skin	subcutaneous
cyan(o)-	denotes a blue colour	cyanosis
cyst(o)-, cyst(i)-	of or pertaining to the urinary bladder	cystotomy
cyt(o)-	cell	cytokine
-cyte	cell	leukocyte
-dactyl(o)-	of or pertaining to a finger, toe	dactylology, polydactyly
dent-	of or pertaining to teeth	dentist
dermat(o)-, derm(o)-	of or pertaining to the skin	dermatology
-desis	binding	arthrodesis
dextr(o)-	right, on the right side	dextrocardia
di-	two	diplopia
dia-	through, during, across	dialysis
dif-	apart, separation	different
digit-	of or pertaining to the finger (rare as a root)	digit
-dipsia	suffix meaning '(condition of) thirst'	polydipsia, hydroadipsia, oligodipsia
dors(o)-, dors(i)-	of or pertaining to the back	dorsal, dorsocephalad
duodeno-	duodenum	duodenal atresia
dynam(o)-	force, energy, power	hand strength dynamometer
-dynia	pain	vulvodynia
dys-	bad, difficult, defective, abnormal	dysphagia, dysphasia
ec-	out, away	ectopia, ectopic pregnancy
-ectasia, -ectasis	expansion, dilation	bronchiectasis, telangiectasia
ect(o)-	outer, outside	ectoblast, ectoderm
-ectomy	denotes a surgical operation or removal of a body part; resection, excision	mastectomy
-emesis	vomiting condition	haematemesis
encephal(o)-	of or pertaining to the brain; also see cerebr(o)-	encephalogram
endo-	denotes something as 'inside' or 'within'	endocrinology, endospore
enter(o)-	of or pertaining to the intestine	gastroenterology
epi-	on, upon	epicardium, epidermis, epidural, episclera, epistaxis
erythr(o)-	denotes a red colour	erythrocyte
ex-	out of, away from	excision, exophthalmos
exo-	denotes something as 'outside' another	exoskeleton
extra-	outside	extradural haematoma
faci(o)-	of or pertaining to the face	facioplegic
fibr(o)	fibre	fibroblast

Prefix or suffix	Meaning	Example(s)
fore-	before or ahead	forehead
fossa	a hollow or depressed area; trench or channel	fossa ovalis
front-	of or pertaining to the forehead	frontonasal
galact(o)-	milk	galactorrhoea
gastr(o)-	of or pertaining to the stomach	gastric bypass
-genic	formative, pertaining to producing	cardiogenic shock
gingiv-	of or pertaining to the gums	gingivitis
glauc(o)-	denoting a grey or bluish-grey colour	glaucoma
gloss(o)-, glott(o)-	of or pertaining to the tongue	glossology
gluco-	sweet	glucocorticoid
glyc(o)-	sugar	glycolysis
-gnosis	knowledge	diagnosis, prognosis
gon(o)-	seed, semen; also, reproductive	gonorrhoea
-gram, -gramme	record or picture	angiogram
-graph	instrument used to record data or picture	electrocardiograph
-graphy	process of recording	angiography
gyn(aec)o-	woman	gynaecomastia
haemangi(o)-	blood vessels	haemangioma
haemat(o)-, haem-	of or pertaining to blood	haematology
halluc-	to wander in mind	hallucinosis
hemi-	one-half	cerebral hemisphere
hepat- (hepatic-)	of or pertaining to the liver	hepatology
heter(o)-	denotes something as 'the other' (of two), as an addition, or different	heterogeneous
hist(o)-, histio-	tissue	histology
home(o)-	similar	homeopathy
hom(o)-	denotes something as 'the same' as another or common	homosexuality
hydr(o)-	water	hydrophobe
hyper-	denotes something as 'extreme' or 'beyond normal'	hypertension
hyp(o)-	denotes something as 'below normal'	hypovolaemia
hyster(o)-	of or pertaining to the womb, the uterus	hysterectomy
iatr(o)-	of or pertaining to medicine, or a physician	iatrogenic
-iatry	denotes a field in medicine of a certain body component	podiatry, psychiatry
-ics	organised knowledge, treatment	obstetrics
ileo-	ileum	ileocaecal valve
infra-	below	infrahyoid muscles
inter-	between, among	interarticular ligament

Prefix or suffix	Meaning	Example(s)
intra-	within	intramural
ipsi-	same	ipsilateral hemiparesis
ischio-	of or pertaining to the ischium, the hip joint	ischioanal fossa
-ismus	spasm, contraction	hemiballismus
iso-	denoting something as being 'equal'	isotonic
-ist	one who specialises in	pathologist
-itis	inflammation	tonsillitis
-ium	structure, tissue	pericardium
juxta- (iuxta-)	near to, alongside or next to	juxtaglomerular apparatus
karyo-	nucleus	eukaryote
kerat(o)-	cornea (eye or skin)	keratoscope
kin(e)-, kin(o)-, kinesi(o)-	movement	kinaesthesia
kyph(o)-	humped	kyphoscoliosis
labi(o)-	of or pertaining to the lip	labiodental
lacrim(o)-	tear	lacrimal canaliculi
lact(i)-, lact(o)	milk	lactation
lapar(o)-	of or pertaining to the abdomen wall, flank	laparotomy
laryng(o)-	of or pertaining to the larynx, the lower throat cavity where the voice box is	larynx
latero-	lateral	lateral pectoral nerve
-lepsis, -lepsy	attack, seizure	epilepsy, narcolepsy
lept(o)-	light, slender	leptomeningeal
leuc(o)-, leuk(o)-	denoting a white colour	leukocyte
lingu(a)-, lingu(o)-	of or pertaining to the tongue	linguistics
lip(o)-	fat	liposuction
lith(o)-	stone, calculus	lithotripsy
-logist	denotes someone who studies a certain field	oncologist, pathologist
log(o)-	speech	logopaedics
-logy	denotes the academic study or practice of a certain field	haematology, urology
lymph(o)-	lymph	lymphoedema
lys(o)-, -lytic	dissolution	lysosome
-lysis	destruction, separation	paralysis
macr(o)-	large, long	macrophage
-malacia	softening	osteomalacia
mammill(o)-	of or pertaining to the nipple	mammillitis
mamm(o)-	of or pertaining to the breast	mammogram
manu-	of or pertaining to the hand	manufacture

Prefix or suffix	Meaning	Example(s)
mast(o)-	of or pertaining to the breast	mastectomy
meg(a)-, megal(o)-, -megaly	enlargement, million	splenomegaly, megameter
melan(o)-	black colour	melanin
mening(o)-	membrane	meningitis
meta-	after, behind	metacarpus
-meter	instrument used to measure or count	sphygmomanometer
metr(o)-	pertaining to conditions of the uterus	metrorrhagia
-metry	process of measuring	optometry
micro-	denoting something as small, or relating to smallness	microscope
milli-	thousandth	millilitre
mon(o)-	single	infectious mononucleosis
morph(o)-	form, shape	morphology
muscul(o)-	muscle	musculoskeletal system
my(o)-	of or relating to muscle	myoblast
myc(o)-	fungus	onychomycosis
myel(o)-	of or relating to bone marrow or spinal cord	myeloblast
myri-	ten thousand	myriad
myring(o)-	eardrum	myringotomy
narc(o)-	numb, sleep	narcolepsy
nas(o)-	of or pertaining to the nose	nasal
necr(o)-	death	necrosis, necrotising fasciitis
neo-	new	neoplasm
nephr(o)-	of or pertaining to the kidney	nephrology
neur(i)-, neur(o)-	of or pertaining to nerves and the nervous system	neurofibromatosis
normo-	normal	normocapnia
ocul(o)-	of or pertaining to the eye	oculist
odont(o)-	of or pertaining to teeth	orthodontist
odyn(o)-	pain	stomatodynia
-oesophageal, oesophag(o)-	gullet	gastro-oesophageal reflux
-oid	resemblance to	sarcoidosis
-ole	small or little	arteriole
olig(o)-	denoting something as 'having little, having few'	oliguria
-oma (sing.), -omata (pl.)	tumour, mass, collection	sarcoma, teratoma
onco-	tumour, bulk, volume	oncology
onych(o)-	of or pertaining to the nail (of a finger or toe)	onychophagy

Prefix or suffix	Meaning	Example(s)
oo-	of or pertaining to an egg, a woman's egg, the ovum	oogenesis
oophor(o)-	of or pertaining to the woman's ovary	oophorectomy
ophthalm(o)-	of or pertaining to the eye	ophthalmology
optic(o)-	of or relating to chemical properties of the eye	opticochemical
orchi(o)-, orchid(o)-, orch(o)-	testes	orchiectomy, orchidectomy
-osis	a condition, disease or increase	ichthyosis, psychosis, osteoporosis
osseo-	bony	osseous
ossi-	bone	peripheral ossifying fibroma
ost(e)-, oste(o)-	bone	osteoporosis
ot(o)-	of or pertaining to the ear	otology
ovo-, ovi-, ov-	of or pertaining to the eggs, the ovum	ovogenesis
pachy-	thick	pachyderma
paed-, paedo-	of or pertaining to the child	paediatrics
palpebr-	of or pertaining to the eyelid (uncommon as a root)	palpebra
pan-, pant(o)-	denoting something as 'complete' or containing 'everything'	panophobia, panopticon
papill-	of or pertaining to the nipple (of the chest/breast)	papillitis
papul(o)-	indicates papulosity, a small elevation or swelling in the skin, a pimple, swelling	papulation
para-	alongside of, abnormal	paracyesis
-paresis	slight paralysis	hemiparesis
parvo-	small	parvovirus
path(o)-	disease	pathology
-pathy	denotes (with a negative sense) a disease, or disorder	sociopathy, neuropathy
pector-	breast	pectoralgia, pectoriloquy, pectorophony
ped-, -ped-, -pes	of or pertaining to the foot; -footed	pedoscope
pelv(i)-, pelv(o)-	hip bone	pelvis
-penia	deficiency	osteopenia
-pepsia	denotes something relating to digestion, or the digestive tract	dyspepsia
peri-	denoting something with a position 'surrounding' or 'around' another	periodontal
-pexy	fixation	nephropexy
phaco-	lens-shaped	phacolysis, phacometer, phacoscotoma
-phage, -phagia	forms terms denoting conditions relating to eating or ingestion	sarcophagia

Prefix or suffix	Meaning	Example(s)
-phago-	eating, devouring	phagocyte
-phagy	forms nouns that denotes 'feeding on' the first element or part of the word	haematophagy
pharmaco-	drug, medication	pharmacology
pharyng(o)-	of or pertaining to the pharynx, the upper throat cavity	pharyngitis, pharyngoscopy
phleb(o)-	of or pertaining to the (blood) veins, a vein	phlebography, phlebotomy
-phobia	exaggerated fear, sensitivity	arachnophobia
phon(o)-	sound	phonograph, symphony
phot(o)-	of or pertaining to light	photopathy
phren(i)-, phren(o)-, phrenico	the mind	phrenic nerve, schizophrenia
-plasia	formation, development	achondroplasia
-plasty	surgical repair, reconstruction	rhinoplasty
-plegia	paralysis	paraplegia
pleio-	more, excessive, multiple	pleiomorphism
pleur(o)-, pleur(a)	of or pertaining to the ribs	pleurogenous
-plexy	stroke or seizure	cataplexy
pneumat(o)-	air, lung	pneumatocele
pneum(o)-	of or pertaining to the lungs	pneumonocyte, pneumonia
-poiesis	production	haematopoiesis
poly-	denotes a 'plurality' of something	polymyositis
post-	denotes something as 'after' or 'behind' another	post-operation, post-mortem
pre-	denotes something as 'before' another (in [physical] position or time)	premature birth
presby(o)-	old age	presbyopia
prim-	denotes something as 'first' or 'most important'	primary
proct(o)-	anus, rectum	proctology
prot(o)-	denotes something as 'first' or 'most important'	protoneuron
pseud(o)-	denotes something false or fake	pseudoephedrine
psor-	itching	psoriasis
psych(e)-, psych(o)	of or pertaining to the mind	psychology, psychiatry
-ptosis	falling, drooping, downward placement, prolapse	apoptosis, nephroptosis
-ptysis	(a spitting), spitting, haemoptysis, the spitting of blood derived from the lungs or bronchial tubes	haemoptysis
pulmon-, pulmo-	of or relating to the lungs	pulmonary
pyel(o)-	pelvis	pyelonephritis

Prefix or suffix	Meaning	Example(s)
py(o)-	pus	pyometra
pyr(o)-	fever	antipyretic
quadr(i)-	four	quadriceps
radio-	radiation	radiowave
ren(o)-	of or pertaining to the kidney	renal
retro-	backward, behind	retroversion, retroverted
rhin(o)-	of or pertaining to the nose	rhinoplasty
rhod(o)-	denoting a rose-red colour	rhodophyte
-rrhage	burst forth	haemorrhage
-rrhagia	rapid flow of blood	menorrhagia
-rrhaphy	surgical suturing	nephrorrhaphy
-rrhexis	rupture	karyorrhexis
-rrhoea	flowing, discharge	diarrhoea
-rupt	break or burst	erupt, interrupt
salping(o)-	of or pertaining to tubes, e.g. Fallopian tubes	salpingectomy, salpingopharyngeus muscle
sangui-, sanguine-	of or pertaining to blood	exsanguination
sarco-	muscular, flesh-like	sarcoma
scler(o)-	hard	scleroderma
-sclerosis	hardening	atherosclerosis, multiple sclerosis
scoli(o)-	twisted	scoliosis
-scope	instrument for viewing	otoscope
-scopy	use of instrument for viewing	endoscopy
semi-	one-half, partly	semiconscious
sial(o)-	saliva, salivary gland	sialagogue
sigmoid(o)-	sigmoid, S-shaped curvature	sigmoid colon
sinistr(o)-	left, left side	sinistrocardia
sinus-	of or pertaining to the sinus	sinusitis
somat(o)-, somatico-	body, bodily	somatic
-spadias	slit, fissure	hypospadias, epispadias
spasmo-	spasm	spasmodic dysphonia
sperma(to)-, spermo-	semen, spermatozoa	spermatogenesis
splen(o)-	spleen	splenectomy
spondyl(o)-	of or pertaining to the spine, the vertebra	spondylitis
squamos(o)-	denoting something as 'full of scales' or 'scaly'	squamous cell
-stalsis	contraction	peristalsis
-stasis	stopping, standing	cytostasis, homeostasis

Prefix or suffix	Meaning	Example(s)
-staxis	dripping, trickling	epistaxis
-stenosis	abnormal narrowing in a blood vessel or other tubular organ or structure	restenosis, stenosis
stomat(o)-	of or pertaining to the mouth	stomatogastric, stomatognathic system
-stomy	creation of an opening	colostomy
sub-	beneath	subcutaneous tissue
super-	in excess, above, superior	superior vena cava
supra-	above, excessive	supraorbital vein
tachy-	denoting something as fast, irregularly fast	tachycardia
-tension, -tensive	pressure	hypertension
tetan-	rigid, tense	tetanus
thec-	case, sheath	intrathecal
therap-	treatment	hydrotherapy, therapeutic
therm(o)-	heat	thermometer
thorac(i)-, thorac(o)-, thoracico-	of or pertaining to the upper chest, chest; the area above the breast and under the neck	thorax
thromb(o)-	of or relating to a blood clot, clotting of blood	thrombus, thrombocytopenia
thyr(o)-	thyroid	thyrocele
thym-	emotions	dysthymia
-tome	cutting instrument	osteotome
-tomy	act of cutting; incising, incision	gastrotomy
tono-	tone, tension, pressure	tonometer
top(o)-	place, topical	topical anaesthetic
tort(i)-	twisted	torticollis
tox(i)-, tox(o)-, toxic(o)-	toxin, poison	toxoplasmosis
trache(a)-	trachea	tracheotomy
trachel(o)-	of or pertaining to the neck	tracheloplasty
trans-	denoting something as moving or situated 'across' or 'through'	transfusion
tri-	three	triangle
trich(i)-, trichia, trich(o)-	of or pertaining to hair, hair-like structure	trichocyst
-tripsy	crushing	lithotripsy
-trophy	nourishment, development	pseudohypertrophy
tympan(o)-	eardrum	tympanocentesis
-ula, -ule	small	nodule
ultra-	beyond, excessive	ultrasound

Prefix or suffix	Meaning	Example(s)
un(i)-	one	unilateral hearing loss
ur(o)-	of or pertaining to urine, the urinary system; (specifically) pertaining to the physiological chemistry of urine	urology
uter(o)-	of or pertaining to the uterus or womb	uterus
vagin-	of or pertaining to the vagina	vagina
varic(o)-	swollen or twisted vein	varicose
vasculo-	blood vessel	vasculotoxicity
vas(o)-	duct, blood vessel	vasoconstriction
ven-	of or pertaining to the (blood) veins, a vein (used in terms pertaining to the vascular system)	vein, venospasm
ventricul(o)-	of or pertaining to the ventricles; any hollow region inside an organ	cardiac ventriculography
ventr(o)-	of or pertaining to the belly; the stomach cavities	ventrodorsal
-version	turning	anteversion, retroversion
vesic(o)-	of or pertaining to the bladder	vesical arteries
viscer(o)-	of or pertaining to the internal organs, the viscera	viscera
xanth(o)-	denoting a yellow colour, an abnormally yellow colour	xanthopathy
xen(o)-	foreign, different	xenograft
xer(o)-	dry, desert-like	xerostomia
zo(o)-	animal, animal life	zoology
zym(o)-	fermentation	enzyme, lysozyme

Abbreviations used in prescriptions

Abbreviation	Latin	English
a.c.	ante cibum	Before food
ad lib.	ad libitum	To the desired amount
b.d. or b.i.d.	bis in die	Twice a day
c.	cum	With
o.m.	omni mane	Every morning
o.n.	omni nocte	Every night
p.c.	post cibum	After food
p.r.n.	pro re nata	Whenever necessary
q.d.	quaque die	Every day
q.d.s.	quaque die sumendum	Four times daily
q.i.d.	quater in die	Four times daily

Abbreviation	Latin	English
q.q.h.	quater quaque hora	Every four hours
R.	recipe	Take
s.o.s.	si opus sit	If necessary
stat.	statim	At once
t.d.s.	ter die sumendum	Three times daily
t.i.d.	ter in die	Three times daily

Chapter 1

Introduction to pharmacology

Suzanne Evans and Tanya Somani

Aim

The aim of this chapter is to provide an introductory overview of the aspects of pharmacology that are important for paramedic practice.

Learning outcomes

After reading this chapter, the reader will:

1. Be aware of the potential for error in every stage of drug administration, and strategies to avoid medication error.
2. Be able to distinguish the generic and trade names of drugs, and know the conventions for generic names of drugs in the same class.
3. Know the range of sites at which the majority of drugs act to produce their effects.
4. Understand the importance of correct choice, dosing and administration of a drug.

Test your knowledge

1. Which medicines are considered to be completely safe?
2. How can the risk of accidental harm from medicines be reduced?
3. When taking a medication history, what should you prompt a patient to include?
4. What is the generic name and what is the trade name of a medication and where is each name located on the packaging?

Pharmacology is the study of medications. It includes the study of how and when to use them safely and effectively, as well as the search for and the development of new and more effective medications. Although in paramedicine, the term 'medication' is often used in reference to therapeutic agents and the term 'drug' in reference to illicit agents, in this chapter we will use the term

Fundamentals of Pharmacology for Paramedics, First Edition. Edited by Ian Peate, Suzanne Evans, and Lisa Clegg.
© 2022 John Wiley & Sons Ltd. Published 2022 by John Wiley & Sons Ltd.

'drug' with the broader meaning of 'any substance that produces a change in physiological function' when discussing the pharmacology of the active substances rather than formulated preparations.

Health practitioners have at their disposal a formidable armoury of powerful pharmacological agents which have the ability to save lives and relieve suffering. These same agents, used incorrectly, are equally capable of causing death, suffering and irreparable damage. The use of these powerful tools comes with a responsibility to know how to use them safely, and to have a deep understanding of what they can do. Paramedics, often called on to select and correctly use medications in uncontrolled environments with the additional pressures of time and stress, have an even greater need to be experts in the medicines they will administer, performing, as they do, the roles of physician, pharmacist and nurse in the field. Add to this a constantly evolving scope of practice in paramedicine, and it can be seen that the expectations placed on paramedics in the practice of pharmacotherapeutics are very high.

Medication errors in healthcare generally are a significant problem, accounting for a large number of hospitalisations and deaths per year. In prehospital care in particular, medication errors are thought to be significantly under-reported (Batt, 2016; Hobgood et al. 2006; Lammers et al. 2014; Nguyen, 2008). Data from a number of studies on medication errors in Australian hospitals suggested that between 5% and 10% of administrations may be made in error (Roughead et al., 2013), and in England alone, more than 237 million medication errors are made every year (Elliott et al., 2018). Medication errors made in all areas of healthcare are a similar concern in the United States, the European Union, and in most countries of the world. In recognition of the problem, in 2017 the World Health Organization launched a global initiative to reduce severe, avoidable medication-associated harm worldwide by 50% over 5 years.

Medication errors in paramedicine can include the general misuse of a medicine, such as administering the wrong dose, using the wrong administration route, or failing to identify contraindications. But, because the paramedic is responsible for all phases of the administration of the medication, including the selection of the appropriate medication and the decision about whether and when to use it, two other types of error can also occur: under- or overuse of medicines. The failure to use a medication that could be of benefit to a patient, such as failing to give aspirin for acute coronary syndrome, would be considered an error of underuse, while using an unnecessary medication, or using a second medication to treat a side-effect produced by the first medication, could be considered errors of overuse (Batt, 2016).

The Institute of Safe Medication Practices (ISMP) Canada, in its 2020 safety bulletin, reported on a multi-incident analysis of medication incidents involving paramedicine. This analysis identified the following five main themes in medication errors in paramedicine:

1. The clinical assessment and management of patients, including taking a complete medical and medication history.
2. Therapeutic product use, including misreading of labelling or mistaking products with similar packaging.
3. Intravenous dosing and administration, including calculating dose and setting up pumps.
4. Handover communications, including communication to hospital personnel.
5. Inventory management, including correct restocking of the ambulance with medication and correct positioning of drugs.

These themes serve to reinforce the multiple responsibilities of paramedics when it comes to administering medicines – paramedics are responsible for taking a complete patient history, calculating a correct dose and administering the medication correctly, right through to ensuring the medication is in the ambulance in the correct place before going out on the road. The scope for medication error increases with each layer of responsibility.

A number of authors have suggested standard methodologies to ensure that the correct approach to medicines use is followed every time, especially under high-stress conditions. The following mnemonic for the assessment of patients was developed by ISMP Canada:

SAMPLE
Signs
Allergies
Medication
Past pertinent history
Last oral intake
Events leading to injury

Students of paramedicine are usually familiar with the golden rules of safe administration of medicines, published as 10 golden rules (McGovern, 1992) but also appearing in shortened forms. These rules stipulate that when giving any medication:

1. Give the right drug
2. To the right patient
3. In the right dose
4. Via the right route
5. At the right time
6. Explain about the medication to your patient
7. Take a complete medication history
8. Find out about any allergies
9. Know about potential drug interactions
10. Document each medication administration.

These rules serve as a guide for safe administration of medicines in the field, but they can also be a useful guide to learning pharmacology. Learning what drugs do and how they do it; who they can be given to and when caution should be exercised; what dose ranges they should be used in; by what routes they can be administered and the correct timing of their administration via these routes; what drugs they cannot be combined with and why, are all part of the pharmacology every student of paramedicine must learn and continue to add to as they gain professional experience and as new medicines become available. The need to be a lifelong learner is never more pressing than in the field of clinical pharmacology.

Companies selling medicines are required by law to provide basic information about the medicine for patients before it is made available to them. In the UK, this information is known as the Patient Information Leaflet (PIL), and in Australia it is the Consumer Medicines Information (CMI). The aim of this information is to educate patients about their medicines so that they can ensure they are taking them safely and effectively.

This information includes:

- What the medicine is used to treat (the **indications** of the medicine)
- Warnings about when the medicine should not be taken (the **contraindications** of the medicine)
- Warnings about when the medicine should be taken with caution
- Other medicines that should not be combined with the medicine (known as **interactions**)
- Possible side-effects (known as **adverse effects**)
- The dose to take and any special instructions regarding how to take the medicine
- What to do in the case of an overdose of the medicine
- How to store the medicine.

The language used in these documents has been chosen to make the information accessible to any patient, hence the avoidance of too much technical language, but it is nonetheless the same information that health professionals need in order to ensure the safe and effective administration of medicines to their patients.

Skills in practice

The decision about whether to administer or withhold a medication requires a process of clinical reasoning, based on your assessment of the patient, their medical and medication history and the indications and contraindications of the medication.

An indication for a medication is a particular symptom or sign reported or displayed by a patient. An indication should not be confused with a definitive diagnosis. In paramedicine, a primary assessment and history taking should be carried out if possible, prior to establishing an indication. Administering an indicated medication should only occur if the potential benefit of the medication is judged to out-weigh the risk to the patient, such as in the following examples:

- An unconscious child who is hypoglycaemic is indicated for glucose 10% administration. The signs used here as indications for the medication are both the finding of hypoglycaemia and the child's level of consciousness.
- A 50-year-old male patient who is experiencing crushing left-sided chest pain has an indication for aspirin administration, provided you have established that he has no abnormal bleeding tendencies.

Sometimes, despite there being an indication for a medication, you will not be able to administer it because of a contraindication. A contraindication is a reason to withhold medication because it might cause harm to the patient, as in the following examples:

- Aspirin is contraindicated for analgesia and fever in paediatric patients who are under 16 years of age because of the risk of Reye's syndrome. The syndrome is quite rare and only occurs in children, but is very serious.
- Ipratropium, a bronchodilator commonly used with salbutamol for the treatment of bronchos-pasm, is usually contraindicated in patients who have glaucoma, as a known side-effect is an increase in intraocular pressure.
- Amiodarone is an antiarrhythmic indicated for tachyarrhythmias (cardiac arrhythmias which involve an increased heart rate), but contraindicated in torsades de pointes, a potentially fatal tachyarrhythmia which can result from long QT syndrome, because amiodarone will result in fur-ther protraction of the QT interval.

As data about medications are gathered, indications and contraindications may change, so it is important to remain abreast of these changes in your practice as a paramedic.

Episode of care

You attend a 49-year-old male patient complaining of left-sided central chest pain. He is diaphoretic, pale and short of breath.

You ask him about his medical history. He reports he has a 'high blood pressure problem'. You glance at his medication list and do not recognise any common antihypertensive medications.

Your check his observations and gain a detailed history, while preparing him for a 12-lead ECG. The ECG suggests a lateral myocardial infarct. Your provisional diagnosis is acute coronary syndrome and you proceed with administering aspirin and a vasodilator.

En route he rapidly becomes hypotensive with a decreased level of consciousness. At hospital, you discover he has recently commenced on a vasodilator for aggressive management of his pulmonary hypertension. This medication was not on his medication list.

You may see medications that patients are taking for indications other than the listed indications. Vasodilators such as sildenafil (Viagra®) and vardenafil (Levitra®) are often prescribed to males for erectile dysfunction, but can also be used to treat pulmonary hypertension.

Patients may be unsure what they are taking medications for and it is imperative to gain a detailed history prior to administration of any medication to ensure contraindications are not encountered. Medications can be used for purposes other than their primary indication.

Naming and classifying drugs

Every drug will have a number of names. Knowing the correct name of a drug is vital in the prevention of medication errors, and becomes even more important when drugs can be identified by several different names. All drugs will have an individual chemical name which conveys very accurately (at least to a chemist!) the drug's molecular structure. These names are usually long, difficult to say and impossible to remember, and they are usually left to research chemists. Many drugs can also be known by the name of the chemical class they belong to, such as opioids or benzodiazepines. But it is the generic, or official, name of the drug that health practitioners should always recognise a drug by. This name should be sufficiently different from any other drug name to minimise the risk of any drug being mistaken for another. With a few exceptions, generic names are usually the same regardless of where in the world you are, and they often derive in some way from the name of the chemical class of the drug, which is often convenient as it makes it easy to identify the class a drug belongs to by its generic name. The generic names of drugs belonging to the statin class of drugs, for example, end in -statin, with agents such as atorvastatin, rosuvastatin, fluvastatin and simvastatin. Generic names of drugs belonging to the beta-blocker class end in -olol and include propranolol, atenolol, pindolol and nebivolol.

Many drug formulations will also have a trade name given to the particular drug formulation by the company that produced it. These names may relate to the generic name or they may relate more closely to their therapeutic use, but because of the multiple formulations available and multiple companies producing them, the trade names of drugs will vary widely depending on where the drug is sold and what it is sold for. Needless to say, these names are not a reliable way to identify the drugs but unfortunately, they are often the most prominent and eye-catching name on the packaging, which will mean that patients will usually refer to drugs by the trade name, unless they are receiving a generic version of the drug. To try and reduce confusion, the Australian government, for example, passed a law, effective February 1, 2021, that requires prescribers to write the generic name of the medication first on any prescription, either without a trade name or with the trade name in brackets after it. Combined with requirements for drug manufacturers to make the generic name of the active drug in the medication more prominent on the packaging than the trade name, the aim is to increase awareness of the active ingredients in medications and to reduce confusion.

With the huge range of drugs currently licensed for use, there are often multiple individual drugs available for any particular indication, so it is important that we also classify our drugs to make talking about them easier. We can classify drugs based on their chemical structures, mechanism of action or broader area of therapeutic use. The functional classifications (those relating to what the drugs do or what they are used for) are the most widely used, as they reflect the clinical uses of the drugs, but we often refer to certain groups of drugs by their chemical classification, as usually all agents belonging to a certain chemical class also have a predictable effect on function. Table 1.1 gives some examples of the ways in which drugs are named and categorised.

Look-alikes and sound-alikes

Mistaking one medication for another because the two names (either generic or trade names) sound alike or the packages look alike is a common cause of medication error. Errors due to look-alike sound-alike (LASA) medications have become so widespread that the World Health Organization launched a worldwide effort to reduce medication errors that come about in this way (WHO, 2007), and many governments have made changes to their medication labelling and naming The addition of 'tall man' writing in the name of a drug has been introduced in the UK, Canada, Australia and the US to make the differences between drug names clearer. This technique involves capitalising the parts of the name that are most likely to be misread, for example:

AmiloRIDE, AmlodiPINE, BuPROPion, BupreNORphine.

The mix of capitalised lettering in the name disrupts rapid reading and forces a more careful observation of the name.

The main element in reducing medication errors, however, continues to be careful cross-checking of LASA medications prior to administration, and ensuring that look-alike medications are not stored in close proximity to each other. Because the packaging and appearance of medications can change, the generic name of the medication should always be checked, and the identity of a medication should never be assumed from its appearance without checking the label. For example, a 500 mL or 1000 mL bag of clear fluid could be Hartmann solution, sodium chloride or glucose 10%.

Table 1.1   Categorisation of drugs based on clinical usage, general action or specific mechanism of action.

Generic name	Trade names	Chemical class	Therapeutic use	General action	Specific mechanism of action
Diazepam	Valium® Valpam® Antenex®	Benzodiazepines	Anxiolytics	Central nervous system depressants	GABA agonists
Atorvastatin	Lipitor® Torvastat®	Statins	Cholesterol synthesis inhibition	Lipid-lowering agents	HMG Co-A reductase inhibitors
Candesartan	Candesan® Adesan® Atacand®	-	Antihypertensives	Blood pressure-lowering agents	Angiotensin receptor antagonists
Salmeterol	Serevent®	-	Acute asthma control	Bronchodilators	Long-acting beta-2 agonists
Diclofenac	Voltaren® Voltarol® Difenac® Clonac®		Analgesic, anti-inflammatory	Non-steroidal anti-inflammatories	Cyclo-oxygenase inhibitors

GABA, gamma-aminobutyric acid; HMG-CoA, 3-hydroxy-3-methylglutaryl coenzyme A.

How drugs bring about their actions

With only one or two exceptions (such as drugs which absorb other substances, e.g. charcoal or resins), drugs act by binding chemically to specific binding sites. It is this fact which explains the various observed characteristics of a drug, for example, the relationship between the shape of a drug molecule and its actions; the relationship between how readily it binds to its site of action and the concentration of drug needed at the site of action to bring about a therapeutic effect; the relationship between the number of different binding sites the drug can bind to and the number of different effects it produces; the strength with which it binds to the site and length of time for which it exerts its effects, and so on.

The site at which a drug binds to have its effects is known as the receptor for that drug, and it may be a receptor normally used by endogenous signalling molecules, such as hormones or neurotransmitters, or a binding site on an enzyme, ion channel or transport molecule. A substance binding at any of these sites would be able to alter physiological function when the structure to which the drug is binding is itself responsible for producing various physiological changes.

How are we able to manipulate physiological function using drugs?

Physiological systems make use of hundreds of specific signalling chemicals to carry out their own signalling function and this provides an opportunity to use drugs to mimic or block the effects that those endogenous signalling chemicals would produce. By employing drugs with chemical structures similar to those of endogenous chemicals, we gain an opportunity to 'operate the levers' of the human machine. Not surprisingly, therefore, the vast majority of the drugs used act by altering the function of one of these key pieces of signalling and transport machinery:

- Receptors
- Enzymes
- Ion channels
- Transport molecules

Drugs used as therapeutic agents act by manipulating physiological mechanisms, which reinforces the importance of having an understanding of human physiological responses as the basis for understanding pharmacology. Without a sound knowledge and understanding of how physiological systems respond, it is impossible to make sense of how drugs will interact with those systems.

Receptors as sites of drug action

An opioid drug such as morphine acts by binding to the receptors for endogenous opioids and, by activation of those receptors, produces similar actions to those generated by the endogenous opioids, including analgesia and a range of other effects. Similarly, bronchodilator drugs such as terbutaline and salbutamol, used during an episode of acute asthma, produce their bronchodilator effect by activating adrenergic beta receptors on the airways. These receptors would be activated physiologically by adrenaline and noradrenaline secreted during the fight or flight response, and the binding of adrenaline or noradrenaline to the beta receptors in the airways would produce a dilation of the airways, allowing a more rapid ventilation of the lungs. A drug which is able to produce this effect without producing the rest of the fight or flight response is a very useful therapeutic agent during an episode of acute asthma (Figure 1.1).

Enzymes as sites of drug action

Enzymes are the large proteins that catalyse the thousands of biochemical reactions that maintain physiological function. An enzyme carries out the catalysis (speeding up) of a particular reaction by binding the reacting molecules and making it 'easier' for the reaction to occur (Figure 1.2). Drugs which have enzymes as their targets tend to be inhibitors of those enzymes, preventing the normal reacting substances from binding with the enzyme for catalysis.

Drugs such as non-steroidal anti-inflammatory drugs (NSAIDs), the prototype of which is aspirin, act by inhibiting the enzyme cyclo-oxygenase, which is responsible for speeding up the reaction producing a range of important signalling molecules known as prostaglandins. It is the reduced level of prostaglandins as a result of blockade of cyclo-oxygenase that produces the range of effects associated with NSAIDs. Another example of a widely used class of drugs which act by blocking an enzyme is the statin class, including atorvastatin and fluvastatin. These drugs lower cholesterol levels by inhibiting the enzyme HMG-CoA reductase, responsible for the production of cholesterol in living cells.

Ion channels

Ion channels represent the only means for ions to cross cell membranes, and all cells contain multiple species of ion channel in their membranes. These channels can be gated in a number of ways, and drugs which can bind to specific channels can alter cellular activity profoundly by altering the passage of ions across the membrane, thereby altering the cell's membrane potential. Most drugs that act in this way block ion channels rather than open them.

The local anaesthetic lidocaine, for example, acts by binding to and inhibiting voltage-gated sodium channels in neuronal cell membranes, preventing the generation of action potentials by the affected neurons. Sensory neurons detecting touch, pressure and pain stimuli therefore become less responsive to those stimuli, resulting in anaesthesia.

The benzodiazepine class of drugs, including agents such as midazolam and diazepam, act by binding to a chloride ion channel in neuronal membranes.

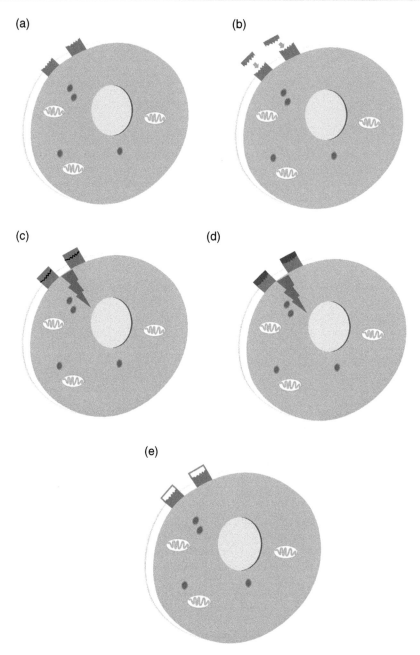

Figure 1.1 Drugs which act at receptors. (a) A cell has receptors for a specific signalling compound (e.g. a neurotransmitter or hormone) located on the cell membrane. (b) The endogenous signalling molecule binds to its receptors, fitting the receptor perfectly. (c) The binding triggers a series of actions inside the cell. These actions would be the normal response to that signalling compound. (d) If the molecular structure of a drug is sufficiently similar to that of the endogenous signalling compound, the drug will also be able to bind to the receptor and produce the same actions in the cell. This drug would be known as an agonist at this receptor. (e) If a drug has a molecular structure vaguely similar to that of the endogenous signalling compound, it may still be able to bind to the receptor, but not fit it perfectly enough to produce the same actions in the cell. This drug could prevent the endogenous signalling compound (and the agonist) getting to the receptor, thereby blocking their actions. This drug would be known as an antagonist at the receptor.

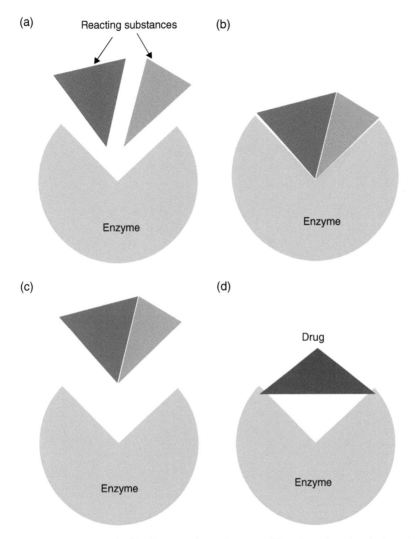

Figure 1.2 Enzymes operate by binding reacting substances (a) and accelerating their reaction – in this case the reaction is a combination of two molecules (b), then releasing the product from the enzyme's binding site (c). A drug which can also bind to this site can prevent the catalytic function of the enzyme, thereby reducing the level of product (d).

This channel is opened normally by the inhibitory neurotransmitter GABA (gamma-aminobutyric acid). Opening a chloride channel in the membrane allows the influx of negatively charged chloride ions to the cell, which hyperpolarises the cell, making it less likely to produce action potentials. The benzodiazepine class of drugs also act at this ion channel, albeit at a different site to GABA, but when they bind, they enhance the inhibitory actions of GABA, and add to the hyperpolarisation of neurons and the resulting nervous system depressant effect (Figure 1.3).

Transport molecules
The large, complex proteins responsible for active transport of substances across cell membranes represent another valuable drug target for manipulation of physiological function.

There are active transporters or pumps in all cell membranes for sodium, potassium and calcium ions, and these are activated when those ions have to be transported across the cell membrane against their concentration gradient, i.e. from a lower to a higher concentration of ions. Ions can

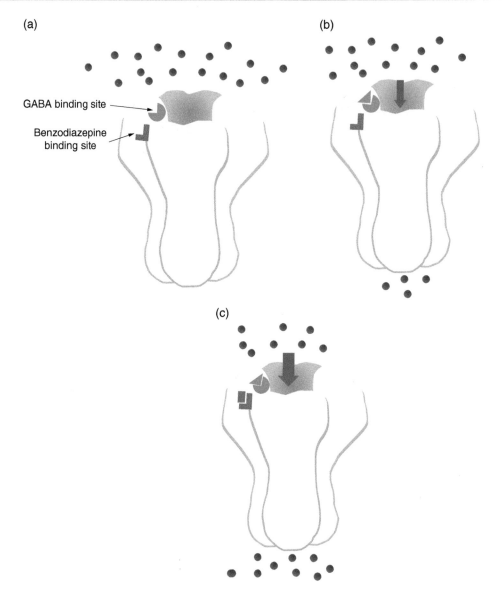

(a)

GABA binding site

Benzodiazepine
binding site

(b)

(c)

Figure 1.3 Benzodiazepines act by binding to a chloride channel. (a) The inhibitory neurotransmitter GABA has its receptor on the ligand-gated chloride ion channel in neurons. The channel also has a binding site for drugs of the benzodiazepine class. (b) Binding of GABA to its receptor opens the channel, allowing chloride ions to flow into the neuron and hyperpolarise the membrane, inhibiting further neuronal activity. (c) Binding of a benzodiazepine to its site will, in the presence of GABA, further increase the flow of chloride ions into the cell by keeping the channel open for longer, thereby further inhibiting neuronal activity.

move through open ion channels if they are travelling down their concentration gradient, but will need active 'pumping' if they are to move the other way.

As with enzymes and ion channels, the drugs that bind transport molecules tend to inhibit the transport when they bind. This alters cell function by interfering with the distribution of ions across the cell membrane, thereby altering membrane potential. The cardiac glycoside drug digoxin, used to treat cardiac failure, acts by binding to a transport molecule – the sodium/potassium ATP-ase or sodium/potassium pumps on the cell membranes of cardiac muscle cells. Digoxin inhibits the function of the sodium/potassium pumps, leading to an accumulation of sodium ions inside cardiac muscle cells, which in turn results in an accumulation of calcium ions in the cells (the additional intracellular sodium ions stimulate another transporter, which pumps sodium ions out of the cell in exchange for calcium ions). The increased level of calcium ions inside the cardiac muscle cells results in stronger contractions, which translates to a stronger, more forceful heartbeat.

Selectivity of binding and its effect

Some drugs are very selective in their binding sites, and can bind to a very limited number of sites, or only one site, but most drugs will be able to bind to more than one site. For example, a bronchodilator medication that acts as an agonist at adrenergic beta receptors may bind at only beta-2 receptor subtypes, in which case it would be a selective beta-2 agonist, but is more likely to bind to both beta-1 and beta-2 receptors, because of the degree of chemical similarity between the two receptor subtypes. The more selective a drug is for a single receptor, the fewer effects it is likely to bring about, so a more selective drug is likely to be one with fewer side-effects. On the other hand, a less selective drug which activates two or three related receptors may have more therapeutic uses, but it will also have more side-effects. The selectivity of a drug will tend to decrease as the dose increases, because binding to other receptor types will become more likely as the concentration of the drug increases. This helps to explain the dose dependency of many side-effects of medications.

Clinical considerations

Salbutamol, also known as albuterol, is a beta-2 receptor agonist and is frequently administered in the out-of-hospital setting for management of bronchospasm. It can also be used in the management of hyperkalaemia because it stimulates the transport of potassium ions from the blood into skeletal muscle cells. This effect is also mediated by the action of salbutamol on beta-2 receptors.

Many patients who have been prescribed salbutamol may have already self-administered their own 'puffer' prior to your arrival and may be tachycardic as a result. This is due to binding to beta-2 receptors in cardiac muscle after absorption of salbutamol into the bloodstream. Tachycardia may predispose the patient to arrhythmias, so regarding these patients as high risk for a cardiac event is warranted.

Muscle tremors may also occur in these patients, due to binding of the drug to beta-2 receptors in skeletal muscle. Although the drug is quite selective for beta-2 receptors, it will also bind to beta-1 receptors at high doses, so if the patient has used their puffer very extensively prior to your treatment, there may be additional tachycardia due to an action on beta-1 receptors in the heart, increasing cardiac risk.

The drug–body interaction is a dynamic process

The interaction between any administered drug and the person it is administered to is dynamic. From the moment it is administered, the drug will be moving from its administration point to other compartments of the body, being absorbed into the bloodstream, and leaving the blood to enter other tissues or other body compartments, so the concentration of the drug in the blood and in various tissues and body compartments will be changing. As the drug passes through the liver, it will be acted on by metabolic enzymes which will convert it to a different form, which may be more or less pharmacologically active, but certainly more water soluble. The drug travelling in the blood will also be filtered by the kidneys, and the water-soluble form of the drug will be trapped there and excreted in the urine.

As the drug is being carried around the body, some of it will arrive at and bind to its sites of action, producing its effects. Even the binding of the drug to its receptors is a dynamic process, akin to molecules playing musical chairs with the receptors – molecules of the drug will bind and detach and bind again rather than simply binding and remaining in place. Each time the molecule detaches from its binding site, it may be whipped away and metabolised, and its place on the receptors may be taken by another, competing molecule. This constantly changing relationship between the drug and the living system it has been introduced into explains a great deal about how drugs have their effects. The delay between administration and action of a drug, the duration of action of the drug, and the ability to reverse or overcome the actions of one drug by giving another drug are all the result of this dynamic interaction between drug and living system.

For the paramedic administering drugs into a system which may be free of other drugs but more likely already contains some pharmacological agents, this constantly changing effect of the drug on the patient will require you to have a good enough grasp on what these agents can do, either alone or in combination, to be able to predict and maintain some control over their actions.

One challenge we are always faced with is getting enough of a drug from its site of administration to its site of action for it to have a therapeutic effect. The drug is effectively in a race to reach its site of action and have its effect before it is chemically degraded and removed from the body. A drug which has a highly desirable therapeutic action may turn out to be useless from a clinical point of view if it cannot be delivered to its site of action. So, a drug that is going to stand a chance of being useful would usually possess characteristics which allow it to be easily absorbed into the blood-stream, preferably after oral administration, which in turn would mean that the drug would not be destroyed by the acid of the stomach or digestive enzymes. And although it would probably be subject to metabolism by the liver, the metabolism should not be so rapid that it is almost completely gone after a single pass through the liver (a phenomenon known as first-pass metabolism), as this would mean that very little of the active drug remained in the bloodstream to circulate after absorption. Other routes of administration might avoid the problem of first-pass metabolism, but each administration route will have its own advantages and disadvantages.

Clinical considerations

Administration of medications in the out-of-hospital setting can be challenging due to poor lighting, uncontrolled environment or a chaotic scene. Practising all steps of safe medication administration is key to reducing the risk of error (Chapter 4 discusses medicines management and the role of the paramedic). Ensuring the same routine is exercised every single time you administer any medications will embed safe practice so you do not overlook a crucial step during a high-acuity incident.

Hand hygiene is important to prevent introduction of harmful pathogens in the out-of-hospital environment. Access to running water may not be practical in the out-of-hospital setting, so utilisation of alcohol-based hand rub is the gold standard in this setting. Healthcare-associated infections generate significant comorbidity and burden for the patient, the community and the healthcare system. Healthcare-associated infections are avoidable and simple hygienic practice and aseptic technique are crucial in breaking the chain of transmission from community, to patient and into care settings such as hospitals.

Intravenous cannulation is a key source for bloodstream infections and risk mitigation efforts, such as use of alcohol-based hand rub and not touching the area between cleaning the skin and immediately prior to cannulation, should be exercised.

Other routes of administration which are common in the out-of-hospital setting include intravenous, intramuscular, topical, intranasal, endotracheal and intraosseous. See Chapter 6 for further discussion.

Once absorbed into the bloodstream, a drug needs to be able to penetrate to its sites of action relatively quickly. If the drug was an antimicrobial being used to treat an infection of the blood, then getting enough drug into the bloodstream for long enough would be all that was required. However, if the drug were required to penetrate the central nervous system, for example, or get into joint spaces or some other protected body compartment, then it would also have to be able to move out of the bloodstream and travel through the cellular walls that form those body compartments. This presents another challenge to a molecule; in order to get through cell membranes, a drug molecule either needs to be soluble in lipids (lipophilic) or, if it is more water soluble (hydrophilic), then it would have to be a very small molecule. Drugs that are highly lipid soluble are generally able to move readily through cellular compartments without difficulty, and will therefore leave the bloodstream and enter the tissues, often concentrating there. Drugs that readily cross the blood–brain barrier, such as those used in general anaesthesia, are highly lipid soluble, allowing them to pass very rapidly into the protected environment of the brain, which explains their ability to produce general anaesthesia in a matter of seconds after being introduced into a vein.

13

The dose, route and timing of administration will all play key roles in the effectiveness of the drug. This is discussed in greater detail in Chapter 5.

Episode of care

You are treating 94-year-old Nelida, who has fallen in her residential aged care facility while going to the bathroom. She has a large bruise on the side of her head (temporal region) and a shortened and rotated left leg, as well as a deep laceration to her left upper thigh caused by the shard of a mirror that broke during the fall. Staff report that the patient has dementia but can still converse appropriately most days. The patient is in extreme pain but her heart rate is not elevated. You realise this is probably due to her being on a beta-blocker for hypertension. You administer intranasal fentanyl repeatedly en route to hospital to treat her pain. On arrival, her level of consciousness has decreased. Reflecting on what might have caused this, you consider that the combination of blood loss and a blunted compensatory response due to the beta-blockers, along with a reduced renal capacity due to her age, and the fact that the repeated fentanyl doses have not been cleared as rapidly as expected has resulted in an accumulation of medication, leading to adverse effects.

While this is not a contraindication of fentanyl, it is important to remember that older patients often clear medications much more slowly than younger patients, and dosing may need to be adjusted to account for this, to avoid adverse effects.

Skills in practice

Medications can come in varying concentrations and formulations for different modes of delivery. Adrenaline is a naturally occurring catecholamine hormone produced by the adrenal glands and is often also administered in the management of life-threatening presentations such as cardiac arrest, anaphylaxis and croup.

The concentration of adrenaline can be expressed as 1:1000 or 1:10 000. This is expressed verbally as 'one in one thousand' and 'one in ten thousand' respectively. This ratio refers to the medication mass per volume of solution:

$$1:1000 = 1\,gram\ of\ adrenaline\ per\ 1000\,mL$$

$$1:10\,000 = 1\,gram\ of\ adrenaline\ per\ 10000\,mL$$

Adrenaline concentrations can and do vary, but the following is a guide to concentrations and routes of administration for various indications:

Concentration	Route of administration	Indication
Adrenaline 1:1000	Intramuscular Nebulised	Anaphylaxis Croup Asthma
Adrenaline 1:10 000	Intravenous	Cardiac arrest Cardiogenic shock

Administering medication to children

Historically, children were considered small adults, with the same physiology and metabolic requirements as an adult, but on a smaller scale. This is now known not to be the case, but many medications are still not tested on children, so safe doses in this patient group are not established empirically. A basic understanding of the differences between adult and child anatomy and physiology will ensure safer administration of medication to children. For example, the child's heart does not have the same capacity to raise cardiac output by increasing its force of contraction and relies on increasing the heart rate to compensate for increased demand. As a result, peripheral vasoconstriction usually occurs more readily, in order to maintain blood pressure.

Medications which cause peripheral vasoconstriction need to be used with extra caution in children because of this. Adrenaline will cause peripheral vasoconstriction when used to treat anaphylaxis or asthma, and the beta-2 agonist salbutamol (albuterol) is also often contraindicated in children because of the possibility of tachycardia. Using medications that cause tachycardia will place further demands on a child's heart, possibly at a time when it is already working hard to compensate. These medications have to be dosed and administered with extreme care in children, and some may be contraindicated.

Reflection

How is dosing calculated for children? If you don't know the weight of the patient and there is no one to give you the weight, how would you estimate it, to ensure you give a safe and effective dose?

What special considerations need to be borne in mind when giving medications intranasally to children?

When administering medications to a child, ensure consent is gained from the parent, caregiver or a response given by the child is appropriate for their age and presentation. Ensure your approach to treating a child extends to providing oversight to the parent/caregiver as well.

Conclusion

The out-of-hospital setting is not the same as the controlled environment of the hospital and the unpredictable and uncontrolled nature of paramedicine requires that the practising paramedic performs the work that would be done by three different health professionals in a hospital. This places a great responsibility on the paramedic when it comes to the safe and effective use of medicines. The paramedic must be an expert in both the correct choice and administration of medications. In addition, because the environment in which the paramedic is operating is particularly conducive to making errors, the paramedic must also be constantly vigilant and ensure the stringent and consistent checking of medication route, dose, time, expiration date and patient. As the scope of paramedic practice increases and more medications are administered in the prehospital setting, the need for paramedics to have a mastery of medicines becomes even greater.

Glossary

Agonist	A drug that binds to a receptor and produces the same response as the endogenous substance. For example, morphine is an agonist at opioid receptors because it produces the same response as the endorphins produce.
Antagonist	A drug that binds to a receptor and prevents the endogenous substance or an agonist from binding and having its effect. Also known as a blocker, because it blocks the activation of the receptor.
Contraindication	A characteristic or condition which would prevent a patient from being able to receive a certain medication.
First-pass metabolism	The metabolism of a large proportion of an administered dose of a drug by the liver almost immediately after absorption.
Indication	A condition or symptom which a medication is approved to treat.

Pharmacodynamics	The actions of a drug on the body.
Pharmacokinetics	The actions of the body on the drug.
Receptor	The site at which a drug molecule binds to have its action.

References

Batt, A. *Enhancing patient safety education for paramedics with the IHI Open School*. http://prehospitalresearch. eu/?p=6171

Elliott, R.A., Camacho, E., Campbell, F. et al. (2018). *Prevalence and Economic Burden of Medication Errors in the NHS in England*. Sheffield: Policy Research Unit in Economic Evaluation of Health and Care Interventions (EEPRU).

Hobgood, C., Bowen, J.B., Brice, J.H., Overby, B. and Tamayo-Sarver, J.H. (2006). Do EMS personnel identify, report and disclose medical errors? *Prehospital Emergency Care* **10**(1): 21–27.

Institute for Safe Medication Practices Canada. (2020). Multi-incident analysis of incidents involving paramedicine. *ISMP Canada Safety Bulletin* **20**(1): 1–4.

Lammers, R., Willoughby-Byrwa, M. and Fales, W. (2014). Medication errors in prehospital management of simulated pediatric anaphylaxis. *Prehospital Emergency Care* **18**(2): 295–304.

McGovern, K. (1992). 10 Golden rules for administering drugs safely. *Nursing* **22**(3): 49–56.

Nguyen, A. (2008). Bad medicine: preventing drug errors in the prehospital setting. *Journal of Emergency Medical Services* **33**(10): 94–100.

Roughead, L., Semple, S. and Rosenfeld, E. (2013). *Literature Review: Medication Safety in Australia*. Canberra: Australian Commission on Safety and Quality in Health Care.

WHO Collaborating Centre for Patient Safety Solutions. (2007). *Look-Alike Sound-Alike Medication Names. Patient Safety Solutions: Solution 1*. https://cdn.who.int/media/docs/default-source/integrated-health-services-(ihs)/psf/ patient-safety-solutions/ps-solution1-look-alike-sound-alike-medication-names.pdf?sfvrsn=d4fb860b_6&ua=1

Further reading

Australian Medicines Handbook (AMH). 2020 print edition or online: https://amhonline.amh.net.au

British National Formulary (BNF). 2020 print edition or online: www.bnf.org

Multiple-choice questions

1. A medication error occurs when:
   (a) The wrong dose is administered
   (b) A drug that would benefit a patient is not given
   (c) A drug that it not necessary is given
   (d) All of the above.

2. The purposes for which a medication can be used are the:
   (a) Mechanism of action
   (b) Contraindications
   (c) Indications
   (d) None of these.

3. The conditions in which a drug cannot be used are the:
   (a) Mechanism of action
   (b) Indications
   (c) None of these.

4. When drugs such as alprazolam are referred to as benzodiazepines, they are being classified according to their:
   (a) Mechanism of action
   (b) Indications
   (c) Chemical class
   (d) Original trade name.

5. When drugs such as reboxetine are referred to as antidepressants, they are being classified according to their:
   (a) Mechanism of action
   (b) Indications
   (c) Chemical class
   (d) Original trade name.

6. A medication which is prescribed for an indication other than its listed indications is being used:
   (a) Illegally
   (b) Off-label
   (c) Even though it is contraindicated
   (d) None of the above.

7. The drugs known as specific serotonin reuptake inhibitors, which include fluoxetine (Prozac®), would act by binding to:
   (a) A receptor for a neurotransmitter
   (b) An ion channel
   (c) An enzyme
   (d) A transport molecule.

8. In general, the more selective a drug is in its binding sites:
   (a) The fewer side effects it will have
   (b) The more easily it will reach its site of action
   (c) The more potent it will be
   (d) The more it will interact with other drugs.

9. When administering adrenaline intravenously, which dilution is most appropriate?
   (a) 1:100
   (b) 1:1000
   (c) 1:10 000
   (d) 1:100 000

10. A drug that is an antagonist or blocker of a receptor is likely to 'fit' the receptor chemically better than a drug that is an agonist.
    (a) True
    (b) False

11. A drug, such as a general anaesthetic, that can penetrate the blood–brain barrier very rapidly after intravenous administration is likely to be:
    (a) Highly water soluble
    (b) A protein
    (c) Highly lipid soluble
    (d) No drugs can penetrate an intact blood–brain barrier.

12. A medication dose may need to be adjusted down in which of these situations?
    (a) Renal failure
    (b) High first-pass metabolism
    (c) Diarrhoea
    (d) Vomiting

13. The NSAID aspirin has its effects due to action at:
    (a) An ion channel
    (b) A neurotransmitter receptor
    (c) A transport molecule
    (d) An enzyme.

14. You are attending a patient who has suffered trauma and lost a lot of blood. The patient's heart rate is normal, even though their blood pressure is low. Which of the following medications being taken is most likely to be responsible for this?

(a) Ibuprofen
(b) Metformin
(c) Atenolol
(d) Tetracycline

15. If a drug undergoes extensive first-pass metabolism, which of these routes should be avoided as administration routes for this drug?

(a) Intramuscular
(b) Intravenous
(c) Oral
(d) Intranasal

Chapter 2

How to use pharmaceutical and prescribing reference guides

Nigel Conway and Jennifer Dod

Aim

This chapter aims to introduce you to commonly used pharmaceutical and prescribing reference guides and their use in paramedic practice. Specific focus is placed on the Joint Royal Colleges Ambulance Liaison Committee (JRCALC) Clinical Practice Guidelines (2019).

For clarification:

- The JRCALC Clinical Guidelines (2019) full reference book will be referred to throughout this chapter as JRCALC Guidelines
- The JRCALC Clinical Guidelines (2019) Pocket Book will be referred to in this chapter as JRCALC Pocket Book
- The JRCALC Clinical Guidelines digital application (app) will be referred to in this chapter as JRCALC app.

Learning outcomes

After reading this chapter, the reader will:

1. Be aware of the different pharmaceutical and reference guides that may be used in paramedic practice
2. Understand how to navigate the:
   - JRCALC Guidelines (full reference book)
   - JRCALC Pocket Book
   - JRCALC app
3. Be aware of other common pharmaceutical resources available to the paramedic.

Fundamentals of Pharmacology for Paramedics, First Edition. Edited by Ian Peate, Suzanne Evans, and Lisa Clegg.
© 2022 John Wiley & Sons Ltd. Published 2022 by John Wiley & Sons Ltd.

Test your knowledge

- How frequently are the hard-copy JRCALC Guidelines reviewed and republished?
- How many HCPC standards of proficiency are there?
- How many different forms of the JRCALC Guidelines are available?
- What is the unique feature of the 'JRCALC plus' feature?
- What are the core paramedic care approaches to the fundamentals of medicine management?

Introduction

The world of medications is vast and learning about them can be daunting for all allied healthcare and nursing profession students, as well as registered professionals. The people you care for may have extensive past medical history and lists of medications specific to treatment interventions. You need to be able to assess, review, administer, consider interactions, monitor and evaluate the effects of these medications.

Regulatory and professional bodies have specific standards of practice which are designed to be applicable to all areas of a healthcare professional's work. In the United Kingdom, paramedics are accountable to the public and their profession through the Health and Care Professions Council (HCPC). There are two sets of HCPC standards that govern paramedic practice:

- HCPC (2016) Standards of conduct, performance and ethics
- HCPC (2014) The standards of proficiency for paramedics (latest review point 2020 to be published).

These two sets of standards apply to all areas of paramedic practice including medicines and pharmacological management (i.e. knowledge, understanding and clinical application) as related specifically to the paramedic role.

The HCPC (2016) and HCPC (2014) standards are essentially frameworks within which all registered UK paramedics must work. Ambulance services and paramedics outside the UK will be guided by equivalent organisations. Examples of these are:

- Australian Council of Ambulance Authorities (CAA), covering Australia, New Zealand and Papua New Guinea: www.caa.net.au/
- Paramedicine Board, Australia: www.paramedicineboard.gov.au/Professional-standards.aspx
- Australian Clinical Practice Guidelines: Ambulance and MICA Paramedics (2018): www.ambulance. vic.gov.au/wp-content/uploads/2018/07/Clinical-Practice-Guidelines-2018-Edition-1.4.pdf.

HCPC Standards of conduct, performance and ethics

This framework (HCPC, 2016) establishes what the expectations are for all UK-registered paramedics specific to behaviour, public expectation and fitness to practise. The framework covers 10 specific areas of paramedic practice in relation to conduct, performance and ethics which in the context of this book can be applied to the specific area of medicines management as well as all other areas of a paramedic's practice. These are:

- Promote and protect the interests of service users and carers
- Communicate appropriately and effectively
- Work within the limits of your knowledge and skills
- Delegate appropriately
- Respect confidentiality

- Manage risk
- Report concerns about safety
- Be open when things go wrong
- Be honest and trustworthy
- Keep records of your work.

Specific drugs and examples of application to paramedic practice, as well as legal and professional issues, can be read and explored in the chapters that follow.

HCPC Standards of proficiency for paramedics

This framework (HCPC, 2014) establishes what UK-registered paramedics must do specific to their regulated profession, which in the context of this book can be applied to the specific area of medicines management as well as all other areas of a paramedic's practice. There are 15 areas of proficiency covered by these standards with more detailed subsections under each proficiency. All paramedics must comply with the standards of proficiency.

- Practise safely and effectively within their scope of practice.
- Practise within the legal and ethical boundaries of the profession.
- Maintain fitness to practise.
- Practise as an autonomous professional, exercising their own professional judgement.
- Be aware of the impact of culture, equality and diversity on clinical practice.
- Practise in a non-discriminatory manner.
- Understand the importance of and be able to maintain confidentiality.
- Communicate effectively.
- Work appropriately with others.
- Maintain records appropriately.
- Reflect on and review practice.
- Assure the quality of their practice.
- Understand the key concepts of the knowledge base relevant to their profession.
- Draw on the appropriate knowledge and skills to inform practice.
- Understand the need to establish and maintain a safe practice environment

In order to fulfil these requirements, paramedics must have a level of pharmaceutical knowledge and an awareness of how and where to find appropriate information to support clinical practice. Contemporary healthcare regimes have resulted in a breadth of emergent new products and complex treatment regimens. As a paramedic student or clinician, you will need up-to-date, clear and concise information to guide your practice. Examples of this can be found in later chapters in this book as well as external sources such as the JRCALC and numerous other guides, websites, texts and resources that are readily available. However, ensuring a robust and evidence-based or evidence-informed selection of these is paramount. Some resources are web based, some print based and some digital app based.

This chapter aims to introduce you to using pharmaceutical and prescribing reference guides with a specific focus on:

- JRCALC Clinical Guidelines (JRCALC, 2019a)
- JRCALC Pocket Book (JRCALC, 2019b)
- JRCALC app.

Pharmaceutical and prescribing guides are vital and valuable resources to draw upon to ensure safe, accountable and evidence-based paramedic practice and patient care.

Clinical consideration

As an undergraduate paramedic student or practising paramedic, there are core approaches to the fundamentals of medicines administration you should apply.

For example, when administering any drug, the paramedic should make sure they have a full understanding of its mechanism of action and the expected physiological effect it will have on the patient.

When out in practice, make sure you know where to easily access this information in your JRCALC so you can check it quickly in an emergency situation.

Joint Royal Colleges Ambulance Liaison Committee (JRCALC) Clinical Practice Guidelines

The JRCALC Clinical Practice Guidelines are an essential resource for paramedics and other healthcare professionals, in emergency care, on the road and in the community. The JRCALC books and app combine expert advice with practical guidance to ensure uniformity in the delivery of high-quality patient care. The books, available as either the comprehensive reference edition or the pocket guide, cover a wide range of topics, from resuscitation, medical emergencies, trauma, obstetrics and medicines to major incidents and staff wellbeing. They include an extensive UK drugs formulary and Page for Age drugs tables to assist in making medicines administration simple. To date, the hard-copy publication has been revised every 2–3 years. The digital version, via an app, is also available for prehospital clinicians to download. The electronic app version is updated more regularly.

The JRCALC Guidelines make reference to the National Institute for Health and Care Excellence (NICE) where appropriate. NICE guidelines inform the breadth of the National Health Service (NHS) in England and are also subject to regular review, update or withdrawal. Independent providers and ambulance services outside the UK should refer to their equivalent guidelines and institutions informing these.

Paramedics must be aware that any subsequent changes in evidence-based guidance after the date of any publication will not be incorporated within the published document. This emphasises the need for vigilance and awareness of possible emergent variations or changes in clinical practice and continuous professional development, as reflected within the HCPC paramedic standards of proficiency. This also supports the increasing use by paramedics of the more regularly updated digital format of the JRCALC Guidelines.

It is worth noting that the physical, hard-copy JRCALC Guidelines text books are available through bookshops and are on sale separately from the digital app. The app is available to the public via the internet on a subscription basis. Ambulance trusts in the UK can also develop a 'service-specific' version of the JRCALC app. This is referred to as the 'JRCALC plus', with most ambulance trust in the UK opting to use this resource for their employees rather than issuing hard-copy books. Independent providers and ambulance services outside the UK who are interested in the 'JRCALC plus' option should contact the publisher direct. This JRCALC (app) resource offers the most current guidance as the digital format can be more easily updated.

Most of the content of the JRCALC Guidelines is universally applicable to NHS ambulance services. However, some modification of these may be evident in regional/individual ambulance services and independent and non-UK ambulance service providers as approved by relevant clinical committees or equivalents to best meet the needs of local service users. Another area of modification to the JRCALC Guidelines for paramedics to be aware of may arise through research sanctioned by relevant research ethics committees.

JRCALC Update information

It is worth noting that the JRCALC Guidelines contain a section at the beginning of the text called 'Update Analysis – "what's changed?"'. This consists of a table containing update information about changes to specific guidelines since the last edition. It is split into sections which reflect those of the book, making it easy to find if there has been an update within the new JRCALC publication to a specific area of guideline since the previous edition (Figure 2.1).

Clinical considerations

- Always make sure you have a copy of your JRCALC Pocket Book or app with you.
- If you use your Pocket Book, make sure you check regularly for any updates which have happened since your book was printed.
- You may inadvertently administer a medication incorrectly if you have not kept up to date with the latest guideline changes.

The knowledge that informs the paramedic profession and the subsequent complex application of this to clinical skills and treatment interventions are constantly changing and updating in response to new research. It is essential for paramedics to keep up to date with the latest changes in policy and procedure. A paramedic who is already familiar with using the guidelines should read through the updated sections when a new edition is published to check any guideline changes which may affect their practice.

Update Analysis – 'What's changed?'

SECTION 4	
Trauma	**Revisions made in Supplementary Guidelines 2017.**
Trauma Emergencies in Adults – Overview	Updated to cover haemorrhage from renal dialysis arteriovenous graft and fistulas included.
Head Injury	Revised guideline. • Includes guidance for mild to moderate head injury, new conveyance decision tool. • Removal of midazolam for traumatic brain injury – for enhanced care team use only.
Limb Trauma	Additional information on open fractures and re-alignment is included.
Burns and Scalds	The adult and child guidelines have been merged. • NICE Red Flags are added, as is information on NARU Chemical Burns.

Figure 2.1   JRCALC Guidelines – Update Analysis. Source: Reproduced with permission from JRCALC Guidelines (2019a).

How to navigate the JRCALC Guidelines

This is a comprehensive resource book containing a wide variety of clinical guidelines and information for paramedics on a broad range of topics. Such a large reference guide can seem daunting at first; however, the text is laid out in a logical order, making information easy to find and access. The resource book is split into seven main sections.

1. General Guidance
2. Resuscitation
3. Medical Emergencies
4. Trauma
5. Maternity Care
6. Special Situations
7. Medicines

The approach taken by the Guidelines presents information specific to commonly used drugs and the practical administration of these. In addition, the Guidelines build on this by identifying where a particular drug should fit into the patient's management plan in a variety of treatment settings (e.g. emergency situations). As such, pertinent information on a particular drug will appear in the Medicines section (section 7) but also in numerous other sections of the book, and successful navigation of this text by paramedics or other clinicians is essential to get the most out of the resource specific to medicines management and clinical application.

It is worth noting that the drugs are presented in alphabetical order in the Medicines section of the Guidelines.

Skills in practice: example of navigating the JRCALC Guidelines

A paramedic looking for information about morphine sulfate will find relevant information about the drug not only in the Medicines section (section 7) but also in other sections specific to other aspects of clinical application such as General Guidance (section 1), Medical Emergencies (section 3) and Trauma (section 4).

General Guidance section (JRCALC Guidelines, section 1)

This section contains a large amount of general information for paramedics covering a broad range of topics including staff health and wellbeing, pain management in adults and children, sexual assault and safeguarding. Each topic has its own chapter within the section. Paramedics can find specific information relating to medicines and their use in clinical practice in the Pain Management for Adults and Children and End of Life Care chapters. It is essential for the paramedic to use the information in these chapters in conjunction with the specific information found in the Medicines section (section 7). Referring only to information on the Medicines pages may result in missing vital information about special applications or clinical situations relating to a specific drug and lead to its incorrect administration in practice.

Clinical considerations

If administering an analgesic (e.g. morphine) or an opioid antagonist (e.g. naloxone) to a patient at the end of their life, make sure you check the Guidelines in the End of Life Care chapter in the General Guidance section (section 1) as well as the specific drug information contained in the Medicines section (section 7).

The End of Life Care chapter contains more specific medication guidance relating to end-of-life care situations and medications may be administered incorrectly if this special guidance is not adhered to.

Resuscitation section (JRCALC Guidelines, section 2)

The Resuscitation section contains information and guidance on a number of topics relating to various aspects of resuscitation. Chapters in this section include out-of-hospital cardiac arrest, basic and advanced life support, foreign body airway obstruction, return of spontaneous circulation, death verification, death of a child and tracheostomy and laryngectomy management. In addition to the general guidance for each drug found in section 7, specific information about the drugs used in prehospital cardiac arrest situations can be found in the overview section at the beginning of each chapter within this Resuscitation section. For example, the advanced life support and return of spontaneous circulation chapters contain further information about the use of drugs covered in section 7 but applied to a cardiac arrest situation.

Medical Emergencies section (JRCALC Guidelines, section 3)

This section contains a large amount of specific information relating to a breadth of medical emergencies commonly encountered by paramedics in practice. Section 3 starts with two chapters giving an overview of medical emergencies in adults and children which contain general information relating to medical emergencies and patient assessment (see Table 2.1). The text then focuses on a number of specific aspects of medical emergencies in more detail within which drugs identified in section 7 could be applied.

Each of these chapters is then further split into subsections: an introduction, incidence, severity and outcome, pathophysiology and assessment and management. This provides a comprehensive overview of each medical emergency and how it should be managed by paramedics in practice. Paramedics should refer to this section to see whether a particular drug is used to treat a certain condition and where that drug fits into patient management.

Clinical consideration

Both hydrocortisone and adrenaline 1:100 have anaphylaxis listed as an indication in their chapters in the Medicines section (section 7). However, the Allergic Reactions Including Anaphylaxis chapter, in the Medical Emergencies section (section 3), should be referred to for more information about where these drugs fit into the management plan for such patients.

Table 2.1   Examples of emergency conditions covered in section 3.

Acute coronary syndrome	Hyperventilation syndrome
Abdominal pain	Hypothermia
Allergic reactions (including anaphylaxis)	Implantable cardiovascular defibrillator
Altered levels of consciousness	Management of resuscitation of patients with left ventricular assist devices
Asthma in adults and children	Meningococcal meningitis and septicaemia
Cardiac rhythm disturbances	Mental health presentations
Chronic pulmonary disease	Mental Capacity Act
Convulsions in adults	Respiratory illness in children
Convulsions in children	Sickle cell crisis
Dyspnoea	Sepsis
Febrile illness in children	Stroke/transient ischaemic attack
Gastrointestinal bleeding	Traumatic chest pain
Glycaemic emergencies in adults and children	Overdose and poisoning in adults and children
Headache	Paediatric gastroenteritis
Heart failure	Pulmonary embolism
Heat-related illness	

Paramedics need to be aware that just referring to the indications in the Medicines section (section 7) may not give full information about where a drug fits into an ambulance service protocol for management of a certain patient condition, and so the JRCALC guidance in the Medical Emergencies section (section 3) should always be referred to alongside the Medicines section in order to ensure best approach and correct patient management.

Trauma section (JRCALC Guidelines, section 4)

The Trauma section is laid out in a similar structure to the Medical Emergencies section. The initial two chapters give an overview of trauma emergencies in adults and children and the subsequent chapters each contain information about a specific trauma emergency and its paramedic management (see Table 2.2).

All the individual chapters follow a similar format, offering information about the incidence, severity and outcome, pathophysiology and assessment and management of each trauma emergency. In relation to drugs and their use in emergency situations, the Trauma chapter should be used similarly to the Medical Emergencies chapters. Each chapter can be used to find more information about drugs used in the treatment of a given emergency and, more specifically, exactly where a particular drug fits into the treatment and management plan for patients in practice. Paramedics should use this information in conjunction with the Medicines section (section 7) and specific drugs within it, in order to find not only information about when a drug should be used and how it fits into a particular management plan, but also information to ensure the drug is administered correctly, thus reducing the possibility of drug errors.

Maternity Care (JRCALC Guidelines, section 5)

The notion of two lives scenarios (i.e. mother and baby) presents the paramedic with numerous challenges specific to this area of care. This section begins with an overview of obstetric emergencies and contains chapters that guide the paramedic through the management of a range of maternity-related presentations. Similarly to the previous sections, paramedics should refer to and check the protocols for each given maternity situation to confirm whether drug therapy is appropriate for a given maternal presentation. After checking the Maternity Care section, further information about dosage or specific drug actions should be sought in the Medicines section (section 7).

Special Situations (JRCALC Guidelines, section 6)

This section contains chapters about specific situations paramedics may encounter and includes information about major, high-risk and complex incidents such as individuals requiring care interventions but who have been incapacitated by police or other security services. Within this section there are two chapters relating specifically to medicines.

- Atropine for CBRNe (chemical, biological, radiological and nuclear explosives).
- DuoDote® auto-injector (atropine combined with pralidoxime).

These two chapters contain information about the presentation, indications, actions, contraindications, cautions and side-effects of these drugs in relation to organophosphate and nerve agent poisoning.

Table 2.2   Examples of specific trauma emergency conditions and management covered in section 4.

Abdominal trauma	Thoracic trauma
Head injury	Falls in older adults
Limb trauma	Burns and scalds
Spinal injury and spinal cord injury	Electrical injuries
Major pelvic trauma	Immersion and drowning

Medicines (JRCALC Guidelines, section 7)

The Medicines section begins with an overview of medicines and goes on to present more detailed information and particular characteristics about medications which can be administered by registered paramedics, provided they have the correct legal authority (HCPC, 2014; JRCALC, 2019a). Chapter 3 of this text discuses legal and ethical issues further.

Individual ambulance trusts across the UK may have variations to their local protocols and Patient Group Directives (PGDs), meaning that not all medicines listed in the JRCALC Guidelines are necessarily given by all registered paramedics across counties or countries within the UK. Paramedics should be cognisant of such variations in local protocols and check with their employing ambulance service to find out which medicines can be administered by paramedics in their local ambulance trust region.

It is important for paramedics to note that PGDs are also available for drugs which are not in the JRCALC Guidelines. This means in some situations a paramedic may find themselves administering a drug which is not listed in the reference book. In such cases, the PGD will provide guidance on the administration of these medicines specific to the local ambulance service protocols.

The Medicines section is split into a short introductory chapter called Medicines Overview, a separate chapter for each medicine listed and finally a 'Page for Age' section. The introductory chapter contains general information for paramedics about medicines, including safety aspects, prescribing terms, drug routes and paediatric doses. All paramedics should make themselves familiar with the information in this chapter before administering any drugs in practice.

Each specific medicine chapter contains detailed information about the presentation of the medicine, its mechanism of action, indications, contraindications, cautions and a table detailing dosage and administration across the age span. All chapters have a similar layout with the specific drug dosage and administration technique featured in a table. This pragmatic layout allows paramedics to quickly access pertinent drug information in an emergency situation (see Figure 2.2). Before administering a drug in practice, paramedics should always refer to the JRCALC Guidelines page specific to that drug to ensure correct administration.

The JRCALC Pocket Book and digital app, section 2.6, also contain this information. This enables paramedics to quickly and easily check medicines administration information in practice/on the road.

Skills in practice

Be alert and aware of the common factors associated with the selection and administration of drugs. In this example you should locate the medication dexamethasone in the JRCALC Guidelines.

- What are the indications for this drug?
- Are there any contraindications for this drug?
- What are the cautions associated with this drug?
- Are there any side-effects associated with this medication?
- What is the presentation of this drug?
- What is the route of administration and are there any recommendations related to its administration?

Refer to JRCALC Clinical Guidelines (2019), pp. 317, 540, 563-564.

Aspirin

ASP

Presentation

300 milligrams aspirin (acetylsalicylic acid) in tablet. form, Dispersible or chewable.

Indications

Adults with:
- Clinical or ECG evidence suggestive of myocardial infarction or ischaemia.

Actions

Has an antiplatelet action which reduces clot formation.

Contra-indications

- Known aspirin allergy or sensitivity.
- Children under 16 years (see additional) information).
- Active gastrointestinal bleeding.
- Haemophilia or other known clotting disorders.
- Severe hepatic disease.

Cautions

As the likely benefits of a single 300 milligram aspirin outweigh the potential, risks, aspirin may be given to patients with:
- Asthma
- Pregnancy

- Kidney or liver failure
- Gastric or duodenal ulcer
- Current treatment with anticoagulants.

Side Effects

- Increased risk of gastric bleeding.
- Wheezing in some asthmatics.

Additional Information

In suspected myocardial infarction a 300 milligram aspirin tablet should be given regardless of any previous aspirin taken that day.

Clopidogrel may be indicated in acute ST segment elevation myocardial infarction – refer to Clopidogrel.

Aspirin is contra-indicated in children under the age of 16 years as it may precipitate Reye's syndrome. This syndrome is very rare and occurs in young children, damaging the liver and brain. It has a mortality rate of 50%.

Dosage and Administration

Route: Oral – chewed or dissolved in water.

AGE	INITIAL DOSE	REPEAT DOSE	DOSE INTERVAL	CONCENTRATION	VOLUME	MAX DOSE
Adults	300 milligrams	NONE	N/A	300 milligrams per tablet	1 tablet	300 milligrams

Bibliography

British National Formulary. Available from: https://bnf.nice org.uk/drug/aspirin.html, 2018.

Figure 2.2 Example of how specific drug (aspirin) information is presented within the JRCALC Medications section. Source: Reproduced with permission from JRCALC Guidelines (2019a).

Page for Age (JRCALC Guidelines, no section number allocated)

The 'Page for Age' is the last section of text within the Guidelines and has no specific section indicator. This section follows on from the Medicines section (section 7). The pages provide a quick and easy way for paramedics to access key information relating to paediatric patients aged from birth to 11 years. All the information is tabulated and each page is laid out in a logical and straightforward way, making it easy to use in an emergency situation. The tables contain information specific to patients of a particular age group and include normal vital signs, airway device sizing, intravascular fluid doses, drugs for cardiac arrest and the other JRCALC Guidelines.

The drug tables have information about the route, dose, concentration and volume specific to an age group, and provide an easy reference guide for use in practice. Paramedics should note that the Page for Age section does not contain information about indications, contraindications and cautions for a given drug, and these should be double-checked for each patient in the appropriate page of the Medicines section (section 7) before administering any drug (see Figure 2.3).

Page for Age: 9 MONTHS

Vital Signs

	GUIDE WEIGHT 9 kg		HEART RATE 110–160		RESPIRATION RATE 30–40		SYSTOLIC BLOOD PRESSURE 70–90

9 MONTHS

Airway Size by Type

OROPHARYNGEAL AIRWAY	LARYNGEAL MASK	I-GEL AIRWAY	ENDOTRACHEAL TUBE
00	1.5	1.5	Diameter: **4 mm**, Length: **12 cm**

Defibrillation – Cardiac Arrest

MANUAL	AUTOMATED EXTERNAL DEFIBRILLATOR
40 Joules	Where possible, use a manual defibrillator. If an AED is the only defibrillator available, it should be used (preferably using paediatric attenuation pads or else in paediatric mode).

Intravascular Fluid

NAME	ROUTE	INITIAL DOSE	REPEAT DOSE	DOSE INTERVAL	CONCENTRATION	VOLUME	MAX DOSE
0.9% Sodium Chloride (5 ml/kg)	IV/IO	45 ml	45 ml	PRN	0.9%	45 ml	360 ml
0.9% Sodium Chloride (10 ml/kg)	IV/IO	90 ml	90 ml	PRN	0.9%	90 ml	360 ml
0.9% Sodium Chloride (20 ml/kg)	IV/IO	180 ml	180 ml	PRN	0.9%	180 ml	360 ml

Cardiac Arrest

NAME	ROUTE	INITIAL DOSE	REPEAT DOSE	DOSE INTERVAL	CONCENTRATION	VOLUME	MAX DOSE
Adrenaline	IV/IO	90 micrograms	90 micrograms	3–5 minutes	1 milligram in 10 ml (1:10,000)	0.9 ml	No limit
Amiodarone	IV/IO	45 milligrams (After 3rd shock)	45 milligrams	After 5th shock	300 milligrams in 10 ml	1.5 ml	90 milligrams

Quick Reference Table

NAME	ROUTE	INITIAL DOSE	REPEAT DOSE	DOSE INTERVAL	CONCEN-TRATION	VOLUME	MAX DOSE
Activated Charcoal	Oral	N/A	N/A	N/A	N/A	N/A	N/A
Adrenaline - anaphylaxis/asthma	IM	150 micrograms	150 micrograms	5 minutes	1 milligram in 1 ml (1:1,000)	0.15 ml	No limit
Benzylpenicillin	IV/IO	300 milligrams	NONE	N/A	600 milligrams dissolved in 10 ml water for injection	5 ml	300 milligrams
Benzylpenicillin	IM	300 milligrams	NONE	N/A	600 milligrams dissolved in 2 ml water for injection	1 ml	300 milligrams
Chlorphenamine	IV/IO	2.5 milligrams	NONE	N/A	10 milligrams in 1 ml	0.25 ml	2.5 milligrams
Chlorphenamine	Oral (tablet)	N/A	N/A	N/A	N/A	N/A	N/A
Chlorphenamine	Oral (solution)	1 milligram	NONE	N/A	2 milligrams in 5 ml	2.5 ml	1 milligram

650   Medicines

2019

Figure 2.3 Page for Age section. Source: Reproduced with permission from JRCALC Guidelines (2019a).

Page for Age: 9 MONTHS

NAME	ROUTE	INITIAL DOSE	REPEAT DOSE	DOSE INTERVAL	CONCEN-TRATION	VOLUME	MAX DOSE
Dexamethasone	Oral (solution)	1.4 milligrams	NONE	N/A	2 milligrams in 5 ml	3 ml	1.4 milligrams
Dexamethasone	Oral (tablet)	2 milligrams	NONE	N/A	2 milligrams per tablet	1 tablet	2 milligrams
Diazepam	Rectal	5 milligrams	5 milligrams	10 minutes	5 milligrams in 2.5 ml	1 x 5 milligram tube	10 milligrams
Diazepam	IV/IO	3 milligrams	3 milligrams	10 minutes	10 milligrams in 2 ml	0.6 ml	6 milligrams
Glucagon	IM	500 micrograms	NONE	N/A	1 milligram per vial	0.5 vial	500 micrograms
Glucose 10%	IV	2 grams glucose	2 grams glucose	5 minutes	50 grams in 500 ml	20 ml	60 ml (6 g glucose)
Glucose 40% Oral Gel	Buccal	An appropriate amount should be administered, considering the child's size	See initial dose	5 minutes	10 grams in 25 grams of gel	1 tube	An appropriate amount should be administered, considering the child's size
Hydrocortisone	IV/IO/IM	50 milligrams	NONE	N/A	100 milligrams in 1 ml	0.5 ml	50 milligrams
Hydrocortisone	IV/IO/IM	50 milligrams	NONE	N/A	100 milligrams in 2 ml	1 ml	50 milligrams
Ibuprofen	Oral	50 milligrams	50 milligrams	8 hours	100 milligrams in 5 ml	2.5 ml	150 milligrams per 24 hours
Ipratropium Bromide	Neb	125–250 micrograms	NONE	N/A	250 micrograms in 1 ml	0.5 ml–1 ml	125–250 micrograms
Ipratropium Bromide	Neb	125–250 micrograms	NONE	N/A	500 micrograms in 2 ml	0.5 ml–1 ml	125–250 micrograms
Midazolam*	Buccal	2.5 milligrams	2.5 milligrams	10 mins	5 milligrams in 1 ml	0.5 ml pre-filled syringe	5 milligrams
Morphine Sulfate	IV/IO	N/A	N/A	N/A	N/A	N/A	N/A
Morphine Sulfate	Oral	N/A	N/A	N/A	N/A	N/A	N/A
Naloxone	IM	400 micrograms	400 micrograms	3 minutes	400 micrograms in 1 ml	1 ml	2,000 micrograms
Naloxone	IV/IO	800 micrograms	800 micrograms then 400 micrograms	1 minute	400 micrograms in 1 ml	2 ml	2,000 micrograms
Ondansetron	IV/IO/IM	1 milligram	NONE	N/A	2 milligrams in 1 ml	0.5 ml	1 milligram
Paracetamol - Infant suspension	Oral	120 milligrams	120 milligrams	4–6 hours	120 milligrams in 5 ml	5 ml	480 milligrams in 24 hours
Paracetamol	IV infusion/IO	90 milligrams	90 milligrams	4–6 hours	10 milligrams in 1 ml	9 ml	270 milligrams in 24 hours
Salbutamol	Neb	2.5 milligrams	2.5 milligrams	5 minutes	2.5 milligrams in 2.5 ml	2.5 ml	No limit
Salbutamol	Neb	2.5 milligrams	2.5 milligrams	5 minutes	5 milligrams in 2.5 ml	1.25 ml	No limit
Tranexamic Acid	IV	150 mg	NONE	N/A	100 mg/ml	1.5 ml	150 mg

*Give the dose as prescribed in the child's individual treatment plan/Epilepsy Passport (the dosages described above reflect the recommended dosages for a child of this age).

Figure 2.3   (Continued)

Reflection

Take some time to reflect on your reading and think about the following questions.

- How many sections of the main JRCALC Guidelines are there?
- At the end of which section does the Page for Age information appear?
- How many chapters are there in the Maternity Care section? In which section of the JRCLAC Guidelines would you find information about specific trauma emergencies?

JRCALC Pocket Book

This is a condensed version of the JRCALC Guidelines meant to be used as a quick reference guide in practice. It is laid out in a similar format to the main reference book but with nine sections rather than seven. The sections are as follows.

- Resuscitation
- Paediatrics
- Trauma
- Special Situations
- Maternity
- General
- Medical
- Medicines
- Page for Age

The main deviations from the layout of the large reference guide are the addition of a Paediatrics section and the use of a separate section for Page for Age. The Pocket Book is very condensed and contains only a fraction of the information found in the large guide. The first seven sections contain tables, algorithms and flow charts with essential information for paramedics pertaining to a selection of emergency situations commonly encountered in practice. These sections should be referred to in order to find basic essential information in an emergency situation and are in no way meant to be a comprehensive set of Guidelines.

The Pocket Book is a handy reference guide for use in practice and most paramedics will refer to it or the app on a daily basis. Either one should always be referred to when administering any medications to check indications, contraindications, dosage and any other pertinent information relating to the drug in question. This best practice approach reflects the requirements of the paramedic standards of proficiency.

The Page for Age section of the Pocket Book is the only section which is completely unchanged from the large reference guide, with the Pocket Book containing full information for each age group. This enables paramedics to find key information on drug dosing by age group easily in an emergency.

Each drug in the Medicines section contains the same information as in the large guide and the only difference in this section is that the more comprehensive Medicines Overview chapter in the large guide is abridged to the Medicines: Best Practice Checklist in the Pocket Book. The Best Practice Checklist is situated at the beginning of the Medicines section of the Pocket Book (see Figure 2.4).

MEDS

Medicines: Best Practice Checklist

- Before administering any medication check the:
  - Type
  - Strength
  - Integrity of the packaging
  - Clarity of the fluid
  - Expiry date.
- Select the most appropriate route, taking into account:
  - The patient's condition
  - The urgency of the situation.
- Only administer drugs via the routes you have been trained for.
- The drug codes are provided for INFORMATION ONLY.
- Complete documentation.

Figure 2.4 Medicines Best Practice Checklist. Source: JRCALC Pocket Book, 2019.

This checklist should be referred to before giving any medication in practice and gives a list of drug administration checks as well as reminders about drug administration routes and documentation. All the drugs listed in the large guide appear in the Pocket Book and the Pocket Book contains full information on presentation, indications, actions, cautions, contraindications, side-effects and dosage and administration for each drug. This means the Pocket Book alone can be referred to when administering a medication in practice with no need to use the large guide.

Reflection

Take some time to think about your reading so far and make responses to the following questions.

- The Glycaemic Emergencies algorithm in the Glycaemic Emergencies in Adults and Children chapter in the Medical Emergencies section of the JRCALC Guidelines (section 3) contains information about when to administer which two drugs?
- Use your JRCALC Guidelines to find the correct drug dosages for administering morphine sulfate to a 6-year-old patient by the IV/IO route and orally.
- Use your JRCLAC Guidelines to find the initial dose, repeat dose and maximum dose when administering atropine sulfate to an adult patient.
- The Heart Failure chapter in the Medical Emergencies section of the JRCALC Guidelines contains specific information about which three drugs used as therapy for heart failure?

JRCALC Guidelines digital application (app)

The JRCALC Guidelines are also available as an app for smartphones, tablets and laptops. The big difference between the Pocket Book and app is that the app is essentially an electronic copy of the large reference guide and is not abridged like the Pocket Book. Many paramedics now choose to use the app over the Pocket Book as it contains the full reference guide. Another big advantage of the app is that it automatically updates when Guidelines change so it does not end up out of date between editions as the printed versions frequently do.

The app is available in two forms: the basic JRCALC Guidelines app (www.classprofessional.co.uk/digital-products/apps/icpg-the-jrcalc-app-subscriptions/) and the JRCALC Guidelines plus app (www.classprofessional.co.uk/digital-products/apps/jrcalc-plus-app/). The basic app is available for purchase in either android or iPhone format. In contrast, the plus app is only available to employees of ambulance service trusts which have subscriptions to it. The basic app contains all the information held in the main reference guide, while the ' plus app may contain more or less information depending on how it has been customised to reflect the specific requirements of a particular ambulance service trust and its employees. Ambulance trusts which purchase a subscription to the plus app are able to restrict and remove content and can also add their own local guidelines or information as required to best reflect their regional service needs.

The app is easy to navigate and is split into five main tabs: Dashboard, Guidelines, Medicines, Algorithms and Page for Age. The Dashboard is the home page and allows easy access to updates and Page for Age as well as allowing Medicines and Guidelines to be bookmarked for quick reference (see Figure 2.5).

The Algorithms tab is unique to the app and contains all the algorithms from each of the Guidelines displayed together in alphabetical order. This makes finding an algorithm for a particular condition or situation easier, plus there is the option to navigate directly to the related full guidance from each algorithm. Another useful feature of the app is the search function. This is situated at the top of the Dashboard home page and enables users to search more easily.

The Guidelines, Medicines and Page for Age tabs of the app contain all the information that the large reference guide holds. The Guidelines tab is split into the same sections as the large guide and the guidelines within each section are displayed alphabetically (see Figure 2.5). The Meds tab contains full information for each medicine and again is displayed alphabetically. The tabs mean information is easy to access in an emergency and the app is well laid out and very user friendly.

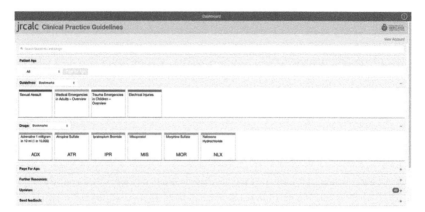

Figure 2.5   Dashboard. Source: South Central Ambulance Service, JRCALC plus.

Test your knowledge

Know where to find this information to help inform your practice.

- The Pain Management in Adults And Children chapters can be found in which section of the JRCALC Guidelines?
- According to the JRCALC Guidelines, for what conditions can paramedics administer adrenaline 1 mg in 1 mL (1 in 1000)?
- Which chapter in the Medical Emergencies section of the JRCALC Guidelines contains information about which drugs to administer for patients having a seizure?
- Which section and chapter of the JRCALC Guidelines contain information for paramedics about the administration of atropine in a CBRNE situation?

Useful additional resources

The JRCAL Guidelines in its different forms offers paramedics a core 'go to' reference point for universal clinical guidance. The next section of this chapter gives an overview of other valuable medication resources to further inform and develop knowledge, understanding and application. These additional resources in both hard-copy and digital formats are commonly used by allied healthcare professional and medical practitioners as evidence-informed texts relevant to their areas of practice.

The range of drugs covered within these additional resources is far broader than the JRCALC Guidelines and may therefore be used by paramedics to develop their knowledge and understanding in relation to broader medications, a patient's medical history, other uses of drugs, drug interactions and contraindications as well as cost. Postqualified paramedics going on to undertake non-medical prescribing courses and clinical roles will need to be more familiar with these additional resources, which include the following.

- *British National Formulary* (BNF)
- *Children's British National Formulary* (CBNF)
- *Monthly Index of Medical Specialities* (MIMS)
- Electronic Medicines Compendium

For an excellent guide to the *British National Formulary* and other resources, we recommend you refer to Pryor and Hand (2021).

British National Formulary (BNF)

Assembled by the Joint Formulary Committee, this is a reliable resource of information on medication. It includes drug information covering individual medication, groups of medication, uses, side-effects and interactions (Young and Pitcher, 2016). The information provided is evidence informed from drug manufacturer/supplier datasheets, literature, consensus guidelines and peer review. The BNF makes use of a grading system of A–E and levels of evidence to help understand the strength of evidence underpinning the associated recommendations given (Joint Formulary Committee, 2019). The BNF is available in hard copy for both the Adult (BNF 2020a) and Children's (BNF 2020b) versions. The resources can also be accessed as a mobile app or online (bnf.nice.org.uk/).

Medication listed within pharmaceutical and prescribing guidance documents can be presented with a generic and brand or trade name. The generic name is used to define:
- The chemical name of a medication
- A term referring to the chemical make-up of a medication rather than to the advertised brand name under which the medication is sold
- A term referring to any medication marketed under its chemical name without advertising
- The medication's active ingredient.

The brand or trade name of a medication is the name given by the pharmaceutical company that manufactures it. It is usually easy to write and say for sales and marketing purposes. An example of this is paracetamol (generic name) which can have the following brand or trade names: Panadol, Calpol.

The brand or trade name is often written more clearly on a medicine's packaging; the generic name will also be written somewhere on the packaging but often in small print. It is also not uncommon to find that some packaging only has the generic name on it.

The production of a given generic medication by individual manufacturers using a different brand or trade name can also result in a medication being presented differently. Examples of this can include a variation in the colour, size and shape of a given medication depending on which company makes it. The paramedic needs to be vigilant and aware of this potentially dangerous issue. It may be that the pharmacist supplying an ambulance service or the patient with a given drug is getting it from a different company, or the prescription has been written in a generic way rather than using a brand name. Paramedics *must* take great care to check and ensure that any medication to be administered is the correct medication.

Monthly Index of Medical Specialities

As you progress through your clinical experience and paramedic career, especially within the primary care setting, you may also come across the MIMS prescribing guide (www.mims.co.uk/). This is an up-to-date prescribing reference for healthcare professionals. MIMS is updated constantly online, to reflect the latest approved prescribing information, along with the addition of new drugs and formulations, and also removes products that are no longer available. MIMS is primarily intended for use by GPs and healthcare professionals undertaking advanced roles working within primary care. All prescribing healthcare professionals wishing to access this resource, including paramedics, will need to subscribe to MIMS to access either the online version or the quarterly print edition.

MIMS is a helpful prescribing resource and provides:

- News on changes that affect medicines and prescribing
- Drug information for branded and generic products, updated daily
- At-a-glance drug comparison tables including dosing and monitoring regimens, available presentations, prices, potential sensitisers and compatible devices
- Quick-reference summaries of key clinical guidance from authoritative national bodies including NICE and the Scottish Intercollegiate Guidelines Network (SIGN)
- Online drugs shortages tracker showing branded and generic medicines that are out of stock
- Online visual guides to help you identify, compare and recommend diabetes and respiratory administration devices.

Electronic Medicines Compendium (EMC)

The EMC contains up-to-date, easily accessible information about medicines licensed for use in the UK. It can be found at: www.medicines.org.uk/emc. The EMC contains more than 14 000 documents, which have been checked and approved by either the UK or European government agencies which license medicines. These agencies are the UK Medicines and Healthcare Products Regulatory Agency (MHRA) and the European Medicines Agency (EMA). The EMC is updated continually and you can browse for medicines or active ingredients using the A–Z buttons. The EMC contains regulated and approved information on medicines available in the UK including the following.

- *Summaries of Product Characteristics (known as SPCs or SmPCs):* an SmPC informs healthcare professionals how to prescribe and use a medicine correctly. It is based on clinical trials that a pharmaceutical company has carried out and gives information about dose, use and possible side-effects. A SmPC is always written in a standard format.
- *Patient Information Leaflets (PILs, Package Leaflets or PLs):* a PIL is the leaflet included in the pack with any medicine. The PIL is a summary of the SmPC and is written for patients.
- *Risk Minimisation Materials (RMMs):* RMMs are resources for healthcare professionals which aim to optimise the safe and effective use of a medicine. RMMs can come in a number of forms, such as educational programmes, prescribing or dispensing guides, patient brochures or alert cards.
- *Safety Alerts:* these are issued by the regulator and/or marketing authorisation holder and contain important public health messages or safety-critical information about a medicine.
- *Product Information:* this is any additional information about a product. It may include important information such as change of packaging or issues related to stock levels.

Within the EMC there are audio and video resources that provide additional information in a user-friendly format, promoting the safe and effective use of a medicine. For example, a video clip may demonstrate how to administer a certain medicine correctly.

Conclusion

This chapter has provided an overview of the main pharmaceutical and prescribing reference guides used within paramedic practice. Guidance has been given to encourage you to start to navigate the

Associated medications

The following are medications commonly used by paramedics in practice.

- Take some time to look these up in the JRCALC Guidelines, section 7, and find the appropriate dose for an adult patient.
- Make sure you can find the appropriate dose for a range of paediatric patients from 0 to 11 (if applicable).

Think about the medications, how they are used in practice, route of administration, cautions and contraindications. Make some notes about your own experiences of administering these drugs in practice, thinking about how you used a reference guide to find the correct drug information. If you are making notes about people you have offered care and support to, you must ensure that you have adhered to the rules of confidentiality.

Medication	Your notes
Morphine sulfate	
Diazepam	
Furosemide	
Salbutamol	
Adrenaline	

JRCALC Guidelines in hard-copy, digital and app format. This guidance will help to ensure you know where to find all the information needed about a medicinal product or device to guide safe and effective paramedic practice. The differences between paper-based and online versions have been highlighted to ensure you are aware where to access the most up-to-date and accurate drug information. An introduction to additional resources has also been given.

Disclaimer

JRCALC is referenced within this chapter. Joint Royal Colleges Ambulance Liaison Committee guidance is subject to regular review and may be updated or withdrawn. JRCALC has not checked the use of its content in this chapter to confirm that it accurately reflects JRCALC publications.

References

British National Formulary. (2020a). *Adult BNF*. London: Pharmaceutical Press.

British National Formulary. (2020b). *Children's BNF*. London: Pharmaceutical Press.

Health and Care Professions Council (HCPC). (2016). *Standards of conduct, performance and ethics*. www.hcpc-uk. org/standards/standards-of-conduct-performance-and-ethics/

Health and Care Professions Council (HCPC). (2014). *The standards of proficiency for paramedics*. www.hcpc-uk. org/standards/standards-of-proficiency/paramedics/

Joint Formulary Committee. (2019). *How BNF publications are constructed: assessing the evidence*. https://bnf.nice. org.uk/about/how-bnf-publications-are-constructed.html

Joint Royal Colleges Ambulance Liaison Committee (JRCALC). (2019a). *Clinical Guidelines*. Bridgwater: Class Professional Publishing.

Joint Royal Colleges Ambulance Liaison Committee (JRCALC). (2019b). *Clinical Guidelines Pocket Book*. Bridgwater: Class Professional Publishing.

Joint Royal Colleges Ambulance Liaison Committee (JRCALC). Basic app. www.classprofessional.co.uk/digital-products/apps/icpg-the-jrcalc-app-subscriptions/

Joint Royal Colleges Ambulance Liaison Committee (JRCALC). Plus app. www.classprofessional.co.uk/digital-products/apps/jrcalc-plus-app/

Pryor, C. and Hand, A. (2021). How to use pharmaceutical and prescribing reference guides BNF/cBNF/MIMS. In: *Fundamentals of Pharmacology for Nursing and Health Care Students* (eds I. Peate and B. Hill). Oxford: Wiley.

Young, S. and Pitcher, B. (2016). *Medicine Management for Nurses at a Glance*. Oxford: Wiley.

Further reading

Australian Clinical Practice Guidelines: Ambulance and MICA Paramedics. www.ambulance.vic.gov.au/wp-content/uploads/2018/07/Clinical-Practice-Guidelines-2018-Edition-1.4.pdf

Australian Council of Ambulance Authorities (CAA): www.caa.net.au/

Australia, Paramedicine Board: www.paramedicineboard.gov.au/Professional-standards.aspx

Electronic Medicines Compendium: www.medicines.org.uk/emc

Joint Royal Colleges Ambulance Liaison Committee (JRCALC): www.jrcalc.org.uk/

National Institute for Health and Care Excellence (NICE). Information on medicines and prescribing: www.nice.org. uk/about/nice-communities/medicines-and-prescribing

Scottish Intercollegiate Guidelines Network (SIGN): www.sign.ac.uk

UK Drug Tariff: www.nhsbsa.nhs.uk/pharmacies-gp-practices-and-appliance-contractors/drug-tariff

Multiple-choice questions

1. What is the correct dose for the administration of benzylpenicillin sodium for a 9-year-old child?
   (a) 1.2 grams
   (b) 600 milligrams
   (c) 300 milligrams
   (d) 1 gram

2. According to the JRCALC Guidelines, paramedics can administer dexamethasone for which respiratory condition?
   (a) Croup
   (b) Asthma
   (c) COPD
   (d) Bronchiolitis

3. What does PGD stand for?
   (a) Parental guidance drug
   (b) Prescription-guided drug
   (c) Patient group directive
   (d) Patient-guided directive

4. Paramedics administer diazepam for the treatment of seizures and which other condition?
   (a) Tachycardia
   (b) Anxiety
   (c) Symptomatic cocaine toxicity
   (d) Nausea and vomiting

5. When should a medication labelled p.c. be taken?
   (a) After food
   (b) Before food
   (c) Every night
   (d) Every morning

6. Which of the following is not a potential side-effect of clopidogrel?
   (a) Dyspepsia
   (b) Nausea
   (c) Abdominal pain
   (d) Diarrhoea

7. When administering GTN, paramedics should check whether the patient has already taken which other drug?
   (a) Sildenafil
   (b) Aspirin
   (c) Bisoprolol
   (d) Clopidogrel

8. What is the maximum adult dose of morphine sulfate which can be administered via the IV/IO route?
   (a) 10 mg
   (b) 20 mg
   (c) 30 mg
   (d) 40 mg

9. Which section of the JRCALC Guidelines features information about specific medical emergencies?
   (a) Section 1
   (b) Section 2
   (c) Section 3
   (d) Section 4

10. The average heart rate of a child aged 6 years old is:
    (a) 60-100 BPM
    (b) 80-100 BPM
    (c) 90-110 BPM
    (d) 80-120 BPM

Chapter 3

Legal and ethical issues

Claire Leader, Emma Senior, Deborah Flynn and Paul Younger

Aim

The aim of this chapter is to examine the legal and ethical considerations that are related to pharmacology and medicines management in contemporary paramedic practice.

Learning outcomes

By the end of this chapter the reader will be able to:

1. Define commonly used legal and ethical concepts
2. Identify situations where legal and ethical considerations are required to make defensible decisions
3. Explain how legal and ethical considerations influence the decision-making process
4. Apply legal and ethical considerations to a variety of scenarios likely to be encountered in modern healthcare settings.

The legal issues discussed in this chapter are predominantly related to the law in the UK. It is essential that you keep to the laws of the country in which you are practising. You are required to have knowledge of and keep to the relevant laws, policies, regulations and guidance about the advice you give people in relation to prescribing, supplying, dispensing or administering medicines within the limits of your training and competence.

Test your knowledge

1. According to law, what must be established in order to prove a case of negligence?
2. Can a wife consent to treatment on behalf of their wife who lacks capacity?
3. What is the meaning of beneficence in relation to ethics?
4. Can a paramedic or other healthcare professional provide treatment for children without the consent of their responsible parent in an emergency situation?
5. What is a professional body's primary function?

Fundamentals of Pharmacology for Paramedics, First Edition. Edited by Ian Peate, Suzanne Evans, and Lisa Clegg.
© 2022 John Wiley & Sons Ltd. Published 2022 by John Wiley & Sons Ltd.

Introduction

This section will introduce readers to fundamental ethical principles relating to paramedic practice and the provision of healthcare, as well as some of the key legal concepts with which those studying paramedicine should become familiar in order to ensure that decisions around pharmacology have a legal and ethical basis.

Any decisions made about pharmacology require consideration of various issues: what you are legally obliged to do, what you are professionally guided to do and what is in the best interests of the person within the situation. In practice, the three usually exist together, but before considering them as a whole, let's start with the fundamentals and look at them separately.

This chapter will consider the three components that underpin high-quality decision making in pharmacology:

- The law
- Ethical principles and theories
- Regulatory bodies.

The law

Laws exist to protect patients and the public. Recent years have seen changes in the culture within healthcare in the UK, with a notable rise in litigation; this is much the same in other countries. Unlike some countries where there is a 'no blame' process for medico-legal cases, the UK system operates a 'fault criterion' whereby fault has to be established for the complainant to prove a case. In the UK clinical negligence claims quadrupled between 2007 and 2017 (National Health Service Improvement (NHSI), 2019) leading to an exponential growth in the number of cases involving healthcare professionals who are forced to defend their practice in a court setting. Failing to monitor a particular drug therapy, failure to recognise the prescription of a contraindicated drug, failure to warn patients of adverse effects and neglecting to protect a patient from harm are all examples of pharmacology cases whereby blame could be laid. As our professional remit grows, so does the legal expectation. Given the amount of resources and information paramedics have access to, the defence of lack of knowledge is wholly insufficient.

UK laws originate from two sources: common law, sometimes referred to as 'case' law, and statute law known as 'Act of Parliament'.

Common law or case law refers to cases that are tried in courts of law whereby a judge will give rule to a set of legal precedents. Common law is constantly changing due to the ways in which judges interpret the law and use their knowledge of legal precedent and common sense as well as applying the facts of the case. Common law safeguards that the law remains common throughout the land and can be divided into either criminal or civil law.

Statute law or Act of Parliament is law which is written down and codified into law. Acts begin as bills which then become Acts once the bills have been heard and possibly amended in the House of Commons and House of Lords before receiving Royal Assent. The Acts can either be private or public. Private Acts may apply to detailed locations within the UK or they may grant specific powers to public bodies such as local authorities. Public Acts are the laws that affect the whole of the UK or one or more of its constituent countries: England, Wales, Scotland and Northern Ireland.

Healthcare and the law in the UK are strongly entwined. The laws created to protect the health of an individual can be seen when under the care of the hospital and its medical team, through to public health and the legal requirements of health and safety. Across the UK, the laws and charters that exist have been created to ensure that the rights and health interests of the individual are protected throughout the duration of their medical care. Paramedics therefore have a legal duty to act with reasonable care when providing services. This 'duty of care' is defined as a 'legal obligation imposed on individuals or organisations that they take reasonable care in the conduct of acts that could foreseeably result in actionable harm to another' (Samanta and Samanta, 2011, p.89). This includes prescribing drug therapy and drug administration as well as consent,

Clinical consideration: the Bolam test

The majority of litigation in relation to medical malpractice comes under the category of negligence.

When considering cases of clinical negligence, courts will assess whether the health professional or organisation in question acted in line with the practice accepted as proper by a body of health professionals specialising in the specific field under scrutiny. This is known as the Bolam test. The case (Bolam v Friern Hospital Management Committee 1957) involved a patient who had suffered a fractured hip during electroconvulsive therapy (ECT). No relaxant or other restraint had been given to the patient in preparation for the treatment. The case explored this, along with the information the patient had been offered. The question was asked of a group of similar professionals and it was assessed that the practitioner had not been negligent as he had acted in accordance with accepted practice at that time. This set the standard and the Bolam test is now utilised in cases of negligence as a benchmark for whether the professional concerned acted in a reasonable manner. However, a judge can still make the assessment that the body of opinion is not reasonable.

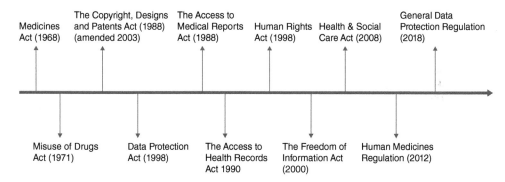

Figure 3.1   Acts and laws relevant to medical practice.

negligence and confidentiality, to name but a few. Failure to act with reasonable care could result in a paramedic being held responsible in both criminal and civil courts as well as being called to account by their regulatory body.

There are several Acts or laws that affect the provision of medicines which are illustrated in Figure 3.1.

Ethical principles and theories

Making ethical decisions is about deciding on the right way to act in a given situation, which is underpinned by the moral values held by an individual or group. In 1979, Beauchamp and Childress (2009) developed a four-point theoretical framework to be used as a method of analysing ethical dilemmas in clinical medicine. The framework included beneficence, non-maleficence, autonomy and justice. These principles remain in healthcare along with the addition of a further two principles. Today the following ethical principles apply.

- Beneficence
- Non-maleficence
- Autonomy
- Justice
- Veracity
- Fidelity

The principles outlined here are commonly felt to underpin judgements health professionals believe to be right. Firstly, *beneficence*, whereby we should endeavour to do good. This extends to protecting others and defending their rights, preventing harm and helping others. It is argued by some such as Pellegrino (1988) that beneficence is the only fundamental principle within healthcare ethics and that the sole purpose of medicine should be to heal. By this assumption, medicines such as contraception and treatments for conditions such as infertility, erectile dysfunction or aesthetics could fall beyond its purpose. However, the notion of 'healing' is complex and dynamic, referring to more than just the rectifying of an immediate physical ailment or condition. Contraception, fertility treatment and plastic surgery support health and wellbeing in many direct and indirect ways, physically as well as psychologically, which is why the endeavour of beneficence is not as straightforward as it would first appear.

In practice, in order to do good, the medical interventions and treatments can often carry a risk of harm and therefore require justification. *Non-maleficence* means that by our actions, we should do others no harm. The principle of non-maleficence therefore cannot be absolute and must be balanced against beneficence. For example, when treating patients with cytotoxic chemotherapy drugs for cancer, we balance beneficence (the potential to do good and eradicate the cancer) against non-maleficence and the risk of the chemotherapy itself to cause the patient's condition to deteriorate, possibly leading to death.

It is also generally believed that people should have the right to make decisions about what is right for them, provided they have sufficient capacity or understanding to do so. This principle is a respect for the *autonomy* of the individual and relates to enabling patients to make self-determined decisions regarding their care. Consent to treatment is a fundamental component of ethical patient care in addition to a legal requirement. It involves a genuine agreement (verbal or written) to receive treatment under circumstances where the patient has been assessed as competent, has been fully informed and where there is no undue pressure exerted (Herring, 2018). Beauchamp and Childress (2009) have argued that no decision can be truly autonomous, as patients rarely have the relevant knowledge to hold a full understanding of treatment options and as such are vulnerable to the coercion of health professionals such as paramedics who feel that they are best placed to make decisions in the interests of their patients (paternalism).

However, patient groups have sought to increase autonomy for patients through changes in policies and practices which decrease the potential for coercion and increase patients freedom to act (Williamson, 2010). An example of this has been seen in recent years, as a greater emphasis has been placed on models of shared decision making between health professionals and patients. The shared decision-making approach seeks a balance between paternalistic care and the informed consent approach. Paternalistic care is where decisions about care are made by paramedics and other health professionals (doctors, for example) and patients passively receive the care prescribed. This model does not factor in patients' own values and beliefs and can lead to patients feeling greater distress where there is a negative outcome (Stewart and Brown, 2001). The informed consent approach offers patients greater responsibility and will often involve health professionals offering patients all the

Clinical consideration

A shared decision-making approach to care has been shown to benefit patients in terms of their active engagement in the treatment plan or taking the prescribed medications (Edwards and Elwyn, 2009). As such, it is an ethical approach to care which has also been shown to reduce the incidence of medicolegal claims where there is a negative outcome (Studdert et al., 2005). The paramedic should always aim to fully involve patients in decisions about drug treatments to maximise engagement and increase the potential for success.

information required and then leaving them to make the decision unsupported. This can lead to patients feeling abandoned and unsure, creating anxiety and distrust (Corrigan, 2003; Deber et al., 2007). The shared decision-making approach involves health professionals and patients working together to devise a plan of care that is in line with the best available evidence as well as the values and beliefs of the individual patient, aligning to the principle of true autonomy.

Health professionals also abide by the principle of *justice* which is the belief that people should be treated fairly, equally and reasonably. At its heart, justice is about equality but how equality is determined can be ambiguous and problematic in healthcare. An example of the difficulties posed within this principle is often seen in relation to the fair and equal distribution of resources, 'distributive justice'. A drug for a specific condition may be available within one healthcare organisation but not available to patients with the same or similar condition in another organisation. Sometimes colloquially labelled the 'postcode lottery', this occurs as a result of differing priorities among those who make difficult commissioning decisions about resources on a local level.

The paramedic should also be honest and tell the truth to enable someone to have the full information relevant to them in order to make full rational choices about their care. This is known as *veracity* and involves conveying accurate and objective information to the patient. Giving patients full information regarding treatment options is the most common application of the veracity principle. Disclosures of medication errors are also an example of veracity and the introduction in the UK of the 'duty of candour' guidance for health professionals (GMC, 2014) highlights the importance of the veracity principle. Informing patients when something has gone wrong, apologising and offering a remedy were measures that were advised in a report on the failings of the Mid-Staffordshire Health Trust. Francis (2013) stated that candour and transparency were key components of a safe and effective culture for patient care. However, in reality true veracity is a complex notion. Returning to the example of the drug that is available in one healthcare organisation and not another, health professionals engage in such rationing 'inconspicuously' (Williamson, 2010, p.201) without necessarily informing patients that they are being denied something that could benefit them. Aside from the greater ethical issues concerned with who makes the decisions and how they are implemented, there is the more immediate concern relating to veracity and the decision whether to inform patients.

Finally, the principle of *fidelity* requires loyalty and trustworthiness; it involves keeping our prom-

Clinical considerations: consent to treatment (adults)

Adults with capacity: the authority to treat comes solely from the patient. In UK law, consent by proxy is not permitted for the care or treatment of adults who have the capacity to make an informed decision.

Adults lacking capacity: where a patient does not have the mental capacity to make an informed decision regarding their care due to an impairment or disturbance to the functioning of the mind, e.g. acute confusional state, dementia, brain injury, being unconscious, then under the Mental Capacity Act (MCA, 2005), the health professional can decide upon the treatment that is deemed in the best interests of the patient without the consent of the next of kin.

Section 3(1) of the MCA (2005) sets out the following benchmarks by which to assess an adult's capacity.

- They are unable to understand the information given to them relating to the decision.
- They are unable to retain the information.
- They are unable to weigh the information as part of the decision-making process.
- They are unable to communicate their decision.

ises, performing our duties and doing what is expected of us within our relationships with patients. This principle can be conflicted where the health professional's loyalty or obligation may be torn between their patients and colleagues or the organisation for which they work. Conflict may also arise as a result of the patient lacking capacity to make an informed choice and the health professional being compelled to over-ride the wishes of their patient in their best interests.

You are required to keep to all relevant laws about mental capacity that apply in the country in which you are practising, ensuring that the rights and best interests of those who lack capacity are still at the centre of the decision-making process.

When ethical dilemmas in practice are encountered, consideration needs to be given to which principles are in conflict and then consider which is more important. In helping to resolve ethical dilemmas, ethical theories are called upon. Several exist, including:

- Utilitarian/consequentialism
- Deontological ethics
- Virtue ethics.

Clinical consideration: consent to treatment (children)

16–17 year olds with capacity: according to section 8(1) of the Family Law Reform Act (1969), consent can be sought from the child for medical and dental treatment. However, those with parental responsibility may still consent on the child's behalf.

16–17 year olds lacking capacity: anyone with parental responsibility can consent on behalf of a child who lacks capacity. In situations where those with parental responsibility do not consent to treatment, but treatment is felt to be in the best interests of the child, a court order may be obtained. In an emergency situation, treatment may still be provided without parental consent where it is deemed a necessity (Glass v United Kingdom 2004).

Under 16 years of age: an assessment of the child relating to 'Gillick' competence (Gillick v West Norfolk and Wisbech Area Health Authority 1986) would determine whether the child has sufficient maturity and understanding of what is involved to enable them to make a decision to consent to treatment or not.

Utilitarian or consequentialism theory considers the rightness of an act as that which, when considering the costs and benefits, creates the greatest good for the greatest number. For example, the issue of immunisation is currently a controversial one with a minority of parents deciding to opt out of immunisation programmes for their children. This puts children and other vulnerable members of society at risk of developing some diseases that were previously eradicated, such as measles (Public Health England, 2019), with the associated implications for individuals, wider society and the health service. The utilitarian perspective would be that all eligible children should be immunised irrespective of the views/wishes of their parents. Utilitarianism would not be concerned with the autonomy of the individual (the right to refuse consent for the vaccine) as this is arguably in conflict with the greater good.

Deontological ethics or deontology is an approach to ethics that determines goodness or rightness from examining acts rather than consequences of the act, as in utilitarianism. Deontologists look at rules and duties. For example, the action may be considered the right thing to do, even if it produces a bad consequence, if it follows the *rule* that 'one should do unto others as they would have done unto them'. According to deontology, we have a *duty* to act in a way that does those things that are inherently good. In this approach, the duty of care to the individual takes priority over any other considerations. Going back to our example of immunisations, children are, in reality, not forced to have immunisations where parents have opted out. A paramedic has a duty to ensure that any care given is consented to, within the parameters of the MCA (2005) as outlined above. Without this consent, we cannot inject a live vaccine into a child no matter what the potential implications might be for wider society. So the act itself is good (abiding by rules of consent) but the consequence may be a negative one (the child contracting measles and passing this on to others). For deontologists, the ends or consequences of our actions are not important nor are our intentions. Duty is the key consideration. However, it is not always clear what one's duty is. Whilst we may agree that our duty is to 'do no harm', there will be instances where the paramedic will have to over-ride this with their duty of care.

Virtue ethics focuses on how we ought to behave, and how we should think about relationships, rather than providing rules or formulas for ethical decision making. It considers the virtues a 'good' person would have: honesty, compassion, generosity, courage, for example (Velasquez et al., 1988). With the common good in mind, these virtues will be applied to actions and decisions. A group of virtues can be accredited to particular roles or professions, and it could be argued that nurses are attracted to the profession because they already function according to these virtues.

What is deemed to be right is not therefore bound by absolute rules or duty, or purely the greatest good, but also considers the virtues that individuals and society value. The ethical views held by society affect healthcare laws and how they are implemented. As society's moral values alter, legislation follows. An example of this was in 1967 when UK society's beliefs changed regarding abortions. It became largely accepted that in some cases they were necessary for saving women's lives as well as reducing the potential for suffering (psychologically as well as physically) of the woman and her pre-existing family, and so the Act was introduced (Abortion Act 1967).

Regulatory bodies

In order to practice, healthcare professionals are aligned to a regulatory body such as the Health and Care Professions Council (HCPC), Nursing and Midwifery Council (NMC), Paramedicine Board Australia, or General Medical Council (GMC). The purpose of a regulatory body is primarily to protect the public and as such they are established and based upon a legal mandate. Their function is regulatory and to impose requirements, restrictions and conditions as well as offering a means of support and guidance to professionals. They also set standards in relation to practice activities, securing compliance and enforcement of their practitioners. Regulatory bodies have traditionally provided their practitioners with ethical guidance in the form of a 'code' or an 'oath' such as the HCPC Standards of Conduct, Performance and Ethics, NMC Code of Conduct (2018), Paramedicine Board Australia Code of Conduct (2018) or the Hippocratic Oath for doctors.

Episode of care

Whilst working on a double crewed ambulance (DCA), you are called to a bedsit that is used by young intravenous drug users (IVDU). You notice that ambulances are only called to IVDU when they are in cardiac or respiratory arrest or have bradypnoea. So the patient's friends only call for help when the patient's condition becomes life threatening. You notice that this patient group does not seek medical help in the same way many other patient groups do. You begin to think about why this is the case, using the principles of ethical professional practice, beneficence (do good) and non-maleficence (do no harm).

Within healthcare, regulatory bodies have a duty to protect, promote and maintain the health and safety of the public. They do this by ensuring proper standards are in place in order to practice. Such standards define the overarching goals and expected role and duties of their practitioners through listing the obligations associated with their individual responsibilities and skill set. The overarching goals are aspirational and represent an optimal position ethically, thus encouraging the individual to strive towards the optimal position. Paramedics, like the public and their patients, possess their own values and beliefs which in turn influence their practice.

Within this scenario, there is a possibility the patients or service user's care has been affected by the HCP's implicit bias towards certain social groups. Several authors have emphasised that a well-meaning, egalitarian (fair-minded) individual can have implicit biases which demonstrate the imbalance between their unconscious ways of thinking and how they explicitly perceive themselves treating people (Fitzgerald and Hurst, 2018; Lang et al., 2016). The elements of implicit bias (IB) are one's perceived stereotypes (a mental picture of what one thinks, knows and expects) and prejudices (feelings) associated with certain categories of people, learnt through a shared culture, which over time slip into one's unconsciousness, which means they remain hidden (Lang et al., 2016). As Stone and Moskowitz (2011) explained, this means that HCPs are unaware of their biases which impacts on the quality of care delivered, seen in how they may judge and behave towards particular groups (Kelly and Roedderts, 2008). Merino et al. (2018) highlighted that over 60% of HCPs harbour variants of IB towards marginalised/vulnerable groups. Examples of vulnerable or marginalised groupings can be based on gender, age, weight, homelessness, ethnicity, immigration status, socio-economic status, educational achievement, mental ill health, sexual orientation, intravenous drug use, disabilities and social circumstances or anyone rendered vulnerable in certain situations (Fitzgerald and Hurst, 2018).

There is consensus that stereotyping saves cognitive resources in stressful environments, a situation in which HCPs often find themselves (Hall, 2017). By drawing on these stereotypes, the HCP is able to make timely decisions based on the minimal information available in times of fatigue, tiredness, heavy workload, uncertainty and inadequate support (Stone and Moskowitz, 2011). Nonetheless, there is a clear link between IB and the quality of care delivered and how it potentially influences the HCP's ability to engage in person-centred care (Merino et al., 2018). Fitzgerald and Hurst (2018) stated that a HCP's IB behaviour towards marginalised groups can impact on the service user's access to healthcare service by producing false diagnoses, non-referral to appropriate services, treatment options or withholding of treatment. Goyal et al. (2015) detailed how IB may have contributed to the creation of health disparities as African-American children were less likely to receive adequate pain management post appendectomy than their white counterparts. IB influences within clinical interactions can leave the service user feeling uncomfortable as they pay attention to the HCPs non-verbal mannerisms such as eye contact, physical closeness and speech errors which can demonstrate the HCP's unease when dealing with particular clientele (Stone and Moskowitz, 2011). This in turn may not only impede patient–HCP communication but may affect patient concordance and willingness to seek future care.

Puddifoot (2017) suggested that IB can cause an ethical dilemma, demonstrated earlier, as there is potential to do harm within these client groups through the HCP's judgement and behaviour based on their IB. Positive beneficence requires the HCP to consider benefits for others alongside balancing the risks (Baillie and Black, 2015) which is compromised through the harbouring of IB. Such behaviours are in direct contradiction to the professional regulatory bodies' codes of professional performance, so the HCP should reflect on how they interact with certain client groups to develop awareness of any implicit biases they may have (Lang et al., 2016). Additionally, Stone and Moskowitz (2011) recommend attending courses to expand cultural competence by learning about IB.

There are a number of guidelines set out by various professional bodies in relation to pharmacology. The General Medical Council (GMC) has outlined expectations of doctors' ethical prescribing practices which aim to provide more detailed advice on how to apply ethical principles when prescribing and managing medicines (GMC, 2013). Additionally, the Royal Pharmaceutical Society and the Royal College of Nursing collaborated in developing the 'Professional Guidance

Clinical consideration

All paramedics have a responsibility to ensure that they are familiar with legislation related to the prescribing, storage and administration of medicines within their sphere of practice. A list of key documents that will support you in the development of knowledge in this area is offered in the further reading section.

on the Administration of Medicines in Healthcare Settings' (Royal Pharmaceutical Society and the Royal College of Nursing, 2019). These standards seek to promote patient safety in relation to the administration of medicines by acknowledging the importance of guidance for health professionals that is enabling and supportive while being clear and concise. The document recognises the importance of a commitment to ethics, values and principles which put patients first. It is incumbent upon the individual HCP to ensure that they are familiar with the most current guidance related to their own sphere of practice to ensure that ethical and legal considerations are applied.

Research

The legal and ethical standards which govern research into pharmacological treatments are very specific to the context of clinical drug trials. During the Second World War, Jewish prisoners in Nazi concentration camps were used as subjects in medical experiments against their will, leading to permanent disfigurement, disability, trauma and in many cases death. In response to these atrocities, the Nuremberg Code (1947) was developed as international guiding ethical principles for the conduct of research involving human participants. They include principles of informed consent, non-coercion and the right to withdraw as well as the importance of robust protocols underpinned by beneficence. These principles were later encapsulated within the Declaration of Helsinki (1964, amended in 2008) and further legislation has evolved to ensure the safety of human participants in clinical trials, including the Data Protection Act (2018), Human Tissue Act (2004), the Medicines for Human Use (Clinical Trials) Regulations (2004) and the Human Rights Act (1998).

Research is an important mechanism to ensure that the drug treatments we offer patients are thoroughly tested for safety and efficacy. Additionally, there is strong evidence emerging that research-active hospitals have better patient outcomes, highlighting the responsibility healthcare providers have to offer their service users the opportunity to be involved in clinical trials (Ozdemir et al., 2015). It is essential that legislation enables clinical researchers to conduct clinical trials in the endeavour of medical advancement, while ensuring that participants are fully informed of the potential risks and benefits, are not coerced into consenting to participate and are aware of their right to withdraw from participating at any time. The guiding principle is that the wellbeing and safety of the participants are paramount and take priority over any other consideration.

Research ethics committees (RECs) have the remit to review any proposed research that involves human participants. Made up of a number of lay people and professionals experienced in their own field, it is the responsibility of the REC to interrogate the research protocol and identify any aspects of the research consent and treatment processes which may pose an unacceptable risk to participants or the public. Approval from a REC is essential before a trial can go ahead. As the trial progresses, researchers will also need to seek ethical approval to make any amendments to the protocol, which may be something as minor as a change of wording within a participant information sheet, to something more substantial such as a change in the dose of

Skills in practice: how to use medical ethics

Not all decisions are made easily and, in some cases, there are multiple factors that influence decision making such as personal experience, religious views, regulatory codes, legal issues and so on. In practice, a practitioner will use a combination of all such factors to reach a decision; this is sometimes described as a systematic study of moral choices. In the first instance, the code of behaviour or conduct presented by a regulatory body is considered correct. Within healthcare there are many examples of ethical decision-making processes which include varying numbers of steps to follow. Overall, there is the general adoption of principle-based ethics to guide decision-making practice within healthcare which is evident in this example.

Step 1 – Ability to recognise an ethical issue. Ask yourself, could this scenario or decision cause harm or damage to someone or some group? Are there choices between different alternatives – for example, good and bad alternatives or maybe two bads or two goods? Is this situation bigger than what is efficient? or what is legal? What are your initial gut reactions? By considering the scenario on an emotive level, you can recognise your own assumptions, values and biases so that you can set them aside before analysing the situation critically.

Step 2 – Gathering the facts. What facts are already known? What other relevant facts need to be gathered? Who are the relevant stakeholders within this scenario and its outcome? Has everyone involved been consulted? Are some concerns more important than others?

Step 3 – Evaluation of alternative options or actions. Include questions from a range of approaches. From a utilitarian approach, ask which actions/options do the least harm and produce the most good? Considering the deontological approach, which actions/options best respect all stakeholders' rights?

From a paramedic perspective, which actions/options treat people proportionately or equally? Which actions/options best serve the whole community and not just some if its members? From a virtue perspective, also consider which actions/options lead me based on the type of person I want to be?

Step 4 – Make the decision. When all approaches have been considered, which actions/options best address the scenario? Which actions/options are best based on all the stakeholders' core values? Consider what others might say when you have shared your chosen actions/options – can you justify your choice?

Step 5 – Carry out the actions/options chosen and reflect on the outcome. Plan how your decision can be implemented with the utmost care, paying attention to any concerns raised by stakeholders. Implement your plan and evaluate. Reflect on the results of your choice of decision and what you have learned from this specific scenario. Consider how the ethical problem could be prevented in the future.

Episode of care

As a paramedic on a DCA, you are called to Paul, a 65-year-old man who has been experiencing cardiac chest pain for the last 45 minutes. You are about to administer sublingual glycerine trinitrate (GTN) when the patient discloses that he used sildenafil 2 hours ago. You confer with a colleague about the benefits and risks of administering GTN when the patient has already taken sildenafil. The *British National Formulary* (Joint Formulary Committee, 2019) and JRCALC guidance show that a severe interaction can take place, leading to profound hypotension. While the treatment may be doing 'good' (beneficence), it also has the potential to do 'harm' (maleficence). It is imperative that the paramedic discuss medication plans prior to treatment to ensure that patients are aware of the impact this will have on their daily activities. In Paul's case, although the GTN could lead to vasodilation, decrease in pain, and improved cardiac blood flow, it could also cause his blood pressure to drop, leading to hypotension. You explain to the patient that on this occasion you will not be administering the GTN, as the interaction with the sildenafil could lead to a dangerous blood pressure drop. Always ensure that every decision made fully involves the patient and aligns with their own values and lifestyle.

Episode of care

Maya is an 85-year-old woman who lives alone. She is usually independent with all her activities of living and, although she does not like to leave the house, she is usually in good physical and mental health. Her daughter visits her three times a week and has noticed some increased confusion over the past few days. Today she has visited and felt it necessary to call the GP as Maya is extremely confused, unable to mobilise, pyrexial, and smells strongly of malodorous urine. The GP calls for an ambulance to transport the patient to hospital with a suspected urinary tract infection (UTI). The paramedic assesses Maya and finds that she is dehydrated with a blood pressure of 70/46, dry oral membranes, passing small amounts of urine. They decide to cannulate the patient to administer IV fluids on route to hospital. However, Maya becomes very distressed when the paramedic attempts to cannulate and Maya's daughter states that she does not consent to her mother receiving IV therapy. Maya has been assessed as an adult lacking capacity by health professionals. In accordance with the Mental Capacity Act (2005) and in Maya's best interests, she is cannulated and receives the IV therapy. Over the course of the next 24 hours, her condition improves and her acute confusional state dissipates. The health professionals have acted in accordance with legal standards. They have also balanced their duty to respect Maya's autonomy with their duty of care in ensuring beneficence (doing good by giving the required treatment in Maya's best interests) and non-maleficence (doing no harm by omitting care that was in her best interests).

medication to be administered. These changes will be implemented in line with Good Clinical Practice (GCP) principles (MHRA, 2012).

Despite these safeguards, notable incidences have occurred in recent years related to the conduct of some clinical trials. For example, in 2006, volunteers in an early-phase drug trial at Northwick Park Hospital became seriously ill. The story became headline news after six participants reacted badly to the medication, suffering a severe immune response leading to organ failure and one participant requiring the amputation of his fingers. This led to a full investigation and the resulting report changed a number of practices in the running of drugs trials which sought to prevent this from happening again (Expert Scientific Group on Phase One Clinical Trials, 2006).

Fortunately however, the ethical and legal frameworks which surround clinical research limit these incidences and provide principles and guidance for the safe conduct of research and researchers.

Conclusion

This chapter has sought to outline the fundamental legal and ethical principles relating to pharmacology in healthcare. The three key components that underpin high-quality decision making with and for patients in our care are related to the law, ethical principles and regulatory bodies. A variety of legislation has been discussed to offer an understanding of and insight into how healthcare professionals manage and administer medicines within the confines of the law. The interplay of legislation, ethical principles and professional regulation is a fine balance that health professionals seek to strike in order to optimise the safety and efficacy of treatment. Legislation is country specific and the paramedic must have an understanding of the laws in the country in which they are practising.

Working in healthcare requires an acknowledgement of the areas of ambiguity and conflict that may be encountered and while we seek to always 'do good', there are countless situations where this endeavour may be obstructed by other considerations such as patient capacity or the wider public interest.

Acknowledgement of the issues outlined within this chapter and a deeper understanding of how to apply the knowledge of ethical principles will ultimately improve practice and provide safer and higher quality patient care. It is incumbent upon all paramedics (and students) to act with integrity within these frameworks and to make individualised decisions which are in the patients' best interest and, wherever possible, fully informed.

The following is a list of considerations, guiding legislation and ethical frameworks for safe and effective practice. Find out more about what each of these involves and how this impacts upon the care of patients, and make notes in the space provided.

The consideration	Your notes
Mental capacity	
Burden of proof for negligence	
Human medicines regulation	
Research ethics committee	
Northwick Park drug trials controversy	

Glossary

Accountability	Taking responsibility for actions taken and being able to provide a rationale for courses of action.
Autonomy	Enabling patients to make self-determined decisions regarding their care.
Beneficence	Endeavouring to do good.
Bolam test	Assessment of whether a health professional acted within the scope of accepted practice.
Deontology	The study of the nature of duty and obligation.

Duty of care	Legal obligation for individuals and organisations to take reasonable care in the conduct of actions that could foreseeably result in actionable harm.
Egalitarianism	Principle that all people are equal and deserve equal rights and opportunities.
Fidelity	Provision of care that is honest, responsible and fair.
Implicit bias	Perceived stereotypes associated with certain categories of people which over time slip into one's unconsciousness. (See also unconscious bias.)
Justice	Treating patients fairly, equally and reasonably.
Mental capacity	Being able to make and communicate your own decisions.
Negligence	Failure to provide adequate care.
Non-maleficence	Endeavouring to do no harm.
Paternalism	Health professionals asserting a dominant attitude over patients, making decisions without the full involvement of patients.
Regulatory body	A public organisation or government body which imposes requirements, restrictions and standards for practice.
Utilitarianism	(or consequential) determing the rightness of an act by considering costs and benefits and the greatest good for the greatest number of people.
Veracity	Conveying honest, accurate and objective information to the patient to support them in making a decision around medical care.
Virtue ethics	Focuses on desirable ways of relating to others, including habits, attitudes and emotion as well as conduct.

References

Abortion Act (1967). www.legislation.gov.uk/ukpga/1967/87/contents

Baillie, L. and Black, S. (2015). *Professional Values in Nursing*. Boca Raton: Taylor & Francis Group.

Beauchamp, T.L. and Childress, J.F. (2009). *Principles of Biomedical Ethics*, 6th edn. Oxford: Oxford University Press.

Corrigan, O. (2003). Empty ethics: the problem with informed consent. *Sociology of Health and Illness* **25**(7): 768–792.

Data Protection Act (2018). www.legislation.gov.uk/ukpga/2018/12/contents/enacted

Deber, R., Kraetschmer, N., Urowitz, S. and Sharpe, N. (2007). Do people want to be autonomous patients? Preferred roles in treatment decision-making in several patient populations. *Health Expectations* **10**: 248–258.

Declaration of Helsinki. (2008). *Ethical principles for medical research involving human subjects*. www.who.int/bulletin/archives/79%284%29373.pdf

Edwards, A. and Elwyn, G. (eds). (2009). *Shared Decision-Making in Health Care. Achieving Evidence-Based Patient Choice*. Oxford: Oxford University Press.

Expert Scientific Group on Phase One Clinical Trials. (2006). *Final Report*. https://webarchive.nationalarchives.gov.uk/20130105143109/http://www.dh.gov.uk/prod_consum_dh/groups/dh_digitalassets/@dh/@en/documents/digitalasset/dh_073165.pdf

Fitzgerald, C. and Hurst, S. (2018). Implicit bias in healthcare professionals: a systematic review. *BMC Medical Ethics* **18**(19): 1–18.

Francis, R. (2013). *Report of the Mid-Staffordshire NHS Foundation Trust Public Enquiry*. London: Stationery Office.

General Medical Council. (2013). *Good practice in prescribing and managing medicines and devices*. www.gmc-uk.org/-/media/documents/prescribing-guidance_pdf-59055247.pdf?la=en

General Medical Council. (2014). *The professional duty of candour*. www.gmc-uk.org/ethical-guidance/ethical-guidance-for-doctors/candour---openness-and-honesty-when-things-go-wrong/the-professional-duty-of-candour

Gillick v West Norfolk and Wisbech area Health Authority and Department of Health and Social Security (1984) Q.B as cited in Children's Legal Centre (1985) Landmark decision for children's rights. *Childright*, **22**:11–18.

Glass v United Kingdom. App. No 61827/00, 39 Eur. H.R.Rep. 15 (2004).

Goyal, M.K. Kuppermann, N., Cleary, S.D. et al. (2015). Racial disparities in pain management of children with appendicitis in emergency departments. *JAMA Pediatrics* **169**(11): 996–1002.

Hall, A. (2017). Using legal ethics to improve implicit bias in prosecutorial discretion. *Journal of the Legal Profession* **42**(1): 111–126.

Herring, J. (2018). *Medical Law and Ethics*. Oxford: Oxford University Press.

Human Rights Act (1998). www.legislation.gov.uk/ukpga/1998/42/contents

Human Tissue Act (2004). www.legislation.gov.uk/ukpga/2004/30/contents

Joint Formulary Committee. (2019). *British National Formulary*. https://bnf.nice.org.uk

Kelly, D. and Roedderts, E. (2008). Racial cognition and the ethics of implicit bias. *Philosophy Compass* **3**(3): 522–540.

Lang, K.R. Dupree, C.Y., Kon, A.A. and Dudzinski, D.M. (2016). Calling out implicit bias as a harm in pediatric care. *Cambridge Quarterly of Healthcare Ethics* **25**: 540–552.

Medicines for Human Use (Clinical Trials) Regulations (2004). www.legislation.gov.uk/uksi/2004/1031/contents/made

Medicines and Healthcare products Regulatory Agency (MHRA). (2012). *Good Clinical Practice Guide*. London: Stationery Office.

Mental Capacity Act (MCA). (2005). www.legislation.gov.uk/ukpga/2005/9/contents

Merino, Y., Adams, L. and Hall, W.J. (2018). Implicit bias and mental health professionals: priorities and direction for research. *Psychiatric Services* **69**(6): 723–725.

National Health Service Improvement (NHSI). (2019). *Clinical negligence and litigation*. https://improvement.nhs.uk/resources/clinical-negligence-and-litigation/

Nuremberg Code. (1947). *Trials of War Criminals Before the Nuernberg [sic] Military Tribunals. Volume II. "The Medical Case."* www.loc.gov/rr/frd/Military_Law/pdf/NT_war-criminals_Vol-II.pdf

Nursing and Midwifery Council. (2018). *The Code: Professional standards of practice and behaviour for nurses, midwives and nursing associates*. www.nmc.org.uk/globalassets/sitedocuments/nmc-publications/nmc-code.pdf

Ozdemir, B.A., Karthikesalingam, A., Sinha, S. et al. (2015). Research activity and the association with mortality. *PLoS ONE* **10**(2): e0118253.

Paramedicine Board Australia. (2018). *Code of conduct (interim)*. www.paramedicineboard.gov.au/professional-standards/codes-guidelines-and-policies/code-of-conduct.aspx

Pellegrino, E.D. (1988). *For the Patient's Good: The Restoration of Beneficence in Health Care*. Oxford: Oxford University Press

Public Health England. (2019). *Measles: guidance, data and analysis*. www.gov.uk/government/collections/measles-guidance-data-and-analysis#epidemiology

Puddifoot, K. (2017). Dissolving the epistemic/ethical dilemma over implicit bias. *Philosophical Explorations* **20**(1): S73–S93.

Royal Pharmaceutical Society and Royal College of Nursing. (2019). *Professional Guidance on the Administration of Medicines in Healthcare Settings*. www.rpharms.com/Portals/0/RPS%20document%20library/Open%20access/Professional%20standards/SSHM%20and%20Admin/Admin%20of%20Meds%20prof%20guidance.pdf?ver=2019-01-23-145026-567

Samanta, J. and Samanta, A. (2011). *Medical Law*. Basingstoke: Palgrave Macmillan.

Stewart, M. and Brown, J. (2001). Patient-centredness in medicine. In: *Evidence-based Patient Choice* (eds A. Edwards and G. Elwyn). Oxford: Oxford University Press.

Stone, J. and Moskowitz, G.B. (2011). Non-conscious bias in medical decision-making: what can be done to reduce it? *Medical Education* **45**: 768–776.

Studdert, D.M., Mello, M.M., Sage, W.S. et al. (2005). Defensive medicine among high-risk specialist physicians in a volatile malpractice environment. *JAMA* **293**: 2609–2617.

Velasquez, M., Andre, C., Shanks, T. et al. (1988). *Ethics and Virtue*. www.scu.edu/ethics/ethics-resources/ethical-decision-making/ethics-and-virtue/

Williamson, C. (2010). *Towards the Emancipation Of Patients. Patients' Experiences and The Patient Movement*. Bristol: Policy Press.

Further reading

Department of Health. (2012). *Compassion in Practice*. www.england.nhs.uk/wp-content/uploads/2012/12/compassion-in-practice.pdf

Family Law Reform Act (1969). www.legislation.gov.uk/ukpga/1969/46

Health and Care Professions Council. (2016). *Standards of conduct, performance and ethics*. www.hcpc-uk.org/globalassets/resources/standards/standards-of-conduct-performance-and-ethics.pdf

Joint Royal Colleges Ambulance Liaison Committee (JRCALC). (2019). *Clinical Guidelines*. Bridgwater: Class Professional Publishing.

National Institute of Health and Care Excellence (NICE). (2018). *Guideline 109 Urinary tract infection (lower): antimicrobial prescribing*. www.nice.org.uk/guidance/ng109

Multiple-choice questions

1. Common law is also known as:
   (a) Criminal law
   (b) Case law
   (c) Statute law
   (d) All of the above.
2. Failure to act with reasonable care could result in a paramedic being held responsible in which courts?
   (a) Criminal court
   (b) Civil court
   (c) Civil and criminal court
   (d) All of the above
3. What year did the Medicines Act become statute?
   (a) 1966
   (b) 1967
   (c) 1968
   (d) None of the above
4. Utilitarian theory considers:
   (a) The greatest good for the greatest number
   (b) Your duty of care takes priority over any other considerations
   (c) How we ought to behave and seek relationships
   (d) All of the above.
5. When adopting principle-based ethics to guide your decision making, where do you need to gather the facts from?
   (a) From all the stakeholders involved within the scenario
   (b) From what is already known
   (c) From other facts that are relevant from other scenarios'
   (d) All of the above
6. Sensitive topics such as abortion can lead to the practitioner having _____ dilemma.
   (a) Ethical
   (b) Clinical
   (c) Legal
   (d) All of the above
7. Implicit means:
   (a) Hidden
   (b) Obvious
   (c) Available
   (d) Explicit.
8. Elements of implicit bias include:
   (a) Stereotypes
   (b) Prejudices
   (c) Stereotypes and prejudices
   (d) Impartialities.
9. Healthcare professionals harbour the _____ level of implicit bias as the general population.
   (a) Lower
   (b) Higher
   (c) Same
   (d) None of the above

10. The influences of implicit bias on the practitioner's professional behaviour include:
    (a) Making the client feel uncomfortable
    (b) Helping them access services
    (c) Correct diagnoses and treatment
    (d) Patient concordance.

11. What is the Bolam test?
    (a) A test to assess patient capacity
    (b) The opinion of a professional body as to whether the action was accepted practice
    (c) An assessment of competency of a patient under 16
    (d) All of the above

12. Shared decision making:
    (a) Is an approach to care that increases patient engagement in treatment
    (b) Improves patient engagement with care and treatment
    (c) Reduces medico-legal claims
    (d) All of the above.

13. What is distributive justice in relation to healthcare?
    (a) The fair and equal distribution of health resources
    (b) The 'postcode lottery'
    (c) An assessment of patient need
    (d) All of the above

14. Why is research in healthcare so important?
    (a) To test drugs for safety and efficacy
    (b) To develop better treatments for patients
    (c) To improve outcomes for patients
    (d) All of the above

15. What must professionals do in order to abide by the 'duty of candour'?
    (a) Only tell the patient when a serious incident has occurred
    (b) Inform patients and their families of everything related to the patient's care at all times
    (c) Apologise to patients
    (d) All of the above

Chapter 4

Medicines management and the role of the paramedic

Annette Hand, Carol Wills and Paul Younger

Aim

The aim of this chapter is to provide the reader with an introduction to medicines management and the role of the paramedic.

Learning outcomes

After reading this chapter the reader will:

1. Understand the term 'medicines management' and the role of the paramedic
2. Be able to appraise the paramedic's role in managing medicines safely and effectively
3. Acknowledge the role of regulatory and advisory bodies in the management and optimisation of medicines
4. Be able to apply the principles of medicine optimisation.

Test your knowledge

1. Which Act provides the legal framework governing the use of Controlled Drugs?
2. What do the 9Rs stand for?
3. What activities are included within medicines management?
4. What does the term PGD stand for?
5. How do you verify the identification of a patient prior to medicines administration?

Fundamentals of Pharmacology for Paramedics, First Edition. Edited by Ian Peate, Suzanne Evans, and Lisa Clegg.
© 2022 John Wiley & Sons Ltd. Published 2022 by John Wiley & Sons Ltd.

Introduction

This chapter will support learning in relation to medicines management and the role of the paramedic. Medicines are the most common intervention in healthcare and are vital in treating or managing many illnesses and conditions. As more people are taking more medicines, it is paramount, for patients, healthcare professionals and organisations, that medicines are used appropriately. Population growth and increases in the numbers of older people push up the volume of medicines prescribed, partly due to older people being more likely to have long-term health conditions such as cardiovascular problems, arthritis or diabetes (Duerden et al., 2013). Effective and safe medicines management is a key responsibility for many paramedics, and it is important that individuals keep up to date with new guidelines and regulations within this ever-expanding area of care.

Globally, health and care providers are regulated and monitored using different systems and approaches. Understanding the various approaches that are used in the jurisdiction where you work can help ensure that you are providing care that is legal, safe and patient centred. This chapter focuses on those regulatory systems that are used across the UK and within the National Health Service (NHS).

Currently all health and social care organisations in the UK are assessed and monitored by an Independent Regulator of Health and Social Care to determine if they provide appropriate and safe care; this includes the use of medicines. These regulators will inspect and assess the quality of care and whether it is safe, effective, caring, responsive and well led. For example, the Care Quality Commission (CQC) outlines Inspection Frameworks for NHS and independent ambulance services which details the inspection guidance for Core Services of Emergency and Acute Care as well as Core Services of Patient Transport Services. Each service is then rated as outstanding, good, requires improvement or inadequate. Follow Clinical Consideration 1 to explore the rating of the service you are currently working in. All health professionals have an important role in the provision of quality services.

Clinical consideration 1

Visit your organisation's website or the regulator's website to access its latest inspection report. What was the outcome of the report?

- Were any areas rated as good or requires improvement?
- What is/would your role be within this provision?

Medicines management

Medicines management involves the safe and cost-effective use of medicines in clinical practice, maximising patient benefits while minimising potential harm. NHS spending on medicines was estimated at £17.4 billion in 2016–17 and is said to be increasing at a rate of 5% each year (Ewbank et al., 2018). This has been said to be unsustainable and all health professionals need to explore how this can be managed. The human costs when things go wrong with medications include increased use of health services, preventable admissions to hospital, serious harm and ultimately death. It is estimated that 70% of errors are identified before they reach the patient and essentially all healthcare providers must minimise the risk and incidence of harm.

In the UK and other countries, laws and regulations exist to control medicines, from a number of perspectives, such as the Medicines Act (1968), Human Medicines Regulations (2012), Prescription Only Medicines (Human Use) Order (1997). These are in place to promote safe and effective medicines management at each stage of the medicines journey. Essential elements of this journey include:

- Manufacturing and marketing
- Procurement and sale
- Selection

- Supply
- Prescribing
- Handling and administration
- Medicine optimisation
- Storage and disposal.

It is important to understand country-specific laws governing medicines management. Key elements will be explored in the following sections.

Manufacturing, marketing, procurement and sale

NHS medicine policies in the UK require that either the European Medicines Agency (the European Union regulatory body) or the Medicines and Healthcare products Regulatory Agency (MHRA) (the UK regulatory body) approves products and medical devices before they can be supplied to patients. Safety, effectiveness and quality of the manufacturing process are assessed and must meet stringent requirements before they are approved for sale and assigned a marketing authorisation. The marketing authorisation is assigned according to the licensed indication and degree of risk of the product, the pack size and whether its supply needs to be supervised and monitored by a health professional. The Medicines Act (1968) and subsequent Human Medicines Regulations (2012) allow the product to then be available to the public as:

- a prescription-only medicine (PoM), meaning that the product can only be supplied by a prescription from an appropriate health professional and issued by a pharmacist. A Controlled Drug (CD) is also a prescription-only medicine
- a pharmacy (P)-only product which can be bought in the presence and under the supervision of a pharmacist, e.g. chemist or in-store pharmacy within a supermarket
- a General Sales List product (GSL) which means it can be bought in a retail outlet, e.g. supermarket or garage shop.

Pharmacy and GSL items are often referred to as 'over-the-counter' products, which is a general term meaning they can be purchased in a retail outlet and do not need a prescription.

Following marketing approval, new products may be scrutinised for clinical and cost-effectiveness by, for example, the National Institute for Health and Care Excellence (NICE) or the Scottish Intercollegiate Guidelines Network (SIGN) to determine whether healthcare organisations will provide them. If NICE or SIGN approves them for use, commissioners must make them available for patients. Many new products or changes in the use of a product will be assigned a black triangle like this:

This alerts paramedics that there is limited experience in the use of this product so all suspected adverse reactions must be reported to the MHRA. Not all products and devices require assessment by NICE; some may be considered by NHS commissioners who can decide if they wish to make them available to patients. This may then lead to the procurement or purchasing of products dependent on a variety of factors which include local priorities, budgets and timeliness of NICE approval. Procurement of medicines and medical devices for the NHS is undertaken by regional pharmacy purchasing groups who aim to obtain the best price possible for the NHS and enter into contracts for supply to NHS trusts and other organisations. These will be included in the national drug tariff (a list of medicines and devices that can be prescribed within the NHS) and then agreed for purchase at a local level, usually via drugs and therapeutic committees.

Independent organisations (e.g. non-NHS pharmacies, independent or private ambulance companies) may choose specific products that they wish to offer for sale to the general public. These are restricted to pharmacy only and GSL products, depending on their status as discussed previously, but also may have restrictions on the amount or dosage which can be sold. For example, the MHRA discourages large quantities of analgesia being sold; as an example, paracetamol can result in liver damage if recommended dosages are exceeded. Shopkeepers thus limit purchase of these to 32 or in some cases 16 tablets per pack.

Selection

Where there are many products or devices available to treat a condition, an NHS organisation, or your employer, will decide which of these products are to be prescribed and included in the local formulary. This ultimately means that some products will be available for supply in some parts of the UK but not all. Selection will be based upon a range of measures including the evidence available to support the product's effectiveness and the cost of supplying the product in comparison to similar products.

The Product Licensing (PL) number is a unique code that is given to a pharmaceutical manufacturer to produce a specific drug formulation. This code is unique to the manufacturer and not the drug. Generic manufacturers may therefore produce drugs for various brands using the same PL number.

Some products which have been licensed for several years are often manufactured by several companies with the result that an identical drug which is therapeutically equivalent has several proprietary or trade names. An example of this is ibuprofen; this is its non-proprietary or generic name, but it can also be supplied with a proprietary name of Brufen® or Nurofen®. Not only can this cause confusion and possible medication errors, but it is generally more cost-effective for the NHS to supply or for the patient to buy a generic product. Compare the proprietary and non-proprietary forms of ibuprofen in Clinical Consideration 2 to understand the differences in cost.

Clinical consideration 2

	Nurofen	Brufen	Ibuprofen
Find out how much is a pack of 16 200 mg tablets of each of these products in your local pharmacy or shop.			
Check the product information on the packets; do they contain the same amount of the same active ingredient?			
What is the Product Licensing (PL) number? Are there any that are the same?			
Which is the cheapest?			

The NHS Business Services Authority (NHSBSA) analyses prescribing trends and states that 81% of all drugs in primary care are already prescribed generically which generates significant savings for the NHS (NHSBSA, 2018). However, it also highlights that for medicines optimisation, there are further savings that could be realised to help provide even better value care. This also includes the NHS spending on products which can otherwise be bought by patients from a pharmacy or supermarket, such as paracetamol. The NHS currently spends around £136 million a year on prescriptions for such medicines (NHS England, 2018). Prescriptions are generally not issued for over-the-counter (OTC) medicines which are used to treat a range of minor health conditions but there are those with chronic ill health who may still have OTC medicines prescribed as part of their care pathway (e.g. paracetamol for pain). All healthcare professionals have a responsibility to help the NHS to deliver an effective and value-for-money service.

Supply

Medicines and medicinal products may be supplied to patients in a variety of ways. These are incorporated within legislation under the Medicines Act (1968), the Prescription Only Medicines (Human Use) Order (1997) and subsequent changes to include patient-specific directions, prescriptions, Patient Group Directions and exemptions.

Clinical Consideration 3 asks that you think about how patients are supplied with medicines/medical devices in your current practice.

Clinical considerations 3

Are these provided through patient-specific directions, prescriptions or patient group directions?

1. Tick the boxes below that apply.
2. Give an example product or clinical situation for each process that you identify.

Patient-specific direction

Prescription

Patient Group Direction

Patient-specific directions

Patient-specific directions (PSD) are written instructions by a doctor, dentist or non-medical prescriber for the supply and/or administration of medicines for a named patient. In paramedic practice, this is most often seen in patients receiving palliative care who have been prescribed anticipatory medication, also known as 'just in case' or just in time' medication, where the patient's GP or hospital doctor has left written instructions, often in the form of a Kardex, and the medication has been dispensed from a pharmacy. As this medication has already been prescribed, it may be administered by a paramedic as a registered healthcare professional, even though they cannot administer that drug under an exemption, or Patient Group Direction (PGD).

Prescriptions

A prescription is a written instruction or order for the supply of a product by an appropriately qualified healthcare professional to a named patient and must meet the legal requirements of the Prescription Only Medicines (Human Use) Order (1997). You will be familiar with these if you have been working in a primary care environment. Prescriptions may be handwritten or electronic.

Clinical consideration 4

- What is your organisation's guidance on the administration of anticipatory (just in time or just in case) medication?
- If you encountered a patient with a PSD for palliative medication, would you be confident to administer it? Medication prescribed in a PSD for those receiving palliative care may be given for symptom management that is not often encountered in paramedic practice.
- In palliative care opiates are given for analgesia. What else can they be prescribed for?
- Why would hyoscine butyl bromide be prescribed to a patient receiving palliative care?

Patient Group Directions

A Patient Group Direction (PGD) is a set of written instructions that allow some registered paramedics to supply and/or administer specified medicines to a predefined group of patients, without them having to see a prescriber first (such as a doctor or non-medical prescriber) (MHRA, 2017). Supplying and/or administering medicines under PGDs is reserved for situations in which this offers an advantage for patient care, without compromising patient safety. PGDs are used across a wide variety of healthcare settings. They are particularly useful in primary care for immunisations (for example, the coronavirus vaccine), in sexual health clinics and emergency care environments.

Patient Group Directions are developed by multidisciplinary groups including a doctor, a pharmacist and a representative of any professional group expected to supply the medicines under the PGD. Legal requirements of a PGD are stated within the Human Medicines Regulations (2012). The legal categories of medicines that can be supplied under a PGD are:

- Prescription only (PO)
- Pharmacy (P)
- General Sales List (GSL).

Unlicensed medicines, dressings, appliances and devices are not allowed to be supplied under a PGD. However, a medication can be supplied under a PGD outside its Summary of Product Characteristics, otherwise known as 'off-label', as long as it is justified by best clinical practice (NICE, 2017). Each PGD will reference the area that it covers and provide clear parameters in which it may be used.

Before using a PGD, paramedics should ensure that they:

- have undertaken the necessary initial training and continuing professional development
- have been assessed as competent and authorised to practise by the provider organisation
- have signed the appropriate documentation
- are using a copy of the most recent and in date final signed version of the PGD
- have read and understand the context and content of the PGD.

When supplying and/or administering a medicine under a PGD, paramedics should follow local organisational policies and act within their code(s) of professional conduct and local governance arrangements.

Patient Group Directions are a useful tool for use by paramedic-employing organisations to introduce drugs into use for which there is no paramedic exemption. It can take several years for amendments to be made in the Human Medicines Regulations (2012) for new drugs. Therefore, when a change happens in practice requiring a drug to be administered by paramedics, PGDs allow that practice to be introduced faster than waiting for the drug to be given an exemption. An example of this is from the Clinical Randomisation of an Antifibrinolytic in Significant Haemorrhage 2 (CRASH 2) trial (Shakur et al., 2010) where it was shown that there is an increased survival rate for major trauma patients who receive tranexamic acid. There is no paramedic exemption for this drug but the results of the trial led to ambulance services in the UK using a PGD to bring tranexamic acid into paramedic practice. Although this study was published over a decade ago, and despite the drug being in widespread use in UK paramedic practice, there still is no prescription exemption for paramedics to administer tranexamic acid and a PGD must be used to administer this drug.

Exemptions

A range of healthcare professionals are permitted to administer specified licensed medicines under the Human Medicines Regulations (2012 schedule 17 and amendments 2016). These include (within occupational health schemes) paramedics, midwives and optometrists. Orthoptists, chiropodists and podiatrists can undertake further training to undertake a wider range of exemptions. Schedule 19 of the Human Medicines Regulation (2012) also allows for certain drugs to be administered by anyone in an emergency; for example, it is this schedule that allows non-healthcare professionals to administer intramuscular (IM) glucagon to hypoglycaemic patients, and IM adrenaline 1:1000 to those with anaphylaxis. It is also the mechanism by which paramedics are able to administer antidotes to nerve agents in the prehospital environment. Other exemptions cover a range of situations such as emergency use of asthma inhalers in schools and access to medicines in a pandemic. It is important that you understand your organisation's policies in respect to the administration of specific medicines to save a life in an emergency. Follow Skills in practice 1 to understand your role within an emergency.

Paramedics registered with the HCPC can under the Human Medicines Regulations (2012 schedule 17 and amendments 2016) administer a number of drugs without a prescription to patients 'only for the immediate, necessary treatment of sick or injured persons and in the case of prescription only medicine containing Heparin Sodium shall be only for the purpose of cannula flushing'.

Skills in practice 1

Referring to Schedule 17 and 19 of the Human Medicines Regulations (2012)

- Under which schedule(s) as a paramedic can you administer adrenaline 1:1000 IM to a patient with anaphylaxis?
- Under which schedule(s) can you administer adrenaline to a patient in cardiac arrest?
- Under schedule 17 a paramedic can administer heparin sodium for which purpose?

The following prescription-only medicines can be administered via parenteral administration.

- Diazepam 5 mg per mL emulsion for injection.
- Succinylated modified fluid gelatin 4% intravenous infusion.
- Medicines containing the substance ergometrine maleate 500 mg per mL with oxytocin 5 international units per mL, but no other active ingredient.

The following prescription-only medicines containing one or more of the following substances, but no other active ingredient, can be administered.

- Adrenaline acid tartrate
- Adrenaline hydrochloride
- Amiodarone
- Anhydrous glucose
- Benzylpenicillin
- Compound sodium lactate intravenous infusion (Hartmann solution)
- Ergometrine maleate
- Furosemide
- Glucose
- Heparin sodium
- Lidocaine hydrochloride
- Metoclopramide
- Morphine sulfate
- Nalbuphine hydrochloride
- Naloxone hydrochloride
- Ondansetron
- Paracetamol
- Reteplase
- Sodium chloride
- Streptokinase
- Tenecteplase

In October 2020, a public and patient consultation was launched by NHS England to propose an increase in the drugs that paramedics can administer via exemption under the Human Medicines Regulations (2012). The proposal was for the introduction of the following drugs to the paramedic exception under Schedule 17 of the Regulations.

- Controlled Drugs:
  - lorazepam (by injection)
  - midazolam (by injection)

- Prescription-only medicines (POMs):
  - dexamethasone
  - magnesium sulfate
  - tranexamic acid
  - flumazenil

Paramedics may also as part of their duties administer Pharmacy (P) only medication and hold a supply of these drugs as part of their practice (MHRA, 2014).

Student paramedic exceptions

The Human Medicines Regulations (2012) do not allow for paramedics to delegate their prescription exemption under schedule 17 to others, nor does it allow student paramedics to administer drugs under supervision. The task of the administration is solely held by the registered paramedic (College of Paramedics, 2018). The only instance where a student may administer medication is where a prescriber, including paramedic independent prescribers, directs a student paramedic to administer prescribed medication.

Although schedule 19 of the Human Medicines Regulations allows any person to administer a list of certain medications in an emergency, this is for circumstances where there is no other person present to administer the medication. As students should be supervised at all times in practice, there should be no need for a student to administer a schedule 19 medication.

Prescribing

Doctors and dentists are currently the only healthcare professionals who are able to prescribe on registration. There are a range of healthcare professionals within the UK who have the right to prescribe medications. Since 1992 non-medical prescribing has been permitted within the UK (Cope et al., 2016). Multiple changes in legislation and professional regulation have enabled paramedics, nurses, midwives, pharmacists, physiotherapists, chiropodists, podiatrists and diagnostic radiographers to become independent prescribers, on successful completion of an accredited prescribing programme and registration of their qualification with their regulatory body. This extension of prescribing responsibilities to other healthcare professional groups is likely to continue where it is safe to do so and there is a clear patient benefit (Royal Pharmaceutical Society (RPS), 2016). There are currently two forms of prescribing: independent prescribing and supplementary prescribing.

An independent prescriber is a practitioner who is responsible and accountable for the assessment of patients with undiagnosed or diagnosed conditions and can make prescribing decisions to manage the clinical condition of the patient. Nurse independent prescribers can prescribe any medicine or product listed within the *British National Formulary* (BNF) as well as unlicensed medicines and any Controlled Drugs (within schedules II–V) if they are competent to do. For other healthcare professionals with prescribing rights, such as physiotherapists and paramedics, there are some restrictions, particularly around the Controlled Drugs they can prescribe.

The Misuse of Drugs Act (1971) is the legislation which specifies which Controlled Drugs registered paramedics can supply and administer as part of their duties. This Act works in combination with the Human Medicines Regulations (2012) as to which Controlled Drugs paramedics can hold and administer as part of their exceptions. The only Controlled Drugs paramedics can supply and administer using exemptions are:

- morphine sulfate (for injection and oral)
- diazepam emulsion (Diazemuls®).

Prior to 2019, paramedics and other prescribing allied health professionals only had their own specific 'Standards for prescribing' issued by the HCPC (2019). Due to the increasing number of healthcare professionals involved in medicines management, a more consistent approach was required, that all healthcare professionals could follow. Since January 2019, all healthcare professionals are required to follow the RPS (2018) 'Professional guidance on the safe and secure handling of medicines' and the RPS (2019) 'Professional guidance on the administration of medicines in healthcare settings'. These guidance documents ensure consistent safe and effect medicine administration and handling of medicines. Alongside this guidance, most local NHS trusts and other employers will also have their own guidance or policies which employees should always check and follow when considering their actions related to medicines management.

Handling and administration

The online document 'Professional guidance on the safe and secure handling of medicines' (RPS 2018), accredited by NICE, provides details on the four core governance principles that underpin a framework for the safe and secure handling of medicines. This guidance applies to all healthcare settings and covers all pharmacists and other health professionals whose role involves handling medicines. The document provides comprehensive guidance on obtaining medicines, their transport, receipt, manufacture or manipulation and storage. It also includes information on the issuing of medicines, and their removal or disposal. This guidance also helps organisations to ensure that they adhere to regulations laid down by the Health and Safety Executive, to ensure prevention of work-related death, injury and ill health of employees as some of these elements can expose healthcare practitioners to the risk of harm.

Professional guidance on the administration of medicines in healthcare settings was coproduced by the Royal Pharmaceutical Society (RPS) and the Royal College of Nursing (RCN) (RPS, 2019). This document provides principles-based guidance to ensure the safe administration and transcribing of medicines by registered healthcare professionals. The principles within the guidance can also be applied in any healthcare setting by any person administering medicines.

The guidance recommends that: 'Those administering medicines are appropriately trained, assessed as competent and meet relevant professional and regulatory standards and guidance' (RPS, 2019, p.3, no. 8).

Employers will have their own policies and procedures for the medicines administration process, which may differ slightly, so it is very important that you check these before administering any medication. An example of a medicine administration procedure is outlined in Box 4.1.

Your employing organisation will ensure that any risks associated with handling or administration of medicines have been identified, and procedures should be in place to minimise any risks. Your employing organisation should also ensure that any necessary equipment and devices, required to aid the administration of medicines, are available and well maintained. Follow Clinical Consideration 5 to understand the medicine administration procedure within your organisation.

Box 4.1 Example of a medicine administration procedure

This may include (but is not limited to) the following.

- Checking the identity of the patient.
- The prescription meets legal requirements, is unambiguous and includes where appropriate the name, form (or route of administration), strength and dose of the medicine to be administered.
- That issues around consent have been adhered to.
- Allergies or previous adverse drug reactions have been checked and recorded.
- The directions for administration (e.g. timing and frequency of administration, route of administration and start and finish dates where appropriate) are clear.
- Any ambiguities or concerns regarding the direction for administration of the medicine are raised with the prescriber or a pharmacy professional without delay.
- Any calculations needed are double-checked where practicable by a second person and uncertainties raised with the prescriber or a pharmacy professional.
- The identity of the medicine (or medical gas) and its expiry date (where available) have been checked.
- That any specific storage requirements have been maintained.
- Confirm that the dose has not already been administered by someone else.

Clinical consideration 5

Refer to your organisation's policy or Standard Operating Procedure (SOP) on medicine administration procedure. How does this compare with the example in Box 4.1?

Prior to administering a medicine, you should have an understanding of what the medication is used for and how it works, the route of administration, potential side-effects and circumstances when you should not give the medication. You need to be familiar with resources that will help you to find out this information.

The correct medicine administration procedure must be followed to ensure the right patient gets the right medication at the right time. To support this further, a systematic approach have been developed for medicines administration, referred to as the 9Rs, or nine 'rights' of medication administration (Elliott and Liu, 2010).

1. *Right patient:* The identity of the patient must be verified by checking their name, address and date of birth both with the patient and on their chart. Extra care needs to be taken for patients who are unable to identify themselves, for example the unconscious patient or those with cognitive impairment.
2. *Right drug:* Many drugs look the same, have similar names and even similar packaging. Without careful checking, the wrong medication could be administered by mistake.
3. *Right route:* The same medicine is often available for administration using a variety of routes but dose and onset of action can be different according to which route is used. The correct route of medicine administration needs to be confirmed prior to giving it to the patient.
4. *Right time:* Medication needs to be given at the prescribed time in order to ensure stable levels of drug within the body and avoid unwanted gaps in therapy. If a medication is ordered to be given at particular time intervals, the paramedic should never deviate from this time by more than half an hour (Galbraith et al., 2015). If administration occurs outside this 30-minute window, bioavailability of the medication may be affected (Elliott and Liu, 2010). It is particularly important that critical medications are administered at the prescribed time as a delay could cause potential harm to the patient.
5. *Right dose:* The dose to be administered will be stated on the prescription. Best practice would suggest that you check the dose of the medication in a pharmaceutical guide (see Chapter 2 of this text) to ensure it is the correct dose. Some medications will require you to carry out a dose calculation before administration. Variables such as age, weight, condition or specific biochemical markers need to be considered to determine the dose that needs to be given.
6. *Right documentation:* It is very important that records of administration, or a medication being withheld from or declined by the patient, is completed at the time, or as soon as possible thereafter, and that all records are clear, legible and accurate (RPS, 2019). If a medication is not administered, or has been refused, details of the reason why (if known) should be included in the record and reported to the prescriber, or healthcare team, where appropriate. Look at Clinical Consideration 6 and consider your actions.
7. *Right action:* Before you administer any medication, you must first ensure that it is prescribed for an appropriate reason. This requires knowledge and understanding of the medical condition(s) of your patient and the action of the drug(s) to be administered. Where possible, you should state to the patient the action of the medication and the reason for which it is prescribed, as this may help to avoid a medication error (Elliott and Liu, 2010).
8. *Right form:* Medications are available in different forms such as tablets, capsules, caplets, syrup, suppositories and ampoules for intravenous administration. It is important that the route of administration is clear (e.g. oral) and that the right form of medication is administered to avoid harm to the patient. Specific instructions may need to be given to patients, for example not to chew enteric-coated tablets as they are designed to dissolve in the alkaline environment of the small intestine, and some drugs are enteric coated because the active ingredient will irritate the stomach mucosa if they dissolve there (Adams and Koch, 2010).

9. *Right response:* Once a medication has been administered, patients should be monitored for any side-effects, adverse effects or adverse reactions, which should be managed and documented appropriately if they occur. It is also important to understand that some patients will need to be monitored to ensure the intended effect or efficacy of the medication is achieved, for example assessment of blood glucose level for the patient with diabetes or blood pressure monitoring for patients with hypertension (Bruen et al., 2017).

If you are in any doubt about administering a medication consult the prescriber or pharmacy professional for further information or advice.

Clinical consideration 6

As a paramedic, you are called to see Mrs Doris Speed, a 64-year-old lady with a history of epilepsy. She has been complaining of diarrhoea and vomiting for 2 days. The patient has declined to go to hospital for assessment and has informed you that she has not been taking her prescribed medication. She stopped taking her laxatives, stating she had moved her bowels four times that day already. Mrs Speed has also declined to take her sodium valproate as she says it makes her feel sick.
 In order to care effectively for Mrs Speed, what actions do you need to take for:

- the laxative?
- the sodium valproate?

Special consideration: Controlled Drugs and critical medications

Some medications, due to their potential to be misused and the harm that this can cause, are classified as Controlled Drugs (CDs). There will be additional requirements that you must follow regarding their use. The Misuse of Drugs Act (1971), and its associated regulations, detail the legal framework governing the use of CDs. NICE has produced the guideline *Controlled Drugs: Safe Use and Management* (NG46) (NICE, 2016a) which provides further details on the systems and processes that must be in place in all healthcare environments (except care homes) for managing the use of CDs. Your trust/employer may have additional policies/procedures related to controlled drugs that you will need to follow.
 Any medication should be administered in a timely manner, but there are some medications that must not be omitted, or their administration delayed, as this has the potential to cause harm to the patient. The NHS Specialist Pharmacy Service (2018) has updated the National Patient Safety Agency (NPSA) Rapid Response Report 'Reducing harm from omitted and delayed medicines in hospital' (February 2010). This document highlights the need for rapid access to medications that are critical for patients, with the risks of delay, or omission, for each drug categorised using a traffic light system (Table 4.1). Medications that fall into the Risk 3 category are classified as 'critical medications' due to the consequences to the patient if they are missed or omitted.
 'Critical medicines' include groups of medicines such as:

- antimicrobials
- anticoagulants
- antiepileptic agents
- anti-parkinsonian agents
- immunosuppressants
- insulin.

Any omission or delay in the administration of a critical medicine must be discussed with the prescriber (or relevant physician) and reported as a patient safety incident.

Table 4.1   The potential risks of missed medication.

Risk 1	Risk 2	Risk 3
Nil or negligible patient impact with nil or minor intervention required; no increase in length of stay	Significant short-term patient impact with moderate intervention required; increase in length of hospital stay possible	Significant or catastrophic long-term patient impact with ongoing intervention required; long increase in length of stay possible
• There is no or negligible risk of patient impact • No or minor intervention necessary • There is no possibility of an increase in the length of hospital stay	• There is a risk of significant short-term patient impact Subsequent moderate intervention is required • A resultant long increase (1–15 days) in the length of hospital stay is possible	• There is a risk of significant long-term patient impact • There is a risk of catastrophic patient impact (i.e. death) • Subsequent ongoing professional intervention is required • A resultant very long (>15 days) increase in the length of hospital stay is possible

Groups requiring special considerations

For women who are pregnant or breast feeding and for the older population, special care needs to be taken in the medicines management process to ensure the safety of the patient.

Pregnancy and breast feeding

Administering medicines during pregnancy is complex and can have major consequences if not managed with caution and expertise. It is important to establish whether someone of child-bearing age may be pregnant prior to administration of any medicine. Careful consideration must be given to the benefits and risks of taking medicines, both for the mother and the foetus. Within each edition of the BNF (and online resource), there is an advice section on the specific medicine issues concerning pregnancy and breast feeding. General advice is that drugs should only be prescribed if the benefit for the mother is greater than the risk to the foetus, but all drugs should be avoided where possible during the first trimester (BNF 80).

In life-threatening emergencies, such as cardiac arrest or anaphylaxis, Chu et al. (2020) recommend that pregnant patients should be managed with the same algorithms and drug regimen as specified in the advanced life support and anaphylaxis guidance from the Resuscitation Council (2015).

There is little information available for identifying the safety of medicines for women who are breast feeding. This can cause confusion for health professionals offering information but also for the breast-feeding woman who may cease breast feeding earlier than planned rather than expose her child to unknown risks (McClatchey et al., 2017). The BNF identifies where it is known that medicines are contraindicated or where caution is indicated during pregnancy and breast feeding.

Older people

Special care is required in managing medicines for older people. A large proportion of older people within the UK have multimorbidity, and within this population the use of multiple medicines (polypharmacy) is very common.

Polypharmacy occurs when an individual is taking four or more regular medicines (Patterson et al., 2012). Taking multiple medications greatly increases the risk of drug interactions and adverse reactions and can also affect compliance. It has been estimated that 30–50% of medicines taken for long-term conditions are not taken as prescribed (NICE, 2016b). As a result of this, it is recommended that older people's medications are reviewed regularly and any medicine which is not of benefit should be discontinued.

As an individual gets older, what the body does to a drug (pharmacokinetics) changes. The most important effect of age is reduced renal clearance, meaning that older people excrete drugs more slowly, increasing the risk of side-effects and adverse reactions (Shi and Klotz, 2011). The BNF state the most common adverse reactions to monitor for are:

- confusion
- constipation
- postural hypotension and falls (BNF 80).

As a result of this, the BNF provides some general principles to be followed for the older person.

- *Lower doses:* Lower doses of medicines may be used (usually 50% of an adult dose) and only increased if needed.
- *Review regularly:* Regular medication reviews should be undertaken to determine if the medication is still appropriate/required. It may be necessary to reduce medications of some drugs as renal function declines.
- *Simplify regimens:* Medications should only be given when there is a clear indication to do so (for example, not prescribing antibiotics for a viral infection). If possible, medicines should only be prescribed once or twice daily and confusing dosage intervals should be avoided.
- *Explain clearly:* Each medication should have clear instructions on how to take it with full directions given (BNF 80).

These are some of the issues which need consideration for medicine management; can you think of any more? Clinical Consideration 7 will help you to explore this further.

Clinical consideration 7

Having read this section, are there any other groups in your practice area that require further consideration prior to administering medications under exception, or PGD?

Monitoring for side-effects

All medicines can have side-effects. The European Medicines Agency (EMA) (2017) defines an adverse drug reaction (ADR) as 'a response to a medicinal product which is noxious and unintended'. Part of your role within medicines management is to understand, and identify, any ADR as some can occur within minutes of administration, whereas others can present years after treatment (Ferner and McGettigan, 2018).

Medicines optimisation

Medicines optimisation builds on medicines management, but encompasses all aspects of a patient's medicines journey from the initial prescription through to ongoing review and support. Medicines optimisation is about ensuring that the right patients get the right choice of medicine, at the right time. By focusing on patients and their experiences, the goal is to help patients to:

- improve their outcomes
- take their medicines correctly
- avoid taking unnecessary medicines
- reduce wastage of medicines
- improve medicines safety.

A multidisciplinary approach to medicines optimisation can encourage patients to take ownership of their treatment (RPS, 2013). The RPS (2013) described four guiding principles for medicines management in practice (see Box 4.2).

   Medicines optimisation examines how patients use medicines over time. It may involve stopping certain medicines as well as starting others, and considers opportunities for lifestyle changes and non-medical therapies to reduce the need for medicines. By improving medicine safety, adherence to treatment and reducing waste, the medicines optimisation approach ensures patients are supported to get the best outcomes from their medicines (NICE, 2015).

Box 4.2   Four principles of medicines management

Principle 1	Aim to understand the patient's experience
Principle 2	Evidence-based choice of medicines
Principle 3	Ensure medicines use is as safe as possible
Principle 4	Make medicines optimisation part of routine practice

The key elements of medicines optimisation are that it:

- is patient centred and makes a difference to the patient's outcomes
- is a partnership between healthcare professional and patient
- is about listening to the patient's views and opinions, supporting adherence and self-care
- is the application of clinical and pharmaceutical expertise and understanding
- provides a personalised medication regimen for each patient
- encourages communication with other healthcare professionals to ensure continuity across care settings
- encourages good governance, including safety, quality and better outcomes.

The paramedic therefore has a significant role in ensuring that patients/service users, and their carers, are central to the shared decision-making process in managing their medicines with the ultimate aim of improving health outcomes.

Safety in medicines management

A recent study found that an estimated 237 million medication errors occur in the NHS in England every year (Elliott et al., 2018). These errors resulted in avoidable ADRs, causing 712 deaths and contributing to 1708 deaths. Non-steroidal anti-inflammatory drugs (NSAIDs), anticoagulants and antiplatelets caused over a third of hospital admissions due to avoidable ADRs. Gastrointestinal bleeds were implicated in half of the deaths from primary care ADRs. The report also found that older people were more likely to suffer avoidable ADRs. The cost to the NHS for these avoidable ADRs was £98.5 million per year. This is a huge financial drain on the NHS but the harm and suffering caused to patients and their families are immeasurable. The transfer of patients between primary and secondary care is also an area for potential error where it is estimated that up to 70% of patients may have an unintentional change or medication error (RPS, 2012a). Further risks of errors were identified for people residing in care homes and recommendations for best practice in managing polypharmacy, repeat prescribing and medication reviews as well as training for staff are advised (RPS, 2012b). NHS England (2018) has since outlined guidance to support safe and effective medicine management practices across primary, secondary and tertiary care, outlining the responsibilities of all professionals.

Medication errors are any Patient Safety Incident (PSI) where there has been an error in the process of prescribing, preparing, dispensing, administering, monitoring or providing advice on medicines. These PSIs can be divided into two categories:

- errors of commission (for example, wrong medicine or wrong dose)
- errors of omission (for example, an omitted dose or a failure to monitor).

The National Reporting and Learning System (NRLS) defines a 'patient safety incident' (PSI) as 'any unintended or unexpected incident, which could have or did lead to harm for one or more patients receiving NHS care'.

The Central Alerting System (CAS) (managed by the MHRA) is a web-based cascading system for issuing patient safety alerts, important public health messages and other safety-critical information and guidance to the NHS and others, including independent providers of health and social care. Alerts within this system include Medical Device Alerts (MDA) and Drug Alerts.

Storage and disposal

Medicines are used in all healthcare settings and the safe and secure handling of medicines is essential to ensure patient safety. The Human Medicines Regulations (2012) outline the legal requirements to support this process. Each medicine must be used and stored according to specific instructions known as the Summary of Product characteristics (SPC or SmPC), details of which can be found in the Electronic Medicines Compendium (www.medicines.org.uk/emc).

The RPS 'Professional guidance on the safe and secure handling of medicines' online document (2018) advises that all individuals who handle medicines must be competent, legally entitled, appropriately trained and authorised to do the job. Medicines must be kept secure and safeguarded from unauthorised access and stored at a level of security appropriate to their proposed use.

The Controlled Drugs used by paramedics from schedule 2 or 3 of the Misuse of Drugs Regulations (2001), such as morphine sulfate, midazolam, or ketamine, must when not in use be stored in a metal container or safe, attached to a wall or the floor as specified in the Misuse of Drugs (Safe Custody) Regulations (1973). The Regulation also specifies that when CDs are being carried by a paramedic as part of their practice, they must at all times (where possible) be kept in a locked container to which only they, or someone authorised by them, have access.

Where products need to be stored at cooler temperatures, the cold chain must be maintained to ensure the integrity of the product is maintained. For example, vaccines deteriorate at room temperature and thus must be stored in a refrigerator and in cool conditions right until the moment they are administered. Where this has been compromised, a risk assessment must be undertaken to determine whether the integrity of the product has been affected.

Safe handling and disposal of toxic substances such as cytotoxic drugs are governed by the Health and Safety Executive (HSE) (2019) as they present significant risks for those who handle them. The HSE offers practical guidance on meeting the Control of Substances Hazardous to Health Regulations (COSHH) (2002) and how these substances should be safely handled and disposed of in all health and social care environments, including the patient's home.

Any unwanted or expired medicines in the community need to be returned to a pharmacy or chemist for safe disposal. Inhalers contain gases which can be harmful to the environment so should not be put in waste bins and must also be returned to a pharmacy/chemist where they can be recycled. Pharmacies are obliged to accept any unwanted medicines from patients. The pharmacy must, if required by NHS England or the waste contractor, sort them into solids (including ampoules and vials), liquids and aerosols, and the local NHS England team will make arrangements for a waste contractor to collect the medicines from pharmacies at regular intervals. Additional segregation is also required under the Hazardous Waste (England and Wales) Regulations (2005). Ambulance providers will have their own policy and procedure for their isolation from practice, and safe disposal of expired medications. It is the responsibility of the practising paramedic to be aware of and follow their employer's medicines policies.

Conclusion

This chapter has explored the many strands to managing medicines to provide safe, efficient and cost-effective care. Paramedics have a role in this process to ensure they understand and follow the regulations, policies and practices which govern safe prescribing, administration and monitoring of medicines. Medicines management should be a partnership between patients and all healthcare professionals to ensure good patient-centred outcomes regardless of the health or social care setting.

You must always ensure that you are working within your scope of practice and also adhere to local and national policies and the appropriate aspects of the law so as to practise safely and effectively.

References

Adams, M. and Koch, R. (2010). *Pharmacology: Connections to Nursing Practice*. Hoboken: Pearson.

Bruen, D., Delaney, C., Florea, L. and Diamond, D. (2017). Glucose sensing for diabetes monitoring: recent developments. *Sensors* **17**(8): 1866.

Chu, J., Johnston, T.A., Geoghegan, J. and Royal College of Obstetricians and Gynaecologists. (2020). *Maternal Collapse in Pregnancy and the Puerperium: Green-top Guideline No. 56. British Journal of Obstetrics and Gynaecology* **127**(5): e14–e52.

College of Paramedics. (2018). *Practice Guidance for Paramedics for the Administration of Medicines under Exemptions within the Human Medicines Regulations* 2012. https://collegeofparamedics.co.uk/

Cope, L.C., Abuzour, A.S. and Tully, M.P. (2016). Nonmedical prescribing: where are we now? *Therapeutic Advances in Drug Safety* **7**: 165–172.

Duerden, M., Avery, T. and Payne, R. (2013). *Polypharmacy and medicines optimisation: making it safe and sound.* www.kingsfund.org.uk/publications/polypharmacy-and-medicinesoptimisation

Elliott, M. amd Liu, Y. (2010). The nine rights of medication administration: an overview. *British Journal of Nursing* **19**(5): 300–305.

Elliott, R., Camacho, E., Cambell, F. et al. (2018). *Prevalence and economic burden of medication errors in the NHS in England.* www.eepru.org.uk/prevalence-and-economic-burden-of-medication-errors-in-the-nhs-in-england-2/

European Medicines Agency (EMA). (2017). *Guideline on good pharmacovigilance practices (GVP): Annex I - Definitions(Rev4).*www.ema.europa.eu/en/documents/scientific-guideline/guideline-good-pharmacovigilance-practices-annex-i-definitions-rev-4_en.pdf

Ewbank, L., Omojomolo, D., Sullivan, K. et al. (2018). *The rising cost of medicines to the NHS.* www.kingsfund.org.uk/sites/default/files/2018-04/Rising-cost-of-medicines.pdf

Ferner, R.E. and McGettigan, P. (2018). Adverse drug reactions. *British Medical Journal* **363**: k4051.

Galbraith, A., Bullock, S., Manias, E., Hunt, B. and Richards, A. (2015). *Fundamentals of Pharmacology: An Applied Approach for Nursing and Health.* Cambridge: Routledge.

Health and Care Professions Council (HCPC). (2019). *Standards for prescribing.* www.hcpc-uk.org/globalassets/standards/standards-for-prescribing/standards-for-prescribing2.pdf

Health and Safety Executive. (2019). *Control of Substances Hazardous to Health.* www.hse.gov.uk/coshh/index.htm

Human Medicines Regulations. (2012). https://www.legislation.gov.uk/uksi/2012/1916/contents/made

McClatchey, A.K., Shield, A., Cheong, L.H., Ferguson, S.L., Cooper, G.M. and Kyle, G.J. (2017). Why does the need for medication become a barrier to breastfeeding? A narrative review. *Women and Birth* **31**(5): 362–366.

Medicines and Healthcare products Regulatory Agency (MHRA). (2014). *Rules for the sale, supply and administration of medicines for specific healthcare professionals.* www.gov.uk/government/publications/rules-for-the-sale-supply-and-administration-of-medicines/rules-for-the-sale-supply-and-administration-of-medicines-for-specific-healthcare-professionals

Medicines and Healthcare products Regulatory Agency (MHRA). (2017). *Patient group directions: who can use them.*www.gov.uk/government/publications/patient-group-directions-pgds/patient-group-directions-who-can-use-them

NHS Business Services Authority (NHSBSA). (2018). *Medicines optimisation – generic prescribing.* www.nhsbsa.nhs.uk/epact2/dashboards-and-specifications/medicines-optimisation-generic-prescribing

NHS England. (2018). *Responsibility for prescribing between primary and secondary/teriary care.* www.england.nhs.uk/publication/responsibility-for-prescribing-between-primary-and-secondary-tertiary-care/

NHS England. (2020). *Consultation on proposed amendments to the list of medicines that paramedics are able to administer under exemptions within the Human Medicines Regulations 2012 across the United Kingdom.* www.england.nhs.uk/wp-content/uploads/2020/10/paramedic-consultation-summary.pdf

NHS Specialist Pharmacy Service. (2018). *Medicines Matters.* www.sps.nhs.uk/wp-content/uploads/2018/10/Medicines-Matters-september-2018-1.pdf

NICE. (2015). *Medicines optimisation: the safe and effective use of medicines to enable the best possible outcomes [NG5].* www.nice.org.uk/guidance/ng5

NICE. (2016a). *Controlled drugs: safe use and management [NG46].* www.nice.org.uk/guidance/ng46

NICE. (2016b). *Multimorbidity: clinical assessment and management [NG56].* www.nice.org.uk/guidance/ng56

NICE. (2017). *Patient group directions.* www.nice.org.uk/guidance/mpg2/chapter/Recommendations#training-and-competency

Patterson, S.M., Hughes, C., Kerse, N., Cardwell, C.R. and Bradley, M.C. (2012). Interventions to improve the appropriate use of polypharmacy for older people. *Cochrane Database of Systematic Reviews* **5**: CD008165.

Resuscitation Council. (2015). *Adult advanced life support.* www.resus.org.uk/resuscitation-guidelines/adult-advanced-life-support

Royal Pharmaceutical Society (RPS). (2012a). *Keeping patients safe when they transfer between care providers – getting the medicines right: final report.* www.rpharms.com/

Royal Pharmaceutical Society (RPS). (2012b). *Improving pharmaceutical care in care homes.* www.rpharms.com/

Royal Pharmaceutical Society (RPS). (2013). *Medicines Optimisation.* www.rpharms.com/Portals/0/RPS%20document%20library/Open%20access/Policy/helping-patients-make-the-most-of-their-medicines.pdf

Royal Pharmaceutical Society (RPS). (2016). *A Competency Framework for all Prescribers.* www.rpharms.com/Portals/0/RPS%20document%20library/Open%20access/Professional%20standards/Prescribing%20competency%20framework/prescribing-competency-framework.pdf?ver=2019-02-13-163215-030

Royal Pharmaceutical Society (RPS). (2018). *Professional guidance on the safe and secure handling of medicines*. www.rpharms.com/

Royal Pharmaceutical Society (RPS). (2019). *Professional guidance on the administration of medicines in healthcare settings*. www.rpharms.com/

Shakur, H., Roberts, I., Bautista, R. et al., CRASH-2 trial collaborators. (2010). Effects of tranexamic acid on death, vascular occlusive events, and blood transfusion in trauma patients with significant haemorrhage (CRASH-2): a randomised, placebo-controlled trial. *Lancet* **376**(9734): 23–32.

Shi, S. and Klotz, U. (2011). Age-related changes in pharmacokinetics. *Current Drug Metabolism* **12**(7): 601–610.

Further reading

Adam, M.P., Polifka, J.E. and Friedman, J.M. (2011). Evolving knowledge of the teratogenicity of medications in human pregnancy. *American Journal of Medical Genetics* **157**: 175–182.

Aronson, J.K. and Ferner, R.E. (2005). Clarification of terminology in drug safety. *Drug Safety* **28**: 851–870.

Care Quality Commission. (2019). *Issue 5: Safe management of medicines*. www.cqc.org.uk/guidance-providers/learning-safety-incidents/issue-5-safe-management-medicines

Clemow, B., Nolan, J.D., Michaels, D.L., Kogelnik, A.M., Cantrell, S.A. and Dewulf, L. (2015). Medicines in Pregnancy Forum: proceedings on ethical and legal considerations. Ethic Special Section Meeting Report. *Therapeutic Innovaion and Regulatory Science* **49**(3): 326–332.

Department of Health. (2013). *The Medicines Act 1968 and the Human Medicines Regulations (Amendment) Order*. London: Department of Health.

HMSO. (1973). *The Misuse of Drugs (Safe Custody) Regulations 1973*. London: HMSO.

HMSO. (1997). *Prescription Only Medicines (Human Use) Order 1997. Statutory Instrument No. 1830*. London: HMSO.

HMSO. (2001). *The Misuse of Drugs Regulations 2001*. London: HMSO.

Jones, S.W. (2009). Reducing medication administration errors in nursing practice. *Nursing Standard* **23**: 40–46.

Murk, W. and Seli, E. (2011). Fertility preservation as a public health issue: an epidemiological perspective. *Current Opinion in Obstetrics and Gynecology* **23**: 143–150.

NHS. (2019). *Medicines optimisation*. www.england.nhs.uk/medicines/medicines-optimisation

NICE. (2009). *Medicines adherence: involving patients in decisions about prescribed medicines and supporting adherence [CG76]*. www.nice.org.uk/guidance/cg76

Northern Ireland Department of Health. (2019). *Medicines Management*. www.health-ni.gov.uk/articles/medicines-management

Nursing and Midwifery Council and Royal Pharmaceutical Society. (2019). *Professional Guidance on the Administration of Medicines in Healthcare Settings*. www.rpharms.com/Portals/0/RPS%20document%20library/Open%20access/Professional%20standards/SSHM%20and%20Admin/Admin%20of%20Meds%20prof%20guidance.pdf?ver=2019-01-23-145026-567

Resuscitation Council. (2012). *Emergency treatment of anaphylactic reactions: guidelines for healthcare providers*. www.resus.org.uk/library/additional-guidance/guidance-anaphylaxis/emergency-treatment

Rezaallah, B., Lewis, D.J., Zeilhofer, H.F. and Ber, B.I. (2019). Risk of cleft lip and/or palate associated with anti-epileptic drugs: postmarketing safety signal detection and evaluation of information presented to prescribers and patients. *Therapeutic and Regulatory Science* **53**(1): 110–119.

Royal College of Nursing. (2018). *Medicines Management: prescribing in pregnancy*. www.rcn.org.uk/clinical-topics/medicines-management/prescribing-in-pregnancy

World Health Organization. (2007). *Promoting Safety of Medicines for Children*. Geneva: World Health Organization.

Multiple-choice questions

1. Medicines management could be best described as:
   (a) Senior managers controlling medicines
   (b) Safe, efficient and cost-effective use of medicines
   (c) People managing to open their medicines.
2. A PoM is:
   (a) The Price of the Medicine
   (b) The Purpose of the Medicine
   (c) A Prescription only Medicine.
3. Patient Group Directions are:
   (a) Maps of the hospital to direct patents
   (b) A list of medicines that can be given to a patient without a prescription

(c) Written instructions directing registered health professionals to supply/
(d) administer specified medicines to a predefined group of patients.
4. Medicines are regulated by the:
   (a) Medicines Regulatory Body
   (b) Medicines and Healthcare products Regulatory Agency
   (c) Regulatory Agency for Medicines.

5. A black triangle is applied to:
   (a) Cheaper medicines
   (b) Products where there is limited experience of use
   (c) Medicines which should not be used.
6. A generic medicine is:
   (a) A non-proprietary medicine
   (b) A medicine which can be used for any condition
   (c) A proprietary medicine.
7. The legal framework for medicines includes:
   (a) The Human Medicines Regulations 2012
   (b) The Medicines Law 2000
   (c) The Regulations for Medical Use 2012.
8. Which of the following is a non-proprietary drug?
   (a) Brufen
   (b) Ibuprofen
   (c) Nurofen
9. Critical medicines:
   (a) Are important medicines
   (b) Need special care
   (c) Must not be omitted or delayed.
10. Before administering a medicine, the paramedic must:
    (a) Consult with the prescriber for every patient
    (b) Understand the medicine being administered and seek advice from the prescriber or pharmacy professional if required
    (c) Contact the pharmacist to check the prescription.
11. Which of the following Royal Pharmaceutical Society guidance should paramedics adhere to for the administration of medicines?
    (a) A competency framework for all prescribers
    (b) Professional guidance for the administration of medicines in healthcare settings
    (c) Professional guidance on the safe and secure handling of medicines
12. Common adverse reactions in older people include:
    (a) Confusion, constipation, postural hypotension and falls
    (b) Chest pain, headaches and constipation
    (c) Earache, stomach pains and dizziness.
13. The Central Alerting System:
    (a) Issues alerts to organisations about healthcare staff
    (b) Alerts healthcare professionals about patients
    (c) Issues patient safety alerts.
14. Which of the following bodies analyse the use of NHS medicines?
    (a) The NHS Business Authority
    (b) The NHS Medicines Authority
    (c) The NHS Supply of Medicines Authority
15. Optimising medicines:
    (a) Focuses on the medicine cost
    (b) Focuses on the patient
    (c) Focuses on the healthcare professional.

Chapter 5

Pharmacodynamics and pharmacokinetics

Dan Davern

Aim

The aim of this chapter is to provide the reader with an introduction to pharmacokinetics and pharmacodynamics as they relate to prehospital emergency care.

Learning outcomes

After completing this chapter the reader should be able to:

1. Define pharmacokinetics and pharmacodynamics
2. Explain the factors involved in medication absorption and distribution
3. Describe biotransformation
4. Explain how medications are eliminated from the body and factors that affect elimination.

Test your knowledge

1. Describe the phases of pharmacokinetics.
2. Describe first-pass metabolism.
3. Define pharmacodynamics.
4. Using an example from prehospital pharmacology, explain the term affinity.
5. List five common factors that affect elimination.

Introduction

This chapter explores the fundamentals of pharmacokinetics and pharmacodynamics as they apply to prehospital emergency care.

Fundamentals of Pharmacology for Paramedics, First Edition. Edited by Ian Peate, Suzanne Evans, and Lisa Clegg.
© 2022 John Wiley & Sons Ltd. Published 2022 by John Wiley & Sons Ltd.

Professional regulatory council

The Health and Care Professions Council (HCPC) is the body responsible for protecting the public by regulating 15 health and care professions in the UK, including paramedicine. There are other regulatory bodies globally which are also charged with the regulatuion and setting of standards for paramedics. The HCPC approves programmes of education and training leading to registration in addition to setting standards of proficiency for paramedics. These proficiency standards set out safe and effective practice for paramedics, to protect members of the public and provide appropriate care. These threshold standards specify that paramedics must 'understand relevant pharmacology and the administration of therapeutic medications, including pharmacodynamics and pharmacokinetics' (HCPC, 2014).

Programmes of education and training

Programmes of education and training leading to registration as a paramedic often involve a modular approach. This may include a specific module on pharmacology and therapeutics or integrate pharmacological learning outcomes through several modules. Regardless of the delivery format, pharmacology comprises an important part of paramedic education.

Paramedics administer medications to patients in order to produce a specific desired effect. Having a detailed understanding of those medications, their effect on the body and the effect of the body on the medication allows the paramedic to practise safely and provide the most appropriate care for patients. The two most common terms paramedics must understand when studying pharmacology are pharmacokinetics and pharmacodynamics.

Pharmacokinetics

Derived from two Greek words, *pharmacon* meaning 'drug' and *kinesis* meaning 'movement', put simply, pharmacokinetics is 'what the body does to the drug'. Strictly defined, pharmacokinetics is the study of the basic processes that determine the duration and intensity of a medication's effect (Bledsoe and Clayden, 2012). These four processes are absorption, distribution, metabolism (sometimes referred to as biotransformation) and elimination (Table 5.1).

Table 5.1   Four stages of pharmacokinetics.

1. Absorption of drugs into the body	How does it get into the body?
2. Distribution of drugs to the tissues of the body	Where does it go?
3. Metabolism (biotransformation) of drugs into the body	How is it broken down?
4. Elimination of drugs from the body	How does it leave?

Source: Young and Pritchard (2016).

The pharmacokinetic processes

The key aspects of pharmacokinetics are what the body does to the drug, how drugs are absorbed by the body, how they are distributed to the body tissues, how drugs are metabolised (the liver is the primary organ for biotransformation), and how the drug is eliminated by the body (primary excretion organs are the kidneys and lungs).

Understanding pharmacokinetics is important to allow paramedics to determine the appropriate route for medication administration (if required) or indeed to simply understand why medications are administered via different routes. For example, why might a drug be administered orally (PO) or intramuscularly (IM), or directly into the circulation by intravenous (IV) injection or by intraosseous infusion (IO)?

Pharmacokinetics gives us an appreciation of the frequency of drug administration, for example why some drugs are administered as a single bolus or why repeat administration is required in some cases. With the liver, kidneys and lungs playing such a vital role, it is clear why diseased or aged organs can have a significant effect on the metabolism of medications.

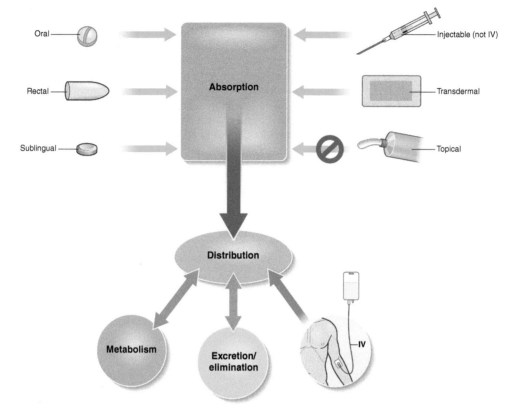

Figure 5.1   Stages of pharmacokinetics and medication administration routes. Source: Reproduced with permission from Young and Pritchard (2016).

Figure 5.1 illustrates the four stages of pharmacokinetics and some common routes of medication administration. It is worth noting that the IV route bypasses the absorption phase and first-pass metabolism; we will discuss this further later in this chapter.

Phase 1: absorption

Medication absorption is the process encompassing a medication's progress from the initial pharmacological dosage administered to a biologically available form which can pass through or across tissues (Bledsoe and Clayden, 2012). It is suggested that drug absorption is determined by several factors including:

- the drug's physicochemical properties
- its formulation
- the route of administration, i.e. enteral or parenteral.

The dosage forms (e.g. tablets, capsules, liquid suspensions), consisting of the drug plus other ingredients, are formulated to be given by a specific route; for example, glyceryl trinitrate (GTN) spray is formulated to be administered via the sublingual route. Another example is midazolam prefilled syringes for buccal administration.

Regardless of the route of administration, drugs must be in solution to be absorbed. Thus, solid forms (e.g. tablets) must be able to disintegrate and disaggregate.

Unless administered directly to the circulatory system (IV/IO), A drug must cross or pass through several semipermeable cell membranes before it reaches the systemic circulation. Cell membranes act as gatekeepers that selectively admit or inhibit the passage of molecules; as such, the site of absorption directly affects the rate at which the medication is absorbed. The area of the absorbing surface also determines the speed of absorption as medications are quickly absorbed from large surface areas; for example, salbutamol administered via nebuliser for inhalation is distributed quickly across the large pulmonary tissue area and is rapidly absorbed into circulation.

Finally, absorption is affected by the blood supply at the site of absorption. Some sites have a rich blood supply while others do not. Medications administered to sites with a rich blood supply will absorb much more quickly; for example, the sublingual route has a rich blood supply to the tissues under the tongue and will absorb rapidly. Areas with a poor blood supply, such as the subcutaneous layer (fatty tissue), will absorb medications much more slowly.

It is essential for paramedics to understand the various rates of absorption from each of the medication administration routes available to them. This enables the paramedic to determine the most appropriate route of administration for specific medications to achieve the desired effect and practise safely.

Reflection – route selection

Epinephrine 1:1000 1 mg/1 mL standard ampoule presentation is a medication used by paramedics for management of anaphylaxis. JRCALC guidelines indicate that the route for administration is intramuscular (IM). Why would paramedics not administer this medication via a quicker route such as intravenous (IV)?

Physiology of transport
Active transport

Active transport requires energy to move a substance. This energy is achieved by the breakdown of adenosine triphosphate (ATP), which is further broken down to adenosine diphosphate (ADP), which releases a considerable amount of energy. An example of this active transport system can be seen in the sodium potassium pump, which actively moves sodium ions into the cell and potassium ions out. As this movement goes against the concentration gradient of the ions, it must use energy. A simpler example of active transport would be a boat's bilge pump, which pumps water from the bottom of the boat back to the body of water; for this pump to work, energy is required.

To be absorbed, orally administered medications must first withstand chemical and bacterial degradation before they are absorbed from the gut. Absorption occurs via diffusion, or transport. Peptide drugs (e.g. insulin) are particularly susceptible to degradation and are not given orally. Absorption of oral drugs involves transport across membranes of the epithelial cells in the gastrointestinal (GI) tract. Absorption is affected by:

- differences in luminal pH along the GI tract
- surface area per luminal volume
- blood perfusion
- presence of bile and mucus
- the nature of epithelial membranes.

The oral mucosa has a thin epithelium layer and is very vascular, both of which favour absorption; however, contact is usually too brief for substantial absorption. A drug such as glucose gel or midazolam placed in the buccal cavity (between the gum and cheek) or glyceryl trinitrate sublingually (under the tongue) is retained longer, enhancing the absorption.

Active transport across the gut epithelium involves drug transporter systems similar to those found in the liver and other organs. Gastrointestinal mucosal epithelium contains many of the metabolic enzymes seen in the liver and other organs, and is the first site of biotransformation for many ingested compounds before they reach the portal circulation. While the gut has a much lower overall enzyme content compared with the liver, the enormous surface area and the obligatory exposure of orally absorbed compounds result in small intestinal intrinsic clearance rates that may be 2–3 times that of the liver.

The small intestine is the place where most orally ingested drugs are taken up. The epithelial cells sit atop a basal membrane and are joined to each other by tight junctions; therefore, drug molecules (and nutrients) have to be taken up across the cell membranes. Like the endothelial cells in the blood–brain barrier, the intestinal epithelia express ABC transporters, which extrude some solutes from the cells back into the gut lumen. Moreover, these cells also express specific enzymes, which metabolise and inactivate many drug molecules (Bledsoe and Clayden, 2012).

Oral administration of drugs is the most common, because it is the most convenient for the patient. However, the obstacles to uptake from the gut into the circulation are formidable; some drugs given orally can fail entirely to be absorbed after administration; an example of this is insulin.

The second most common route of application is intravenous injection or infusion. In this case, the absorption stage is bypassed altogether. This route is used with most protein drugs, as well as with small molecules that fail to be taken up after oral ingestion. In clinical emergencies, intravenous application is usually preferred even with drugs that are suitable for oral application in principle, in order to ensure their rapid and quantitative uptake.

Passive transport

The primary means for drugs to cross the cell membrane is by passive diffusion. Passive transport occurs when drug molecules move from an area of high concentration to an area of low concentration, down the concentration gradient. During this process, no energy is used. There are several factors that determine to what degree and how quickly drug molecules move by passive transport.

- The size of the drug molecules.
- Solubility of the drug molecules.
- The concentration of the drug molecules in various body compartments.

Drug molecules that use passive diffusion are typically small, predominantly lipid soluble and uncharged.

Absorption depends on the route of administration (Table 5.2), which can be classed as: (1) *enteral*, entering the GI tract, either by oral administration or rectal suppositories, or (2) *parenteral*, not into the GI tract, such as via injection (IV, IO, IM) or transdermal (Le, 2017).

Enteral

Medications which are given enterally are absorbed through the GI tract. Enteral medications are taken orally (PO) or rectally (PR), which have several disadvantages in prehospital emergency care. The patient must be conscious and co-operative to swallow oral medications. Medications which are absorbed through the GI tract must first pass through the liver before distribution through the body. Here, the drug can be partially metabolised, which in turn leads to a reduction in the amount of medication available for distribution. This process is called first-pass metabolism. Medications administered via the enteral routes have other disadvantages including a variable absorption rate and irritation of the stomach lining. However, there are advantages to enteral administration; it is considered the safest route of administration and is the most common. Enteral administration often does not require a sterile technique or equipment and its slow uptake to circulation often prevents rapid changes in blood chemistry leading to adverse effects.

Parenteral

The term 'parenteral' is made up of two words – *par* meaning 'beyond' and *enteral* meaning 'intestine'. Hence, we can say that parenteral administration literally means introduction of substances into the body by routes other than the gastrointestinal tract. Parenteral is the second most common route of drug administration and is a significantly quicker route from administration to effect. Parenteral routes of administration can be injectable (Figure 5.2), such as IV, IM, IO or subcutaneous (SC), or non-injectable such as intranasal (IN), topical or inhalation. All of these routes are used routinely in prehospital management.

There are several disadvantages to parenteral administration.

- An increased risk to the patient.
- Injectable routes are invasive and thus can cause pain, tissue damage and potential infection.

Table 5.2   Factors that affect absorption of drugs.

Route	Factors affecting absorption
Intravenous (IV)	None: direct entry into the venous system
Intramuscular (IM)	Perfusion of blood flow to the muscle Fat content of the muscle Temperature of the muscle: cold causes vasoconstriction and decreases absorption; heat causes vasodilation and increases absorption.
Subcutaneous (SC)	Perfusion of blood flow to the tissues Fat content of the tissue Temperature of the tissue: cold causes vasoconstriction and decreases absorption; heat causes vasodilation and increases absorption.
Oral (PO)	Acidity of the stomach Length of time in the stomach Blood flow to the gastrointestinal tract Presence of interacting foods or drugs
Rectal (PR)	Perfusion of blood flow to the rectum Lesions in the rectum Length of time retained for absorption
Mucous membranes (sublingual, buccal)	Perfusion or blood flow to the area Integrity of mucous membranes Presence of food or smoking Length of time retained in area
Topical (skin)	Perfusion or blood flow to the area Integrity of skin
Inhalation	Perfusion or blood flow to the area Integrity of lung lining Ability to administer drug properly

Source: Reproduced with permission from Karch (2017).

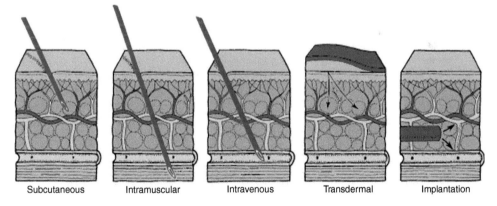

| Subcutaneous | Intramuscular | Intravenous | Transdermal | Implantation |

Figure 5.2   Injectable routes of administration. Source: Reproduced with permission from MSD Manuals: www.msdmanuals.com/home/drugs/administration-and-kinetics-of-drugs/drug-administration

- The preparation time is increased and sterile techniques must be used.
- Training is required for use of the parenteral route.

There are several advantages to using a parenteral route. Parenteral routes are far more effective with medications that absorb poorly or are unstable in the GI tract, such as insulin or heparin. Parenteral routes can be used in unconscious patients or those actively vomiting who require emergency treatment. The bioavailability of the drug is faster and much more predictable, in addition to avoiding the interference by digestive enzymes or liver metabolism (Le, 2020).

See also Chapter 6 of this text for a more detailed discussion regarding drug formulas.

Phase 2: distribution

Once a drug is absorbed into the bloodstream, it is distributed throughout the body by the circulatory system. Distribution is the process by which a drug passes from the bloodstream to body tissues and organs. It is how a drug moves from intravascular space, e.g. blood vessels, to extravascular space, e.g. body tissues, as it is carried around the body by the circulatory system. Several factors can affect the distribution of a drug.

- Cardiovascular function
- Regional blood flow
- Protein binding
- Physiological factors

Similar to absorption, distribution is dependent on cardiovascular function. When medications are absorbed, they are initially distributed to more highly perfused areas of the body such as the brain, heart, liver and kidneys. Distribution to the skin, muscles or GI tract is much slower. A patient in shock or in congestive cardiac failure (CCF) will have a reduced cardiac output, which leads to a much slower and more unpredictable distribution. Marked reduction of cardiac output can lead to negligible drug delivery in areas of minimal perfusion (Raj and Raveendran, 2019).

A variance in regional blood flow can also affect distribution. Patients in cardiogenic shock, for example, will experience reduced blood flow to organs such as the kidneys; thus, medications such as furosemide which act specifically on the kidneys may not reach the kidneys in a concentration to be effective. In the JRCALC guidelines for paramedics, cardiogenic shock is a contraindication for the administration of furosemide.

Protein binding

Binding to plasma proteins is both a help and a hindrance to the distribution of drugs through the body. Transport in the bloodstream by binding to proteins helps drugs to reach regions remote from the site of administration. When a drug is bound to a protein, it cannot readily leave the capillaries and affect the target tissues. However, the rate of distribution of a drug into the tissues will be controlled by the concentration gradient produced by the concentration of unbound unionised drug. Usually, it is the unbound drug concentration that is considered to be active. The fraction of unbound drug can also influence the rate of drug elimination. Binding does, therefore, affect both the duration and intensity of drug action. Some drugs compete with others for the same protein-binding site, which will change the effectiveness of the drug or cause toxicity when two or more drugs of the same group are administered together (Karch, 2017).

Blood–brain barrier

There are physiological barriers which affect distribution. The blood–brain barrier is an example of this. These barriers inhibit the movement of certain molecules while allowing others to enter. The blood–brain barrier is a collection of capillary endothelial cells within the brain. The make-up of these cells does not allow entry to water-soluble medications, in addition to excluding the most ionised molecules, for example dopamine. However, non-ionised and unbound molecules pass much more easily and reach the central nervous system (CNS), in addition to drugs with a high lipid solubility. The delivery of substances to the brain is limited by the blood–brain barrier, making it a protective mechanism for the brain. A growing body of evidence supports a major role for the blood–brain barrier in the ethology and pathogenesis of multiple vascular and neurodegenerative disorders (Pardridge, 2005).

Placental barrier

The placental barrier is another physiological example (Figure 5.3). The term 'placental barrier' is a misnomer, as the placenta is not a true barrier for the transfer of most drugs and toxicants from mother to fetus. The placenta has been characterised as 'a lipid membrane that permits bidirectional

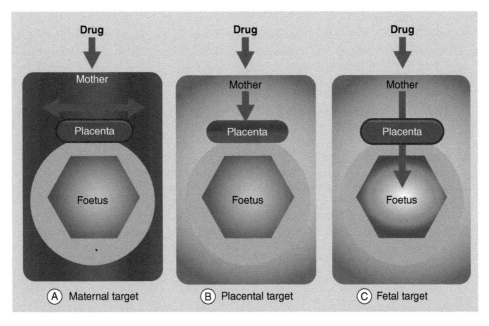

Figure 5.3 The placental barrier and drug administration.

transfer of substances between maternal and fetal compartments' rather than as a barrier. In humans, the placental barrier consists of the trophoblastic epithelium, covering the villi, the chorionic connective tissue and the foetal capillary endothelium. Because medications must traverse the maternal blood supply and cross capillary membranes into the foetal circulation, delivering medications to the foetus requires them to be lipid soluble, non-ionised and non-protein bound.

Phase 3: metabolism (biotransformation)

Metabolism, sometimes referred to as biotransformation, is the recognition by the body that the drug is present and the transformation of the drug into useable parts. Most drugs are metabolised in the liver but other organs include the kidneys and intestines. The blood supply from the GI tract intersects with the liver through the portal vein, so that all medications absorbed in the GI tract pass through the liver. This first pass through the liver has the potential to partially or completely inactivate medications. This first-pass effect is why paramedics may administer medications parenterally to bypass the GI tract and avoid the first-pass hepatic metabolism.

Biotransformation can metabolise a drug into an active or inactive form. Some drugs are fully metabolised before they are eliminated; lidocaine is one such example. Some drugs are partially metabolised before being eliminated, while some are not metabolised at all prior to elimination (Bledsoe and Clayden, 2012). Protein-bound medications cannot be biotransformed. Biotransformation occurs immediately following the administration of the medication. Some medications are biotransformed rapidly while others are not. Epinephrine 1:10 000 is a common medication administered during cardiac arrest which is active upon administration; this medication undergoes a rapid biotransformation to an inactive form before it is eliminated. Because of this rapid biotransformation to inactivity, the medication is repeated every 3–5 minutes as required. Some medications, however, are inactive when administered but when absorbed are converted to their active form. Paramedics administer several medications which must be converted to an active form before a therapeutic effect is achieved. Diazapam is one such example.

Rates of reaction

To understand the processes of pharmacokinetics, the rates of these processes have to be considered. They can be characterised by two basic underlying concepts: a zero-order reaction and a first-order reaction.

Zero-order reaction

Consider the rate of elimination of alcohol (A) from the body. We can say that the rate of decrease in concentration is independent of concentration and depends only on the rate constant (k). So, in a zero-order process, the same amount of drug will disappear in a given amount of time regardless of how much drug is present. For example, if k = 2 mg/L/h, the concentration will decrease by 2 mg/L every hour whether the starting concentration is 10 mg/L or 100 mg/L.

Drugs that have this type of elimination will show accumulation of plasma levels of the drug and hence non-linear pharmacokinetics. Zero-order kinetics are rare and elimination mechanisms are saturable.

First-order reaction

First-order kinetics occur when a constant proportion of the drug is eliminated per unit of time. The rate of elimination is proportionate to the concentration of drug in the body. Most drugs are eliminated in this way and the elimination mechanisms are not saturable. In this reaction, the higher the concentration of drug, the greater the amount eliminated each unit of time. For every half-life that passes, the drug concentration is reduced by 50% (Hallare and Gerriets, 2021). For example, if 10 mg of morphine is administered IV to a patient, after 2 h (approximate half-life of morphine) 5 mg will be eliminated, another 2 h later a further 2.5 mg will be eliminated, after a further 2 h an additional 1.25 mg will be eliminated, and so on until the entire concentration is eliminated from the body.

First-pass metabolism

The first-pass effect is a phenomenon of drug metabolism whereby, specifically when administered orally, the drug concentration is greatly reduced before it reaches the systemic circulation. It is the fraction of drug lost during the process of absorption which is generally related to the liver and GI wall. Notable drugs that experience a significant first-pass effect include morphine, midazolam, diazepam and GTN. An example of this can be seen in Figure 5.4.

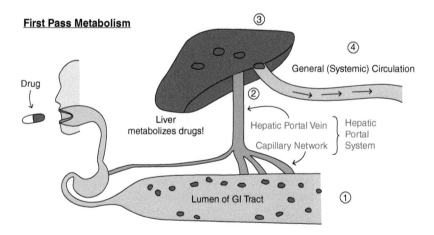

The First Pass Process

1) The drug is absorbed by the GI Tract.

2) Drug absorbed from the gastrointestinal tract travels immediately to the liver through the hepatic portal vein.

3) The first pass effect occurs at this stage. Hepatic first pass occurs when drug absorbed from the gastrointestinal tract is metabolised by enzymes within the liver to such an extent that most of the active agent does not exit the liver and, therefore, does not reach the systemic circulation.

4) The remaining drug is distributed around the body within blood cells and plasma.

Figure 5.4   First-pass metabolism.

Hepatic first-pass effect

Drugs given by the oral route are absorbed from the stomach and the small intestine into the hepatic portal vein, which goes directly to the liver. The process of biotransformation begins and the drug will start to be metabolised in preparation for excretion from the body. The drug molecules in the plasma move through the system. The molecules are now metabolised by the liver enzymes in the normal fashion. This first-pass effect reduces the fraction of the dose administered, which then goes on to reach the systemic circulation and become available for therapeutic effect.

For drugs administered orally, the amount of first-pass metabolism known to occur has been factored into oral dosing regimens and guidelines. This means that the bioavailability, which is a known factor, has been considered when dose and dose ranges are advised. It is important therefore for the paramedic to be aware of any hepatic dysfunction when administering oral drugs. If there is compromised liver function or disease such as cirrhosis, then first-pass metabolism will be compromised. This could lead to more active drug entering the systemic circulation due to the reduced liver enzyme functionality and may cause side-effects, adverse effects or toxicity. Some drugs are destroyed by liver enzyme systems at this first-pass stage and will not enter the general systemic circulation. An example of such a drug is GTN, which is metabolised completely by the liver and inactivated. Consequently, you will find GTN being administered via the sublingual route to bypass this effect.

Not all oral drugs are destroyed by the liver at first pass, but many clinically significant drugs do undergo an extensive first-pass effect. Therefore, the doses of some drugs are considerably higher when given by the oral route compared to their dosing if given IV (Scott and McGrath, 2008).

Phase 4: elimination

Drugs are removed from the body by various elimination processes. Drug elimination refers to the irreversible removal of drug from the body by all routes of elimination. Drug elimination is usually divided into two major components: excretion and biotransformation. Drug excretion is the removal of the intact drug. Non-volatile drugs are excreted mainly by renal excretion, a process in which the drug passes through the kidney to the urinary bladder and ultimately into the urine (Figure 5.5). Other pathways may include the excretion of drug into bile, sweat, saliva, milk (via lactation) or other body fluids. Volatile drugs, such as gaseous anaesthetics, alcohol or drugs with high volatility are excreted via the lungs into expired air. Excretion through the mammary glands is an area of concern when breast-feeding mothers are administered medication.

The rate of elimination can vary depending on the medication and the state of the body. For example, a patient in shock will experience poor perfusion to the kidneys. In these cases, medications which are primarily excreted via the kidneys remain present in the body for a longer period of time. The slower the rate of elimination, the longer the medication remains in the body.

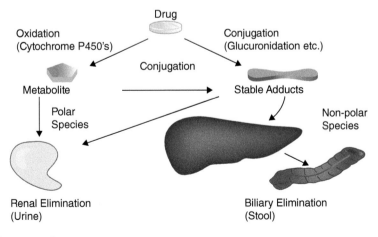

Figure 5.5   Drug excretion process.

Example: pharmacokinetics of paracetamol

Paracetamol is commonly used in prehospital care for pain management and management of pyrexia (a high temperature). It is typically used to relieve mild or moderate pain, such as head-aches, strains or sprains, and reduce fevers caused by bacteria or viruses. Paracetamol is often rec-ommended as one of the first treatments for pain, as it is safe for most people to take and side-effects are rare. Paracetamol can be administered enterally or parenterally, and is available in tablet form, suspension, rectal suppositories or soft pack for infusion. The pharmacokinetics of paracetamol can be seen in Box 5.1.

Box 5.1   Pharmacokinetics of paracetamol

Absorption	Following oral administration, it is rapidly absorbed from the gastrointestinal tract, its systemic bioavailability being dose dependent and ranging from 70% to 90%
Distribution	It distributes rapidly and evenly throughout most tissues and fluids and has a volume of distribution of approximately 0.9 L/kg; 10–20% of the drug is bound to red blood cells
Metabolism	Paracetamol is extensively metabolised (predominantly in the liver), the major metabolites being the sulfate and glucuronide conjugates Large doses of paracetamol (overdoses) cause acute hepatic necrosis as a result of depletion of glutathione and binding of the excess reactive metabolite to vital cell constituents. The plasma half-life ranges from 1.9 to 2.5 h and the total body clearance from 4.5 to 5.5 mL/kg/min. Age has little effect on the plasma half-life, which is shortened in patients taking anticonvulsants. The plasma half-life is usually normal in patients with mild chronic liver disease, but is prolonged in those with decompensated liver disease
Elimination	In healthy subjects 85–95% of a therapeutic dose is excreted by the kidney in the urine within 24 h, with about 4% appearing as unchanged paracetamol and its glucuronide, sulfate, mercapturic acid and cysteine conjugates, respectively

Clinical considerations discussed below should be understood in relation to pharmacokinetics.

Clinical consideration: half-life

The half-life of medication is how long it takes for the medication to be reduced by half of its blood concentration level. This is done through metabolisation. It can be affected by the individual's ability to metabolise, such as if the patient has renal failure and liver damage.

Clinical consideration: steady state

A steady state (SS) is when the amount of drug administered is equal to the amount of drug elimi-nated within one dose interval, resulting in a plateau or constant serum drug level. Drugs with a short half-life reach steady state rapidly, whilst drugs with a long half-life take as long as days to weeks to reach a steady state.

Clinical consideration: termination of action

A termination of action is when the medication has stopped its action at the site of requirement. This may be seen in analgesic control; when the pain returns, the medication has stopped acting.

Clinical consideration: therapeutic range

A therapeutic range is similar to therapeutic index. It is the range area where the medication is effective for the individual. Linking back to analgesic control, it is the period from when pain is blocked to when it returns (Figure 5.6).

This can be seen with medication such as paracetamol, where you can repeat the dose of 1 g every 4–6 h. Greater dosages can be toxic as you have exceeded the therapeutic index.

The example of paracetamol and ibuprofen (subject to any contraindications) can be seen in Figure 5.7 where to maintain a therapeutic level (black line), the two medications are used to complement each other, while not exceeding the recommended dose and thus therapeutic index.

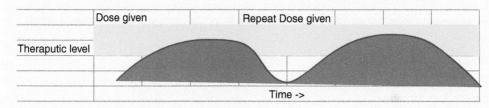

Figure 5.6   Therapeutic range.

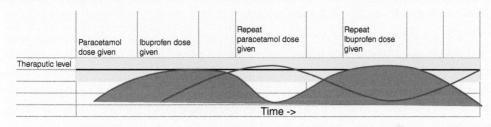

Figure 5.7   Therapeutic level.

Pharmacodynamics

Pharmacodynamics is the study of the mechanisms by which specific medication dosages act to produce biochemical or physiological changes in the body. Put simply, pharmacodynamics explores what the drug does to the body, specifically, how the drug molecules interact within the body, what they interact with and how they cause their effects. Medications act in four different ways They can:

1. bind to a receptor site
2. change the physical properties of a cell
3. combine chemically with other molecules
4. alter a normal metabolic pathway.

Medications predominantly operate by binding to a receptor. Almost all medication receptors are proteins on the cell surface and are part of the body's normal regulatory function. They can be stimulated or inhibited by molecules which interact with them. Receptors are usually named in accordance with the medication that stimulates them; for example, a receptor that is stimulated by an opiate is called an opioid receptor. When a receptor is stimulated by multiple medications, the generic name is used.

The force of attraction between a receptor and a medication is called their *affinity*. The greater the affinity, the stronger the bond between the two. Different medications may bind to the same receptor but the strength of the bond may vary.

The shape of the binding site determines its receptivity to molecules. The receptor sites are quite specific; similar to a door lock, only a specific key will open it. In a similar way, non-opiate medications generally will not affect an opiate receptor; however, a medication with a similar binding site will occasionally cross-react.

One of the key challenges when studying pharmacodynamics is that drugs are affected by a patient's physiological changes such as disease, genetic mutations, ageing and/or by other drugs. These changes are likely to alter the level of binding proteins or decrease receptor sensitivity (Campbell and Cohall, 2017). It is important that paramedics recognise that some drugs acting on the same receptor (or tissue) differ in affinity, the expected responses that they can achieve (i.e. their 'efficacy') and the amount of the drug required to achieve a response (i.e. their 'potency'). It is worth noting that the affinity and efficacy are not directly related. Constant exposure of receptors or body systems to drugs sometimes leads to a reduced response, for example, desensitisation.

Agonists and antagonists

Chemicals that stimulate receptor sites fall into two broad categories: agonists and antagonists. The terms 'agonist' (a molecule that binds to a receptor causing activation and resultant cellular changes) and 'antagonist' (a molecule that attenuates the action of an agonist) apply only to receptors (Figure 5.8).

Agonist

An agonist is a drug that binds to a receptor, activating it and producing a biological response. Agonists can be full, partial or inverse. Some drugs act on a variety of receptors. These are known as non-selective and can cause multiple and widespread effects. A full agonist results in a maximal response by occupying all or a fraction of receptors. A partial agonist results in less than a maximal response even when the drug occupies all of the receptors (Scott and McGrath, 2008).

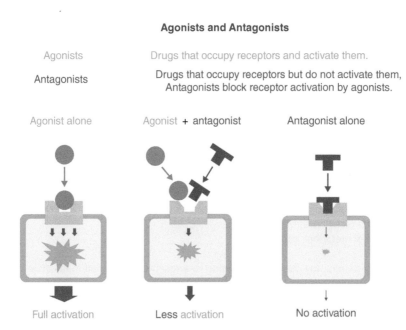

Agonists and Antagonists

Agonists   Drugs that occupy receptors and activate them.

Antagonists   Drugs that occupy receptors but do not activate them,
                 Antagonists block receptor activation by agonists.

Agonist alone   Agonist + antagonist   Antagonist alone

Full activation   Less activation   No activation

Figure 5.8 Agonists and antagonists.

The maximal effect or response an agonist can produce, abbreviated as Emax, is determined both by the number of receptors bound to the agonist, which depends mainly on the amount of the agonist given, also known as the dose, as well as its intrinsic activity, which is the ability of the agonist to fully or partially activate its receptors. So full agonists, upon binding to the receptor at high doses, are capable of producing a maximal response of 100% Emax. This represents the point where all available receptors are bound to an agonist. In contrast, partial agonists, even at very high doses, result in a smaller response, so their Emax will be lower (Pleuvry, 2004). A full agonist is like a really well-made spare key that is just as effective as the original, while a partial agonist is a poorly made spare key that could open the lock, but it takes longer.

An example of a widely used agonist is salbutamol, which is a beta-2 agonist. One easy way to remember the location of beta-1 and beta-2 cells simply and quickly is that humans have 1 heart and 2 lungs. Beta-1 cells are mainly based around the heart (1 heart) and beta-2 cells are mainly based around the lungs (2 lungs). Therefore, salbutamol, being a beta-2 agonist, would have its main effects on the receptors based within the lungs. Beta-1 receptors, along with beta-2, alpha-1 and alpha-2 receptors, are adrenergic receptors primarily responsible for signalling in the sympathetic nervous system. Beta agonists bind to the beta receptors on various tissues throughout the body. Beta-2 agonists are used for both asthma and chronic obstructive pulmonary disorder (COPD), although some types are only available for COPD. Beta-2 agonists work by stimulating beta-2 receptors in the muscles that line the airways, which causes them to relax and allows the airways to widen (dilate). Hence why salbutamol is known as a bronchodilator.

Using opioids as an example, Table 5.3 gives examples of opioid by receptor binding.

Antagonists

In opposition to an agonist is an antagonist. An antagonist is a type of receptor ligand or drug that blocks or dampens a biological response by binding to and blocking a receptor rather than activating it, like an agonist. They are sometimes called blockers; examples include alpha blockers, beta blockers and calcium channel blockers.

Antagonists can be competitive or non-competitive.

- A competitive antagonist binds to the same site as the agonist but does not activate it, thus blocking the agonist's action.
- A non-competitive antagonist binds to an allosteric (non-agonist) site on the receptor to prevent activation of the receptor (Pleuvry, 2004).

Clinical consideration: confidence in the drug

In clinical practice, all drugs have been tested through rigorous drug research trials prior to being made available for safe administration through clinical practice guidelines. These drugs are licensed for use within a recommended dose range. This ensures that patients achieve a good response to the medication administered and remain safe during care. Practitioners should always consider the contraindications and the patient's state prior to drug administration to ensure no additional harm is caused.

Table 5.3 Examples of opioid by receptor binding.

Full agonist	Partial agonist	Mixed agonist	Antagonist (also known as blockers or reversals)
Codeine	Buprenorphine	Buprenorphine	Naloxone
Fentanyl	Butorphanol	Butorphanol	Naltrexone
Heroin	Pentazocine	Nalbuphine	
Hydrocodone	Tramadol	Pentazocine	
Hydromorphone			
Levorphanol			
Meperidine			
Methadone			
Morphine			
Oxycodone			
Oxymorphone			

Episode of care: adult suffering an opiate overdose

Ms Murphy is a 24-year-old female with a past medical history of substance use and depression. Ms Murphy has been a heroin user since the age of 17. She was arrested a year ago for assault and theft and sentenced to 1 year in prison. Ms Murphy was released 2 weeks ago and has been living in temporary accommodation since her release. During her incarceration, she suffered withdrawal symptoms but has been off heroin for 8 months and is currently prescribed methadone daily. One month into her stay, staff find Ms Murphy unconscious with respiratory depression and pinpoint pupils following an opiate overdose. She is administered naloxone by the staff and quickly recovers prior to the arrival of the ambulance crew. Ms Murphy admits to injecting heroin that morning but 'no more than I would usually take'. She is refusing further care and transport to hospital.

Clinical considerations

A significant clinical consideration in cases such as this is the body's tolerance to medications. Tolerance happens when a person no longer responds to a drug in the way they did at first. So it takes a higher dose of the drug to achieve the same effect as when the person first used it. This is why people with substance use disorders use more and more of a drug to get the 'high' they seek. However, when the body has gone through withdrawal, such as during a period of incarceration, the level of tolerance is not what it was prior to incarceration as such the dose required for overdose may be less than the normal dose used prior to withdrawal. Evidence shows former prisoners are at a much higher risk of opiate overdose following release (Binswanger, 2007).

The second clinical consideration in the case of Ms Murphy is the potential for reoccurrence of respiratory depression and overdose symptoms.

Naloxone is a synthetic derivative that antagonises opioids. It has been postulated to antagonise the three different opioid receptors in the brain. The drug onset is related to its rapid entry into the brain, which is affected by the 12–15 times greater brain to serum ratio compared to morphine, primarily due to its high lipophilicity. The distribution half-life for naloxone has been reported to be 4.7 minutes while the elimination half-life averages 65 minutes. Naloxone competitively inhibits most opioids rapidly. The short duration of activity of naloxone may play a role in the reoccurrence of toxicity and respiratory depression due to the high dose of heroin self-administered and its longer half-life. For example, in a study, 16 healthy volunteers received intravenous morphine at 0.15 mg/kg and were reversed with low-dose naloxone (0.4 mg). Interestingly, there was a return to severe respiratory depression within 30 minutes. Paramedics should consider the potential for a return of respiratory symptoms in such patients and ensure an appropriate management plan is instigated.

Drug potency and efficacy

Potency is the concentration or dose of a drug required to produce 50% of that drug's maximal effect. Efficacy is the maximum effect which can be expected from this drug (i.e. when this magnitude of effect is reached, increasing the dose will not produce a greater magnitude of effect) (Figure 5.9). Intrinsic activity is the drug's maximal efficacy as a fraction of the maximal efficacy produced by a full agonist of the same type acting through the same receptors under the same conditions.

Therapeutic index

The therapeutic index is classified as the margin of safety that exists between the dose of a drug that produces the desired effect and the dose that produces unwanted and possibly dangerous side-effects. This relationship is defined as the ratio $LD_{50}:ED_{50}$, where LD_{50} is the dose at which a drug kills 50% of a test group of animals and ED_{50} is the dose at which the desired effect is produced in 50% of a test group. In general, the narrower this margin, the more likely it is that the drug will produce unwanted effects. The therapeutic index has many limitations, notably the fact that LD_{50} cannot be measured in humans and, when measured in animals, is a poor guide to the likelihood of unwanted

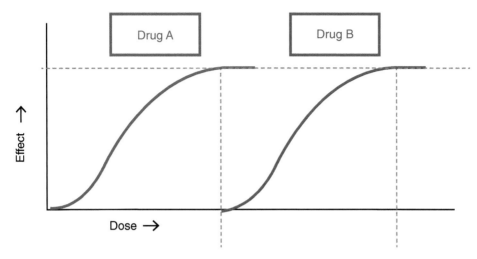

Figure 5.9   Drug potency and efficacy. Both Drug A and Drug B achieve the same maximum effect, i.e. they have equal efficacy. However, drug A achieves this effect at a lower dose. Thus, Drug A has higher potency than Drug B.

effects in humans. Nevertheless, the therapeutic index emphasises the importance of the margin of safety, as distinct from the potency, in determining the usefulness of a drug (Raj and Raveendran, 2019).

Narrow therapeutic index (NTI) drugs are defined as those drugs where small differences in dose or blood concentration may lead to dose- and blood concentration-dependent, serious therapeutic failures or adverse drug reactions. Serious events are those which are persistent, irreversible, slowly reversible or life-threatening, possibly resulting in hospitalisation, disability or even death. Some examples of drugs that are known to have an NTI can be seen in Table 5.4. Slight changes in medication dose or blood concentration level can be dangerous.

Adverse drug reactions

An adverse drug reaction (ADR, or adverse drug effect) is a broad term referring to unwanted, uncomfortable or dangerous effects that a drug may have (IUPHAR, 2019) (Table 5.5 and Box 5.2). Adverse drug reactions can be considered a form of toxicity; however, toxicity is most commonly

Table 5.4   Narrow therapeutic index examples.

Drug	Description
Warfarin	A vitamin K antagonist used to treat venous thromboembolism, pulmonary embolism, thromboembolism with atrial fibrillation, thromboembolism with cardiac valve replacement and thromboembolic events post myocardial infarction
Digoxin	A cardiac glycoside used in the treatment of mild-to-moderate heart failure and for ventricular response rate control in chronic atrial fibrillation
Lithium	A medication used to treat manic episodes of bipolar disorder
Phenytoin	An anticonvulsant drug used in the prophylaxis and control of various types of seizures
Heparin	An anticoagulant indicated for thromboprophylaxis and to treat thrombosis associated with a variety of conditions such as pulmonary embolism and atrial fibrillation
Vancomycin	A glycopeptide antibiotic used to treat severe but susceptible bacterial infections such as methicillin-resistant *Staphylococcus aureus* (MRSA) infections
Amiodarone	A class III antiarrhythmic indicated for the treatment of recurrent haemodynamically unstable ventricular tachycardia and recurrent ventricular fibrillation
Amitriptyline	A tricyclic antidepressant indicated in the treatment of depressive illness, either endogenous or psychotic, and to relieve depression-associated anxiety

Source: Drugsbank 2021.

Table 5.5   Physiological changes in older patients and pregnant/lactating patients (Bledsoe and Clayden, 2012)

Older patients	Pregnant/lactating patients
Decreased cardiac output	Increased cardiac output
Decreased renal function	Increased heart rate
Decreased brain mass	Increased blood volume
Decreased body fat	Decreased protein binding
Decreased serum albumin	Decreased hepatic metabolism
Decreased respiratory capacity	Decreased blood pressure
These changes can lead to altered pharmacokinetics and pharmacodynamics for many medications. The rate of metabolism and elimination can be decreased and there can be an increase in relevant potency of medications. In a clinical scenario, for example managing a CCF patient who also has renal failure, this may require an increased dose of furosemide and a reduced dose of morphine	These anatomical and physiological changes must be considered prior to administering medications or fluids. In addition, the potential of medications crossing the placental barrier and affecting the foetus must be considered. As such, medications should be administered in pregnancy only when the potential benefits outweigh the risks. As with pregnancy, the same risk–benefit approach should be applied with breast-feeding mothers due to the excretion of some medications into breast milk

Box 5.2   Factors altering medication response.

Different patients may have a different response to the same medication. Factors that alter standard medication response include the following.

Age

The liver and kidneys in infants are not fully developed, so their response to medications may be altered. Also, with age, the function of these organs deteriorates. Therefore, infants and geriatric patients are most susceptible to having an altered response to a medication.

Body mass

Drug doses often need adjustment in obese patients. Paramedics should consider the patient's body composition when calculating doses. Drug clearance is greater in obesity and correlates with lean body weight. Body size metrics help guide dose selection, but there are advantages and disadvantages to all of them.

The clinical issue is that calculating drug doses using each body size descriptor will result in a different weight. Consider dosing a 150 kg man who is 170 cm tall. Rounded to the nearest 5 kg, his body size descriptors are:

- total body weight = 150 kg
- lean body weight = 80 kg
- ideal body weight = 65 kg.

Obviously, large variations exist for mg/kg dosing depending on which metric is used. Estimating the optimal dose for obese patients is difficult and, in many cases, ill defined. Basing maintenance doses on total body weight is unlikely to result in a comparable drug response across different body sizes and generally increases the risk of adverse events. Individualised dosing based on the patient's lean body weight is recommended, with accompanying therapeutic drug monitoring and monitoring of the patient's clinical response.

Pathological state

Several disease states alter the medication response relationship. The most common are hepatic and renal dysfunctions. The most common issue with both is the accumulation of medications in the body. Renal failure will probably decrease the elimination of medications, while hepatic failure can inhibit or decrease metabolism and prolong the duration of action.

Genetic factors

Genetic factors such as a specific enzyme deficiency or a lower metabolic rate can alter the absorption and biotransformation of a medication, in turn modifying the response of the patient.

applied to effects of overingestion (accidental or intentional) or to elevated blood levels or enhanced drug effects that occur during appropriate use (e.g. when drug metabolism is temporarily inhibited by a disorder or another drug). You can read more about adverse drug reactions in Chapter 7 of this text.

Conclusion

A fundamental understanding of pharmacokinetics and pharmacodynamics is essential for paramedics and prehospital providers. Anticipating the desired effects as well as potential adverse effects is required to ensure patient safety. Factors such as absorption, distribution, biotransformation and elimination in addition to the therapeutic concentration and toxicity should be considered with the administration of all medications.

References

Binswanger, I.A., Stern, M., Deyo, R. et al. (2007). Release from prison – a high risk of death for former inmates. *New England Journal f Medicine* **356**(2): 157–165.

Bledsoe, B.E. and Clayden, D.E. (2012). *Prehospital Emergency Pharmacology*, 7th edn. New York: Pearson.

Campbell, J.E. and Cohall, D. (2017). Pharmacodynamics – a pharmacognosy perspective. In: *Pharmacognosy: Fundamentals, Applications, and Strategies* (eds S. Badal and R. Delgoda). St Louis: Elsevier Inc.

Hallare, J. and Gerriets, V. (2021). *Half Life*. Treasure Island: StatPearls Publishing.

Health and Care Professions Council. (2014). *Standards of proficiency*. www.hcpc-uk.org/globalassets/resources/standards/standards-of-proficiency---paramedics.pdf?v=637106257480000000

International Union of Basic and Clinical Pharmacology (IUPHAR). (2019). *Pharmacodynamics*. www.pharmacologyeducation.org/pharmacology/pharmacodynamics

Karch, A. (2017). *Focus on Nursing Pharmacology*, 7th edn. Philadelphia: Wolters Kluwer.

Le, J. (2020). *Drug Metabolism*. www.msdmanuals.com/en-gb/professional/clinical-pharmacology/pharmacokinetics/drug-metabolism

Le, J. (2017). *Drug Absorption*. www.msdmanuals.com/en-gb/professional/clinical-pharmacology/pharmacokinetics/drug-absorption

Pardridge, W.M. (2005). The blood–brain barrier: bottleneck in brain drug development. *NeuroRx* **2**(1): 3–14.

Pleuvry, B. (2004). Pharmacology: receptors, agonists and antagonists. *Anaesthesia and Intensive Care Medicine* **5**(10): 350–352.

Raj, G. and Raveendran, R. (2019). *Introduction to Basics of Pharmacology and Toxicology Volume 1: General and Molecular Pharmacology: Principles of Drug Action*. Singapore: Springer Nature.

Scott, W. and McGrath, D. (2008). *Nursing Pharmacology Made Incredibly Easy*. Philadelphia: Wolters Kluwer Health/Lippincott Williams and Wilkins.

Young, S. and Pritchard, B. (2016). *Medicines Management for Nurses at a Glance*. Oxford: Wiley.

Further reading

Bickly, L. (2017). *Bates' Guide to History Taking and Physical Examination*, 12th edn. Philadelphia: Wolters Kluwer.

BNF and NICE. (2019). *Amitriptyline*. https://bnf.nice.org.uk/drug/amitriptyline-hydrochloride.html

BNF and NICE. (2019). *Phenelzine*. https://bnf.nice.org.uk/drug/phenelzine.html

Hale, T.W. (2012). *Medication and Mother's Milk*, 15th edn. Amarillo: Hale Publishing.

Health Education England. (2017). *Advisory Guidance: Administration of Medicines by Nursing Associates*. www.hee.nhs.uk/sites/default/files/documents/Advisory%20guidance%20-%20administration%20of%20medicines%20by%20nursing%20associates.pdf

Kwatra, S., Taneja, G. and Nasa, N. (2012). Alternative routes of drug administration – transdermal, pulmonary and parenteral. *Indo Global Journal of Pharmaceutical Sciences* **2**(4): 409–426.

NHS. (2018). *Antidepressants*. www.nhs.uk/conditions/antidepressants/

NHS. (2018). *Stevens–Johnson syndrome*. www.nhs.uk/conditions/stevens-johnson-syndrome/

Royal Pharmacological Society and Royal College of Nursing. (2019). *What is Pharmacology?* www.bps.ac.uk/about/who-we-are-(2)/history-of-the-society

Talevi, A. and Quiroga, P. (2018). *ADME Processes in Pharmaceutical Sciences: Dosage, Design, and Pharmacotherapy Success*. Basel: Springer.

Multiple-choice questions

1. An accurate definition of pharmacodynamics is:
   (a) The study of how a certain concentration of a drug produces a biological effect by interacting with specific targets at its site of action
   (b) The study of how the body affects the given drug
   (c) The study of how a drug affects the body.

2. Tolerance develops because of:
   (a) Diminished absorption
   (b) Rapid excretion of a drug
   (c) Both of the above
   (d) None of the above.

3. Which of the following is considered a parenteral route?
   (a) Oral
   (b) Rectal
   (c) Intravenous

4. What is meant by medications that have a narrow therapeutic index?
   (a) The gap between effective and toxic effect is large
   (b) The gap between effective and toxic effect is small
   (c) The gap between effective and toxic effect is insignificant

5. Pharmacokinetics is the study of drugs and their corresponding pharmacological, therapeutic, or toxic responses in humans and animals. Is this:
   (a) True?
   (b) False?

6. Which route of drug administration is most likely to lead to first-pass effect?
   (a) Sublingual
   (b) Intravenous
   (c) Intramuscular
   (d) Oral

7. Absorption and distribution are processes of:
   (a) Pharmacodynamics
   (b) Pharmacokinetics
   (c) Pharmacovigilance
   (d) Pharmacotherapeutics.

8. The two principal organs responsible for drug elimination are:
   (a) The spleen and the respiratory system
   (b) The kidneys and the bowel
   (c) The spleen and the bowel
   (d) The kidney and the liver.

9. A drug that may change the acidity of the stomach acid is likely to affect a drug that is dissolved in the stomach.
   (a) True
   (b) False

10. Active transports uses energy (ATP) to transfer molecules and ions in and out of the cell.
    (a) True
    (b) False

11. Drug potency is an expression of:
    (a) How much alcohol is used within the drug
    (b) The activity that judges the therapeutic effectiveness of the drug in humans
    (c) The activity of a drug in terms of the concentration or amount of the drug required to produce a defined effect.

12. Clinical efficacy:
    (a) Judges the therapeutic effectiveness of the drug in humans
    (b) Is the activity of a drug in terms of the concentration or amount of the drug required to produce a defined effect
    (c) Is how ethical it is to administer the drug.
13. Naloxone is an example of an antagonist.
    (a) True
    (b) False
14. Another name for biotransformation is:
    (a) Administration
    (b) Distribution
    (c) Metabolism
15. Drugs that are not lipid soluble:
    (a) Are not able to pass the blood–brain barrier
    (b) Can pass the blood–brain barrier.

Chapter 6

Drug formulations

Sarah Dineen-Griffin and Barbara C. Wimmer

Aim

The aim of this chapter is to review different drug formulations and the points to consider for the administration of medicines to patients via various routes of delivery.

Learning outcomes

1. Identify the different formulations of medicines that are commonly available and used by the paramedic.
2. Understand the administration of medicines via different routes, including potential advantages and disadvantages of these routes.
3. Understand the reasons why a certain drug formulation may be selected.
4. Identify the risks and considerations regarding altering medicine dose form, for instance, by crushing.

Test your knowledge

1. Why are the specific formulations of a medicine important and what implications does this have in the healthcare setting?
2. What are the key issues a paramedic should think about when considering the route of drug administration?
3. What are the benefits and rationale for sublingual drug administration and when would this route be used in practice?
4. What specific oral formulations must not be chewed or broken?
5. Which populations may have problems swallowing conventional oral formulations such as tablets or capsules?

Fundamentals of Pharmacology for Paramedics, First Edition. Edited by Ian Peate, Suzanne Evans, and Lisa Clegg.
© 2022 John Wiley & Sons Ltd. Published 2022 by John Wiley & Sons Ltd.

Introduction

This chapter explores the different formulations of medicines, includes discussion about the administration of medicines via different routes (such as parenteral and enteral) and gives examples of their use and administration in paramedic practice, clinical considerations and implications.

The therapeutic nature of a medicine determines the route of administration. For example, for most gastrointestinal (GI) diseases, oral drug delivery is a logical option. The choice of route will depend on the physicochemical and therapeutic properties of a drug. For example, transdermal drug delivery has several criteria that must be met by the drug in order to be delivered via this route, such as high potency and ready permeability.

91

Routes of drug administration

A route of administration is defined as the path by which a medicine or other substance is taken into the body (MSD Manual, 2020). Routes may be classified by the location to which they are administered or applied, or by the site of action. Intravenous (IV) and oral administration are common examples. Administration may also be enteral (delivered through the GI tract for a system-wide effect, topical (local) or parenteral (delivered via routes other than the GI tract for a systemic effect) (Figure 6.1).

Medicines are introduced via the following routes.

- Taken by mouth (orally).
- Placed under the tongue (sublingually) or between the gums and cheek (buccally).
- Inserted in the rectum (rectally) or vagina (vaginally).
- Applied to the skin (cutaneously) for a local or systemic effect.
- Delivered through the skin by a patch (transdermally) for a systemic effect.
- By injection into a vein (IV), into a muscle (intramuscularly [IM]), into the space around the spinal cord or into the space between layers of tissue around the brain (intrathecally), directly into the marrow of a bone (intraosseous), beneath the skin (subcutaneously [SC]) or into the dermis (intradermal).

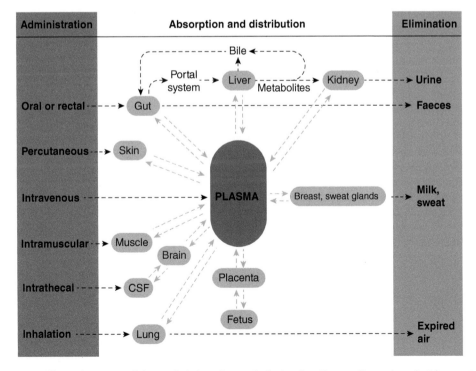

Figure 6.1 The main routes of drug administration and elimination. Source: Reproduced with permission from Rang (2016).

- Applied to the eye (ocular) or the ear (otic).
- Sprayed into the nose and absorbed through the nasal membranes (nasally).
- Breathed into the lungs, through the mouth (by inhalation) or mouth and nose (by nebulization).

The choice of route of drug administration is governed by various factors including:

- physicochemical properties of a medicine, e.g. physical (solid, liquid and gas) and chemical (solubility, stability, pH, irritancy) properties
- desired site of action
- rate of absorption of the drug from different routes
- drug metabolism
- condition of the patient.

In acute situations, for example, medicines are most often given IV. The absorption of medicines from the GI tract and tissues can often be unpredictable in acutely ill patients due to altered blood flow or bowel motility.

Parenteral administration

Parenteral administration refers to any routes of administration that do not involve drug absorption via the GI tract (including IV, IM, SC, intrathecal, intradermal or intraosseous). Reasons for selecting the parenteral route over the oral route may be due to low oral bioavailability of a drug, the need for immediate effect (e.g. in an emergency situation), for patients who are unable to take the drug by mouth, or if there is a need to control the rate of absorption and duration of effect. There are a number of advantages to parenteral administration. These include:

- drugs that are poorly absorbed, inactive or ineffective if given orally, can be given by this route
- the IV route provides a rapid onset of action
- the IM and SC routes can be used to achieve slow or delayed onset of action
- patient compliance issues are largely avoided.

Disadvantages of parenteral administration include cost, pain, appropriately prepared staff to administer and a potential need for supporting equipment, for example, infusion devices.

Intravenous administration

Specific medicines must be given by an IV injection or infusion and are delivered directly into the vein. The IV route is most frequently used. This is because it is flexible regarding the rate of dosing and injection volume (Riebesehl, 2015). However, infusions allow for controlled or constant plasma profiles (Riebesehl, 2015). A drug given by the IV route, however, tends to have a shorter duration of action. As such, some medicines may be administered by continuous infusion. This method overcomes repetitive injections, prevents delays in drug administration and allows for more precise titration and extended duration of effect (McGrath and Brown, 2009; Sinatra, 2003). During an infusion, a solution is moved by an infusion pump or by gravity, through thin tubing and cannula, which is inserted into a vein (MSD Manual, 2020). An IV 'push' or 'bolus' is the rapid administration of a drug in a bolus (a single, large dose of a drug). A bolus injection may be necessary if a patient requires a particular medicine immediately.

Episode of care

Ms Smith is a 59-year-old female with chronic obstructive pulmonary disease (COPD). You are treating her for severe shortness of breath (SOB) associated with an exacerbation, and IV dexamethasone is administered. *Are there any adverse effects of dexamethasone when it is used like this? What if it was used on a daily basis? What else can dexamethasone be used for?*

Dexamethasone may cause adverse effects including headache, oedema, vertigo, fluid retention, nausea, hypertension, hyperglycaemia and congestive heart failure (Australian Medicines Handbook, 2020; Joint Formulary Committee, 2020). Adverse effects are more common with prolonged administration, and include Cushing syndrome (euphoria, fat redistribution around the mid-section and upper back, between the shoulders, moon face, muscle wasting, thinning of the skin, poor wound healing, hypertension, obesity, osteoporosis and increased susceptibility to infections). In an emergency setting, dexamethasone can be used for severe asthma and COPD exacerbations, suspected croup and severe sepsis (Australian Medicines Handbook, 2020; Joint Formulary Committee, 2020). In other settings, dexamethasone can be used for cerebral oedema due to malignancy or postoperative or chemotherapy-induced nausea and vomiting (Australian Medicines Handbook, 2020; Joint Formulary Committee, 2020).

93

Subcutaneous administration

The administration of a SC injection is into the fatty tissues (SC tissue) between the muscle and skin. The SC tissue has small blood vessels (capillaries), which allows a medicine to be more slowly absorbed than if administered via the IV route (Case-Lo, 2018; Shepherd, 2018). The advantages of administering medicines via the SC route are that they are less expensive, sometimes more effective when administering specific drugs, beneficial for medicines that have low oral bioavailability (e.g., insulin) or medicines that require continuous absorption (e.g., heparin) (Case-Lo, 2018; Shepherd, 2018). Solutions are not appropriate to be delivered via the SC route as it is irritating to the tissue and may result in necrosis of the skin. A 16mm long and 25–27 gauge needle is generally used to administer medicines via this route (Department of Health, 2020; Public Health England, 2020). Areas for injection include (1) the abdomen, about 2 inches from the navel, (2) back or side of the upper arm, (3) top of the thigh, or (4) top of the buttocks (Figure 6.2). The site of injection may vary for individuals as each patient has different levels of SC tissue. Separating the SC fat from the muscle underneath by lifting the skin fold may be required (Shepherd, 2018). For those patients requiring frequent injections, the injection sites should be rotated (Villines, 2018).

Intramuscular administration

The IM route is preferred to the SC route when larger volumes of a medicine are required. IM injections are limited to volumes of up to 5 mL. A longer needle is used because the muscles lie below the skin and fatty tissues. Medicines can be injected into the upper arm, thigh or buttock.

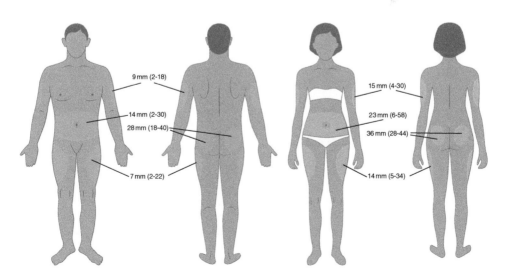

Figure 6.2   Subcutaneous injection sites and the average thickness of the subcutaneous fat.

Drug absorption is influenced by factors (e.g. exercise) that alter blood flow to the muscle. A medicine will be absorbed more quickly where there is greater blood supply. Slower absorption may be achieved by altering the drug vehicle. For example, slower release of a drug can be achieved by using a depot IM injection. Within paramedic practice, glucagon, benzyl penicillin, hydrocortisone and adrenaline are examples of medicines administered via the IM route.

Skills in practice: administration of adrenaline auto-injector (e.g. EpiPen® or EpiPen Jr®) for anaphylaxis or severe allergic reaction

The EpiPen or EpiPen Jr adrenaline auto-injector is a disposable, pre-filled automatic injection device capable of administering adrenaline in the event of anaphylaxis or severe allergic reaction. The emergency administration of adrenaline will assist with relaxing the muscles in the airways to improve breathing and reverse rapid and dangerous decreases in blood pressure (Queensland Ambulance Service, 2019a).

Procedure for administration
1. Lay person flat – do *not* allow them to stand or walk. If unconscious, place in recovery position. If breathing is difficult, allow them to sit.
2. Remove the EpiPen or EpiPen Jr auto-injector from the carrier tube. Inspect and confirm it is within the expiry date and the solution is clear. If it is discoloured, discard and use an alternative device.
3. Form fist around the EpiPen with orange tip pointing downwards and remove blue safety cap by pulling upwards (do not bend or twist).
4. Hold leg still and push the orange tip firmly into the patient's mid-outer thigh (with or without clothing) until a click is heard or felt.
5. Hold onto the patient's thigh for 3 seconds.
6. Remove from the patient's thigh – the orange needle cover will automatically extend to cover the injection needle.
7. Dispose of the auto-injector immediately into a sharps container.

Additional practice points
If required, the EpiPen or EpiPen Jr auto-injector may be injected through the patient's clothing.

When administering an auto-injector to a child, hold the child's leg firmly to minimise risk of injury (e.g. lacerations) to the child or the person giving the dose.

The following doses are recommended by organisations such as the Australasian Society of Clinical Immunology and Allergy (Australian Medicines Handbook, 2020). A repeat dose may be administered if there is no response after 5 minutes.

Adult, child >20 kg – IM 0.3 mg

Child 7.5–20 kg, IM 0.15 mg

Clinical consideration: administration of adrenaline

The IM route is preferred over IV for the administration of adrenaline (Australian Medicines Handbook, 2020). IV administration may be necessary if repeated IM doses of adrenaline do not produce the desired clinical response. IV administration should only be by those experienced in its use. Blood pressure, pulse oximetry and ECG should be continuously monitored. SC administration is not recommended in anaphylaxis as absorption is erratic (Australian Medicines Handbook, 2020).

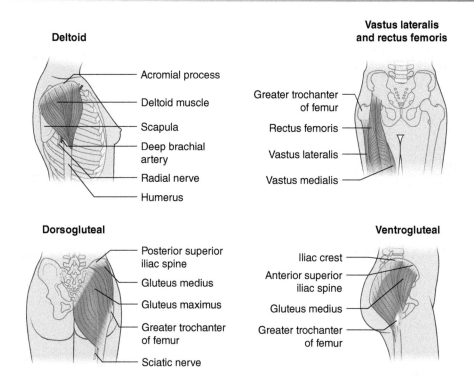

Figure 6.3   Sites identified for IM injection.

Known sites identified for IM injections include ventro-gluteal, deltoid, dorso-gluteal, rectus femoris and vastus lateralis (Figure 6.3) (Kirk, 2018). The Joint Royal Colleges Ambulance Liaison Committee (JRCALC) primarily recommends the anterolateral aspects of the thigh or upper arm for administration for their ease of access and rapid absorption (JRCALC, 2019).

Intraosseous administration

Intraosseous administration is the process of injecting directly into the marrow of a bone and provides a non-collapsible entry point into the systemic venous system. This is an effective route for fluid resuscitation and drug delivery when IV access is not available or not feasible. Intraosseous administration allows for the administered medications and fluids to go directly into the vascular system.

Intrathecal administration

Intrathecal administration is when a needle is inserted into the subarachnoid space (between two vertebrae in the lower spine and the space around the spinal cord), and a medicine is delivered to the cerebrospinal fluid (ScienceDirect, 2008). Intrathecal administration produces rapid or local effects on the brain, spinal cord and meninges (MSD, 2020). Anaesthetics and analgesics (such as morphine) can be administered via this route.

Intradermal administration

Intradermal (ID) injections are shallow or superficial injections of a drug into the dermis, located below the epidermis. This route is relatively rare compared to injections via the SC or IM route. Due to the more complex technique, ID injections are not the preferred route of administration for injections (Shrestha and Stoeber, 2018), and therefore are used for certain therapies only. ID injections are used for sensitivity tests, such as for allergies, whereby a small and very thin needle is used to inject a diluted allergen just below the skin surface. The advantage of these tests is that it is easy to visualise the body's response and the degree of reaction can be assessed.

Skills in practice

Different syringes and needles may be desired for different procedures and should be chosen carefully according to the type of procedure and injection to be administered. It is important to consider the length and gauge of a needle, in addition to, the type of syringe appropriate for the volume of a medicine to be delivered, viscosity and the injection site. The size, age and condition of the person receiving the injection are also important to consider. Site selection and consideration of the appropriate degree of entry are requirements for successful and comfortable administration (Figure 6.4).

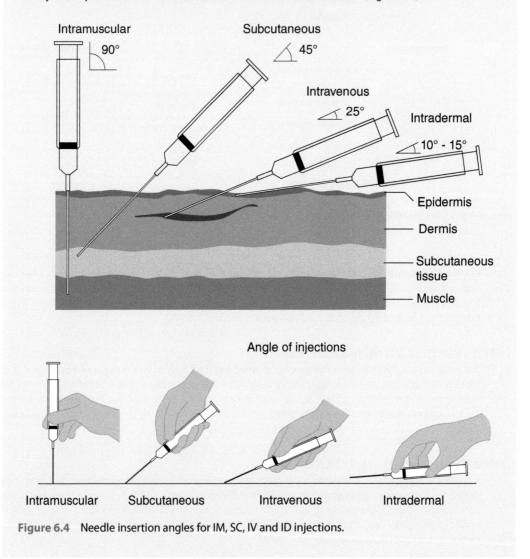

Figure 6.4   Needle insertion angles for IM, SC, IV and ID injections.

It is important for paramedics to evaluate their patient's specific body composition and select the best needle gauge and length accordingly. Becoming familiar with the various injection techniques and developing a positioning approach that works well for both the patient and paramedic will promote optimal outcomes. Regardless of classification, injections require sterile environments and procedures to minimise the risk of introducing pathogens into the body.

Formulations
Localised versus long-acting injectable formulations
Localised injectables

Injections may be administered to produce a local effect and avoid undesirable side-effects if systemically administered. Medicines can be injected directly into the vitreous humour of the eye (known as intravitreal injections) for conditions such as macular degeneration (American Society of Retina Specialists, 2017). Intra-articular injections can also be administered (that is, into the articular space around a joint). As an example, intra-articular corticosteroids can be used for inflammation and pain in osteoarthritis. Evidence suggests that most people, immediately after receiving intra-articular corticosteroids, will experience a significant decrease in pain rating scores (McAlindon et al., 2017). However, while these injections may work to relieve inflammation and pain, the benefits are only short term. Evidence has shown that further damage to the joint cartilage and acceleration of the development of osteoarthritis may result following administration of intra-articular corticosteroids (McAlindon et al., 2017).

Long-acting injectables

Long-acting injectable formulations release medication at a predictable rate over a long period and are not intended to have a rapid effect. Long-acting injectables are often used to increase adherence to a medicine by reducing the frequency of administration. Depot injections are usually oil based or an aqueous suspension and allow for an active drug to be released consistently and gradually absorbed over a long period. For example, depot antipsychotics (e.g. haloperidol decanoate) may be prescribed for patients with a history of non-adherence to oral antipsychotics (Lehman et al., 2003; West et al., 2008).

Topical formulations

Topical administration involves application of the drug primarily to elicit local effects at the site of application and to avoid systemic effects (Bardal et al., 2011). Examples include drugs administered to the eye (e.g. beta-blockers for the treatment of glaucoma [Brooks and Gillies, 1992]), the nasal mucosa or the skin (e.g. topical steroids in the management of dermatitis [Gabros et al., 2020]). There are advantages of topical administration in the management of localised disease including that the drug is able to work predominantly at the intended site of action and a reduction in systemic side effects.

Ocular

Medicines for eye disorders (such as conjunctivitis or glaucoma) may come in the form of a liquid, gel or ointment so they can be applied to the eye. They are almost always used for their local effects. There are advantages and disadvantages. For example, liquid drops may run off the eye before being absorbed however, they are relatively easy to use. Ointments remain in contact with the surface of the eye longer, however, may cause blurry vision. Solid inserts may be hard to put in and keep in place, however, they release a drug continuously and slowly. Some examples of eye drops produce a local effect (acting directly on the eyes) including artificial tears for dry eyes, acetazolamide and betaxolol for glaucoma, or phenylephrine used to dilate pupils.

Clinical consideration: topical beta-blockers

Topical beta-blockers reduce the intraocular pressure (IOP) by blockade of sympathetic nerve endings in the ciliary epithelium, causing a fall in aqueous humour production. Two types of topical beta-blockers are available for use in glaucoma: non-selective, which block both beta-1 and beta-2 adrenoceptors, and cardioselective, which block only beta-1 receptors (Brooks and Gillies, 1992). As topical beta-blockers can be absorbed systemically, there is potential for cardiovascular and respiratory effects (Australian Medicines Handbook, 2020; Joint Formulary Committee, 2020). Topical beta-blockers are contraindicated in bradyarrhythmia, second- or third-degree atrioventricular block or uncontrolled heart failure (Australian Medicines Handbook, 2020). Care should be taken when treating with other drugs that cause bradycardia as this may further decrease heart rate (Australian Medicines Handbook, 2020). As topical beta-blockers may precipitate bronchospasm, they are generally contraindicated in asthma (Australian Medicines Handbook, 2020; Joint Formulary Committee, 2020).

Otic

Ear inflammation and infection can be treated using medicines which are directly applied to the affected ears. Ear drops, as solutions or suspensions, are generally applied to the outer ear canal. Systemic effects are absent or minimal if drugs are given by the otic route, which means little to no drug enters the blood stream. However, systemic effects may be seen if applied too frequently or used for long periods. Examples include ciprofloxacin (for ear infection), benzocaine (to anaesthetise the ear) and hydrocortisone (for ear inflammation).

Nasal

Drug administration via the nasal cavity yields rapid drug absorption and therapeutic effects. If a drug is to be inhaled via the nose and absorbed through the thin membranes of the nasal passages, it must be transformed into tiny droplets in air (atomised). Once absorbed, the drug enters the bloodstream. Drugs that can be administered by the nasal route include sumatriptan (for migraine headaches [Derry et al.,, 2012]), and corticosteroids (for allergies [Chong et al., 2016]). Some peptide hormone analogues (e.g. antidiuretic hormone and gonadotropin-releasing hormone) can also be administered as nasal sprays.

Clinical consideration: topical medications

Paramedics may be called to administer topical medications and creams to patients. As described in this chapter, topical medications come in varying forms depending on patient needs. Topical medications are designed to act locally on the affected area through absorption of the skin. It is therefore required that all health professionals wear gloves when administering topical treatments to prevent the absorption of the medication through their hands. Following hand hygiene techniques and using clean gloves is important when in contact with broken skin to prevent the transmission of microorganisms. At all times, the paramedic must adhere to local policies and procedures.

Transdermal

Transdermal administration is effective for introducing drugs into the systemic circulation through the skin. For example, glyceryl trinitrate may be used for the prophylaxis of angina (Yellon et al., 2018), fentanyl for the treatment of chronic pain (Taylor, 2020), oestrogens for hormone replacement (Beck et al., 2017) or nicotine for smoking cessation (Wadgave and Nagesh, 2016). A drug must be highly lipophilic and may be mixed with a chemical (such as alcohol) to enhance penetration through the skin into the bloodstream.

There are many advantages of transdermal administration including avoiding GI drug absorption, first-pass effects and replacement of oral administration. Patches are beneficial for drugs which are quickly eliminated and may be delivered slowly and continuously for many hours or days to produce long-lasting effects. Disadvantages include local skin reactions, irritation of the skin and issues with adhering the system to the skin. Transdermal delivery systems also require relatively potent drugs for administration in this manner.

Vaginal formulations

Certain medicines may be administered vaginally to women as a solution, cream, gel, pessaries (a tablet inserted into the vagina) or intravaginal rings (soft plastic rings inserted into the vagina). Administering a drug vaginally has the potential advantage of exerting effects primarily in the vagina with limited systemic adverse effects compared to other routes of administration. Medicines primarily delivered via the intravaginal route include oestrogens and progestogens, antibacterials to treat bacterial vaginosis or antifungals to treat vaginal candidiasis. For example, intravaginal hormone replacement therapy (HRT) creams containing the hormone estriol (an oestrogen) can be used in postmenopausal women for relief of symptoms (such as dryness, soreness and redness) occurring after menopause.

Inhaled formulations

Inhalation

The lungs are an effective route of administration. The alveolar epithelium is very thin (approximately 0.1–0.5 mm thick) which permits rapid and complete drug absorption (Colombo et al., 2012). The pulmonary alveoli represent a large surface area. This, in addition to, blood flow to the lungs provides for rapid exchange of drugs and rapid adjustment of plasma concentration. Local (e.g. bronchodilators in the treatment of asthma) and systemic (e.g. inhaled general anaesthetics) effects may be intended.

Inhaled drugs must be atomised into smaller droplets to ensure the drug can pass through the trachea and into the lungs. This results in an increase in the amount of drug absorbed. For example, glucocorticoids such as beclomethasone dipropionate (Singh et al., 2016) and bronchodilators such as salbutamol (Ullmann et al., 2015) are administered to limit systemic effects and achieve high local concentrations. However, drugs are partly absorbed following inhalation and therefore may result in side effects. As an example, tremor may follow salbutamol use (Australian Medicines Handbook, 2020; Joint Formulary Committee, 2020). The process of delivering drugs to the lung is not simple and is related to many factors associated with the inhaled product and the patient.

The lung is a desirable target for drug delivery given that it provides direct access to deliver drugs to the disease site while limiting systemic adverse effects. Local drug delivery through the lung also has the advantage of bypassing absorption in the GI tract and first pass metabolism. Furthermore, the large surface area of the lung can be utilised for the systemic absorption of certain medications, from small molecules to large proteins (Patton et al., 2004). Systemic drug delivery to the lung is non-invasive.

Episode of care: methoxyflurane

You are dispatched to a local park to attend to a 34-year-old male who has fallen down while running. He has injured his ankle and cannot bear any weight on it. He requires pain relief and you offer him methoxyflurane.

Describe the mechanism of action of methoxyflurane. What are its adverse effects? How is it administered?

Methoxyflurane is a general anaesthetic, mainly used for immediate, short-term pain relief in the prehospital setting, e.g. by a paramedic crew. Its overall effects are to enhance the transmission of inhibitory neurotransmitters (e.g. GABA) and inhibit the transmission of excitatory neurotransmitters (e.g. glutamate) (Porter et al., 2018). Methoxyflurane has low blood solubility, meaning it doesn't take long to saturate the blood. It has a fast onset of action and short duration. Onset of pain relief is achieved after 6–10 breaths and continues for several minutes after stopping. It has high lipid solubility, meaning that it is highly potent because it easily crosses the blood–brain barrier to exert its effects. Therefore, low doses are required. Adverse effects include drowsiness, confusion, nausea, headache, decreased heart rate and blood pressure. Methoxyflurane is administered via an inhalation device, as follows (Queensland Ambulance Service, 2019b).

1. Tilt the inhaler to a 45° angle and pour the contents of one 3 mL bottle into the base whilst rotating.
2. Instruct the patient to inhale and exhale gently through the mouthpiece.
3. If stronger analgesia is required, the patient may be instructed to temporarily cover the dilution hole with their own finger to increase concentration.

Nebulisation

A drug must be aerosolised into small particles to reach the lungs if given by nebulisation. Examples of drugs that can be nebulised include tobramycin for cystic fibrosis (NPS MedicineWise, 2019) and salbutamol for symptom-relief associated with an asthma exacerbation (EMC, 2020; Queensland Ambulance Service, 2020). Adverse effects may occur if the drug is deposited directly in the lungs and may include shortness of breath or lung irritation. Importantly, the amount of drug delivered to the lungs will be maximised with proper use of the nebuliser. When the device is reused and inadequately cleaned, contamination may also occur.

Episode of care

You are dispatched for a 40-year-old male having difficulty breathing. On arrival, you find the patient sitting on the deck and are met by a 35-year-old female. The patient is flushed and anxious and is only able to speak short sentences. The male reports a history of asthma which is aggravated by dust, pollen and exercise. He mentioned to you that he suddenly felt chest constriction while mowing the lawn. He normally uses his salbutamol inhaler, however, couldn't find an inhaler when needed. His asthma has been controlled over the last few years with regular use of preventer and symptom controller inhalers. He advises he has never experienced an asthma attack this severe.

How would you initially treat this patient? Describe how the patient's inhaler (salbutamol) works. What are the roles of preventers and symptom controllers in the management of asthma?

This patient appears to be suffering from an acute asthma exacerbation. The patient would initially be treated with salbutamol (via an inhaler or nebuliser with oxygen). Additional treatment options (depending on response, severity and drug availability) include ipratropium, dexamethasone and adrenaline. Salbutamol is a beta-2 receptor agonist (Ullmann et al., 2015). It causes relaxation of bronchial smooth muscle and bronchodilation (as a 'reliever medication' – to be used only when required). Preventers are used on a regular basis to control the underlying inflammation in asthma and prevent or reduce the occurrence of asthma exacerbations. Symptom controllers can be used on a regular basis with preventers to keep the airways open. As long as they are used in conjunction with preventers, they can reduce the occurrence of asthma exacerbations. However, if used without a preventer, they may mask underlying inflammation and may increase the risk of an asthma exacerbation.

Enteral formulations

Enteral administration involves absorption of the drug via the GI tract and includes oral, gastric or duodenal (e.g. feeding tube) and rectal administration. Furthermore, other locations often classified as enteral include sublingual (under the tongue) and buccal (between the cheek and gums/gingiva).

Oral

Oral (PO) administration is the most frequently used route of administration. Drugs administered orally include tablets or chewable tablets, capsules and liquids (MSD Manual, 2020). There are many advantages of oral administration. It is inexpensive and offers convenience and simplicity, all of which improve patient compliance. Tablets and capsules have a high degree of drug stability which allows for accurate dosing. For patients who cannot tolerate tablets and capsules, such as children or older patients who have difficulty swallowing, the use of liquids or soluble formulations is beneficial.

The oral route is nevertheless problematic because of the unpredictable nature of GI drug absorption. Food may impact how rapid a drug is absorbed and how much of a drug is absorbed in the GI tract. Some medicines taken orally are to be taken with food or alternatively, on an empty stomach. Similarly, drugs taken concomitantly may interact or affect how much and how fast the drug is absorbed (MSD Manual, 2020). Additionally, the formulation impacts how quickly the medication is absorbed and gets into the systemic circulation (Figure 6.5).

If a patient is vomiting or is unable to swallow, oral administration is less desirable. Drugs delivered via the oral route need to be stable in gastric acid, otherwise they may be destroyed by acid and digestive enzymes in the stomach and may be poorly or erratically absorbed (World Health Organization, 2011a, b). If the oral route is not suitable (for example, if a patient is nil by mouth, if rapid onset of action is required, or if a drug is poorly absorbed), other routes of administration should be used.

Tablets

Immediate release

Immediate-release medications quickly disintegrate and release the drug rapidly (Maiti and Sen, 2017). This is particularly important in situations where a quick onset of action is required (e.g. sumatriptan, a triptan medication, is a fast-disintegrating tablet indicated for the treatment of acute migraine).

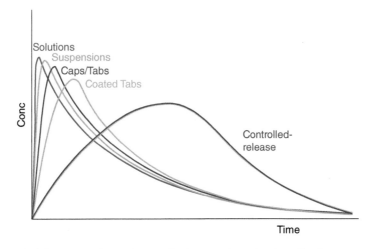

Figure 6.5   Speed of absorption depending on the formulation of oral medications.

Controlled release

Controlled-release formulations deliver a drug at a predetermined rate over a specified period of time, achieving a constant drug plasma concentration (Wen and Park, 2010). This may also be termed modified release, sustained release, extended release or long-acting. The main advantage for individuals taking controlled-release dosage forms is that doses usually only need to be taken once or twice daily. Damage to the release-controlling mechanism, for example, by chewing or crushing a controlled-release tablet, can result in the full dose of drug being released at once rather than over a number of hours. This may increase the risk of toxicity and adverse events, or the medication may not be absorbed at all, leading to suboptimal treatment. Therefore, controlled-release preparations generally must not be crushed or broken at the point of administration.

There are some exceptions, however, such as controlled-release medications that are scored. For example, gliclazide controlled-release scored 60 mg tablets (indicated for type 2 diabetes) have a score line and may be administered as whole or half tablets. To ensure that the controlled-release properties of the product are maintained, the tablets should not be chewed or crushed.

102

Skills in practice: controlled-release medications

Controlled-release medications should not be used to treat acute conditions requiring rapid onset or quick and safe titration.

Enteric coated

Some medications are not stable in the acidic stomach environment. An enteric coating is a polymer barrier applied to oral medication that prevents its dissolution or disintegration in the gastric environment. Medications with enteric coating pass safely through the acidic stomach environment and disintegrate later in the GI system, generally in the small intestine (World Health Organization, 2011a, b). Broadly speaking, there are two forms of enteric-coated tablets: tablets that are coated on their outside and tablets that contain small enteric-coated pellets.

Enteric-coated tablets and patients with swallowing difficulties

Generally, tablets with enteric coating must not be chewed or crushed and should be swallowed as a whole. Breaking the integrity of the tablet would bring the contents in contact with the stomach acid which may destroy the active ingredient(s). Dispersible tablets that contain enteric-coated pellets may be dispersed in water or fruit juice. For example, omeprazole magnesium dispersible tablets can be placed in half a glass of non-carbonated water or fruit juice, should be stirred until the tablet disperses into little pellets, and consumed immediately or within 30 minutes (Australian Medicines Handbook, 2020; EMC, 2021).

Dispersible (soluble/effervescent)

Before an oral medication can be absorbed in the GI tract to exert its effect, it needs to disintegrate into a solution. In the case of dispersible, soluble or effervescent tablets, this process is speeded up and the medication exhibits a quicker effect than conventional tablets. Dispersible or soluble tablets dissolve in water to produce a clear or slightly opalescent solution (World Health Organization, 2011a, b). Effervescent tablets need to be dispersed in water prior to use as they react quickly in water, releasing carbon dioxide.

Chewable

Chewable tablets are usually uncoated and are intended to be processed by chewing to facilitate release of the active ingredient(s) (World Health Organization, 2011a, b). The release of drug happens quicker than with a conventional tablet when swallowed as a whole. Chewable tablets are a versatile dosage form offering several advantages including oral drug delivery without the need for water, ease of swallowing and the stability advantages of solid dosage forms. An example of a dispersible/chewable medication is lamotrigine which is indicated for the treatment of epilepsy and bipolar disorder.

Capsules

Immediate release

Immediate-release capsule formulations need to be swallowed whole and are designed to dissolve as quickly as possible so that the medication can get into solution and be absorbed without delay (Maiti and Sen, 2017). Immediate-release formulations are used when a fast onset of action is desirable.

Controlled release

Controlled-release capsules can have a hard or a soft shell and exhibit a controlled rate of release of their active ingredient(s) in the GI tract. Similar principles apply as with controlled-release tablets – crushing or chewing them could release all the content at once and cause potential overdose or it could lead to the medication not being absorbed and reduced effect.

Enteric coated

Similar principles as for enteric-coated tablets apply here (World Health Organization, 2011a, b). With enteric-coated capsules, either the capsule itself is coated, and therefore protected from the acidic environment, or capsules contain small pellets with individual enteric coating (multi-unit pellet systems [MUPS]). Both capsules and pellets must not be crushed or chewed. In the case of capsules containing individual enteric-coated pellets, the capsule contents may be mixed with a spoonful of yoghurt or apple puree. This option is suitable for people with swallowing difficulties.

Liquid formulations

Solutions/suspensions

Solutions are homogeneous mixtures of two or more components. A suspension is a heterogeneous mixture in which particles do not dissolve but rather remain suspended. That means that particles may still be seen with the naked eye. Solutions and oral liquid suspensions can be very useful particularly for patients with dysphagia, children or older people.

Skills in practice

Suspensions

Suspensions need to be shaken well before each use. This is important to ensure the uniformity of the dose at the time of administration. If a suspension is not shaken well and particles (active ingredient) have settled, the suspension when administered could potentially be less concentrated than expected while the remainder of the stock suspension would then be more highly concentrated.

Oral formulations of morphine

Morphine, an opioid analgesic indicated for severe pain, is an example of a medication with various oral formulations including conventional (immediate-release) tablets, conventional oral liquids, controlled-release tablets (12-h), controlled-release oral liquids (granules, 12-h) and controlled-release capsules (12- or 24-h). Different oral formulations and combinations of immediate- and controlled-release forms can be used to achieve optimal control in acute and chronic pain.

Recommendations for the different oral formulations of morphine
- Controlled-release tablets must be swallowed whole, not crushed or chewed.
- Controlled-release capsules may be opened, pellets sprinkled on soft food or mixed with 30 mL of liquid, and taken within 30–60 minutes depending on the brand used. Pellets must not be crushed or chewed.
- For controlled-release suspension, the contents of the sachet should be added to the recommended amount of water, mixed thoroughly and taken immediately (Australian Medicines Handbook, 2020).

Sublingual and buccal formulations

Buccal and sublingual medications are available in the form of tablets, wafers, films or sprays. Sublingual administration is undertaken by placing the drug under the tongue. Drugs can be rapidly absorbed through the sublingual mucosa, given its high permeability and supply of blood vessels. Peak blood drug levels are usually achieved 3–10 times faster than via the oral route. Glyceryl trinitrate, indicated for the treatment of acute angina, is an example of a drug that is administered sublingually. 'Wafer'-based versions of tablets are also available which dissolve rapidly under the tongue. Rizatriptan, indicated for the acute treatment of migraine, is an example of a drug administered as a wafer. Additionally, wafers may be used where low medication adherence is suspected. Olanzapine, indicated for schizophrenia, is available as a wafer formulation.

Buccal administration is undertaken by placing the drug between the inner lining of the cheek and gums. Buccal tissue is less permeable than sublingual tissue and results in slower absorption.

Skills in practice: glyceryl trinitrate

You are dispatched to an office building for a 49-year-old male patient experiencing chest pain. Upon arrival, you are greeted by a female co-worker. She tells you that the patient took his heart medication, but is still in a lot of pain. You find the patient sitting in a chair. He has a fearful look, is clenching his fist against his chest and is noticeably diaphoretic (sweating). After initial assessment, you determine his pulse to be 75 beats per minute, his blood pressure 134/84 mmHg, his cardiac rhythm and oxygen saturation level normal. His regular medications include atenolol and glyceryl trinitrate (GTN). He has a history of hypertension and angina. GTN is a sublingual medication, which comes in both tablet and spray form and is used to treat acute chest pain, commonly brought on by angina, or by patients experiencing myocardial infarction (MI). GTN is a potent coronary vasodilator, which reduces venous return due to its vasodilating properties, therefore reducing left ventricular load and resulting in pain relief for the patient, if the chest pain is coronary in origin. Advantages of sublingual GTN include that it is rapid acting and provides almost immediate relief of symptoms. Disadvantages are the side-effects, which can be severe in some patients such as hypotension or severe headache.

The following steps should be followed for the administration of sublingual GTN spray (Queensland Ambulance Service, 2019c).

1. Position the patient in a sitting or semi-reclined position.
2. Remove the plastic cover from the GTN spray bottle, thoroughly wipe the entire container, including the nozzle, with an alcohol swab and allow it to dry.
3. If using a new bottle, prime the pump by holding the bottle upright, facing away from the patient, and depress the nozzle five times (do not shake the bottle). If first use for the day, prime by spraying once.

4. Instruct the patient to open their mouth wide and lift their tongue to the roof of their mouth (some patients may have difficulty and may require demonstration).
5. Bring the bottle approximately 3-4 cm from the patient's mouth (without contact) with the nozzle aimed directly under the tongue and steadily depress the nozzle once.
6. After the last administration, thoroughly wipe the entire bottle, including the nozzle, and inside of the cap using an alcohol swab.
7. Recap the bottle.

Rectal formulations

The rectal route is an effective route of administration. Rectal preparations may include creams, ointments, suppositories and enemas. This route allows for rapid and effective absorption given the rectal mucosa is highly vascularised. Medications may be delivered to the distal one-third of the rectum with the aim of partially avoiding first-pass metabolism. This allows for greater bioavailability than some medications which are delivered orally.

A suppository is a solid dosage form for rectal administration. A suppository may be beneficial for patients who are unable to take a medicine orally (for example, in patients who are nil by mouth or are unable to swallow). Paracetamol, diazepam and laxatives are examples of medicines that can be administered rectally. A disadvantage of this route is patient acceptability.

Clinical consideration: dosage differences across formulations

Paracetamol is an analgesic medication commonly utilised as first-line pain relief. Paracetamol is available in different formulations including rectal suppositories, oral tablets, oral liquid and IV. It is therefore vital that paramedics understand the differences in drug dosages across formulations. For example, a standard and maximum adult dose of paracetamol administered orally in tablet form is 1 g every 4–6 h, up to four times daily. However, for adults who weigh less than 50 kg, the maximum IV dose is 15 mg/kg every 4–6 h. For adults who weigh over 50 kg, the dose remains the same as oral recommendations. Recommendations are also in place for patients with known hepatic disorders or those at risk of hepatotoxicity. For example, a maximum daily dose of 3 g can be administered to this patient group. Clinical judgement should be exercised if a patient is deemed at risk of toxicity and the dosage adjusted accordingly. It is also important to check a patient's cumulative paracetamol dose over the previous 24 h, prior to administering the next dose of paracetamol, and to seek guidance on dosages where unsure. Adhere to local policy and procedure.

Conclusion

This chapter provides details of different formulations of medication available and their uses. The reader has been provided with knowledge and guidance concerning the various formulations of drugs, how to administer these safely and correctly and when to consider alternative formulations, and now will have a wider understanding when entering into practice.

Find out more about these conditions

The following is a list of conditions requiring a variety of medications to be administered via a variety of routes using different drug preparations. Take some time to test your knowledge and write some notes about each condition. Think specifically about the different medications, treatments or therapies a patient may require and how these might be administered.

Condition	Notes
Nausea and vomiting	
Epilepsy	
Angina	
Atrial fibrillation	
Opioid overdose	

Glossary

Bioavailability	The degree to which a medication is absorbed into the circulatory system.
Digestion	The breakdown of material in the alimentary canal into substances that can be absorbed by the body.
Plasma concentration	Concentration of a medication or other substance measured in the patient's blood plasma.
Systemic absorption	The process of a medication being directly absorbed through the body for therapeutic effect.
Topical application	Application to body surfaces such as the skin or mucous membranes.

References

American Society of Retina Specialists. (2017). *Intravitreal Injections*. www.asrs.org/patients/retinal-diseases/33/intravitreal-injections

Australian Medicines Handbook. (2020). ,https://amhonline.amh.net.au/

Bardal S.K., Waechter, J.E. and Martin D.S. (2011). Pharmacokinetics. In: *Applied Pharmacology* (eds S.K. Bardal, J.E. Waechter and D.S. Martin). Philadelphia: W.B. Saunders, 17–34.

Beck, K.L., Anderson, M.C. and Kirk, J.K. (2017). Transdermal estrogens in the changing landscape of hormone replacement therapy. *Postgraduate Medicine* **129**(6): 632–636.

Brooks, A.M. and Gillies, W.E. (1992). Ocular beta-blockers in glaucoma management. Clinical pharmacological aspects. *Drugs and Aging* **2**(3): 208–221.

Case-Lo, C. (2018). *What is a Subcutaneous Injection?* www.healthline.com/health/subcutaneous-injection

Chong, L., Head, K., Hopkins, C., Philpott, C., Burton, M.J. and Schilder, A.G.M. (2016). Different types of intranasal steroids for chronic rhinosinusitis. *Cochrane Database of Systematic Reviews* **4**: CD011993.

Colombo, P., Traini, D. and Buttini, F. (2012). *Inhalation Drug Delivery: Techniques and Products*. Hoboken: Wiley.

Department of Health, Queensland Government. (2020). *Management of Subcutaneous Infusions in Palliative Care*. www.health.qld.gov.au/cpcre/subcutaneous/section3

Derry, C.J., Derr,y S. and Moore, R.A. (2012). Sumatriptan (intranasal route of administration) for acute migraine attacks in adults. *Cochrane Database of Systematic Reviews* **2**: CD009663.

EMC. (2020). *Salbutamol 5mg/2.5mL Nebuliser Solution*. (www.medicines.org.uk/emc/product/3214/

EMC. (2021). *Omeprazole magnesium 10 mg dispersible gastro resistant tablets*. www.medicines.org.uk/emc/product/4585/smpc

Gabros, S., Nessel, T.A. and Zito, P.M. (2020). *Topical Corticosteroids*. Treasure Island: StatPearls Publishing.

Joint Formulary Committee. (2020). *BNF 80: September 2020-March 2021*. London: Pharmaceutical Press.

Joint Royal Colleges Ambulance Liaison Committee (JRCALC). (2019). *Clinical Practice Guidelines*. https://aace.org.uk/clinical-practice-guidelines/

Kirk, A. (2018). Best practice technique in intramuscular injection. *Journal of Paramedic Practice*. www.paramedicpractice.com/features/article/best-practice-technique-in-intramuscular-injection

Lehman, A.F., Kreyenbuhl, J., Buchanan, R.W. et al. (2004). The schizophrenia patient outcomes research team (PORT): update treatment recommendations 2003. *Schizophrenia Bulletin* **30**: 193–217.

Maiti, S. and Sen, K.K. (2017). Drug delivery concepts. In: *Advanced Technology for Delivering Therapeutics.* IntechOpen. www.intechopen.com/chapters/54825

McAlindon, T.E., LaValley, M.P., Harvey, W.F. et al. (2017). Effect of intra-articular triamcinolone vs saline on knee cartilage volume and pain in patients with knee osteoarthritis: a randomized clinical trial. *JAMA* **317**(19): 1967–1975.

McGrath, P. and Brown, S. (2009). Pain in children. In: *Pain Management Secrets*, 3rd edn (eds C. Argoff and G. McCleane). St Louis: Elsevier.

MSD Manual. (2020). *Drug Administration.* www.msdmanuals.com/home/drugs/administration-and-kinetics-of-drugs/drug-administration

NPS Medicinewise. (2019). *Tobramycin.* www.nps.org.au/medicine-finder/tobramycin-an-solution-for-inhalation

Patton J.S., Fishburn, C.S. and Weers, J.G. (2004). The lungs as a portal of entry for systemic drug delivery. *Proceedings of the American Thoracic Society* **1**(4): 338–344.

Porter, K.M., Dayan, A.D., Dickerson, S. and Middleton, P.M. (2018). The role of inhaled methoxyflurane in acute pain management. *Open Access Emergency Medicine* **10**: 149–164.

Public Health England. (2020). *The Green Book.* www.gov.uk/government/collections/immunisation-against-infectious-disease-the-green-book#the-green-book

Queensland Ambulance Service. (2019a). *Drug administration: Epipen®/Epipen Jr® adrenaline auto-injector.* www.ambulance.qld.gov.au/docs/clinical/cpp/CPP_EpiPen%20and%20EpiPen%20Jr%20adrenaline%20auto%20injector.pdf

Queensland Ambulance Service. (2019b). *Drug Therapy Protocols: Methoxyflurane.* www.ambulance.qld.gov.au/docs/clinical/dtprotocols/DTP_Methoxyflurane.pdf

Queensland Ambulance Service. (2019c). *Drug Therapy Protocols: Glyceryl Trinitrate.* www.ambulance.qld.gov.au/docs/clinical/dtprotocols/DTP_Glyceryl%20trinitrate.pdf

Queensland Ambulance Service. (2020). *Salbutamol.* www.ambulance.qld.gov.au/docs/clinical/dtprotocols/DTP_Salbutamol.pdf

Rang, H.P. (2016) *Rang and Dale's Pharmacology*, 8th edn. Philadelphia: Elsevier Churchill Livingstone.

Riebesehl, B.U. (2015). Drug delivery with organic solvents or colloidal dispersed systems. In: *The Practice of Medicinal Chemistry*, 4th edn (eds C. Wermuth, D. Aldous, P. Raboisson and D. Rognan). Philadelphia: Elsevier, 699–720.

ScienceDirect. (2008). *Intrathecal Drug Administration.* www.sciencedirect.com/topics/medicine-and-dentistry/intrathecal-drug-administration

Shepherd, E. (2018). Injection Technique 2: administering drugs via the subcutaneous route. *Nursing Times* **114**(9). www.nursingtimes.net/clinical-archive/assessment-skills/injection-technique-2-administering-drugs-via-the-subcutaneous-route-28-08-2018/

Shrestha, P. and Stoeber, B. (2018). Fluid absorption by skin tissue during intradermal injections through hollow microneedles. *Scientific Reports* **8**(1): 13749.

Sinatra, R. (2003). Pain, Postoperative. In: *Encyclopedia of the Neurological Sciences* (eds R. Daroff and M. Aminoff). St Louis: Elsevier.

Singh, A., Nandan, D., Dewan, V. and Sankar, J. (2016). Comparison of clinical effects of beclomethasone dipropionate and budesonide in treatment of children with mild persistent asthma: a double-blind, randomized, controlled study. *Indian Journal of Medical Research* **144**(2): 250–257.

Taylor, K.P. and Goyal, A. (2020). Fentanyl Transdermal. Treasure Island: StatPearls Publishing.

Ullmann, N., Caggiano, S. and Cutrera, R. (2015). Salbutamol and around. *Italian Journal of Pediatrics* **41**(Suppl 2): A74.

Villines, Z. (2018). *Is a subcutaneous injection painful?* www.medicalnewstoday.com/articles/322710

Wadgave, U. and Nagesh, L. (2016). Nicotine replacement therapy: an overview. *International Journal of Health Science* **10**(3): 425–435.

Wen, H. and Park, K. (2010). Introduction and overview of oral controlled release formulation design. In: *Oral Controlled Release Formulation Design and Drug Delivery: Theory to Practice* (eds H. Wen and K. Park). Hoboken: John Wiley & Sons, 1–20.

West, J., Marcus, S., Wilk, J., Countis, L., Regier, D. and Olfson, M. (2008). Use of depot antipsychotic medications for medication nonadherence in schizophrenia. *Schizophrenia Bulletin* **34**(5): 995–1001.

World Health Organization. (2011a). *Revision of monograph on tablets.* (www.who.int/medicines/publications/pharmacopoeia/Tabs-GeneralMono-rev-FINAL_31032011.pdf

World Health Organization. (2011b). *Revision of monograph on capsules.* www.who.int/medicines/publications/pharmacopoeia/Caps-GeneralMono-rev-FINAL_31032011.pdf

Yellon, D.M., He, Z., Khambata, R., Ahluwalia, A. and Davidson, S.M. (2018). The GTN patch: a simple and effective new approach to cardioprotection? *Basic Research in Cardiology* **113**(3): 20.

107

Further reading

eTG complete. Melbourne: Therapeutic Guidelines Limited. www.tg.org.au

Maria, S., Colbeck, M. and Caffey, M. (2020). *Paramedic and Emergency Pharmacology Guidelines*, 2nd edn. Melbourne: Pearson Australia Group.

National Institute for Health and Care Excellence (NICE). British National Formulary (BNF). Available from: https://bnf.nice.org.uk/

108   Multiple-choice questions

1. Enteric-coated tablets:
   (a) Disintegrate in the stomach
   (b) Take longer to dissolve and take effect than regular tablets
   (c) Can be crushed
   (d) Are suitable for patients who have difficulty in swallowing.

2. Modified-release medications:
   (a) Are suitable for crushing/dissolving
   (b) Require less frequent dosages
   (c) Are not suitable for the treatment of chronic pain
   (d) Should be used to treat acute conditions requiring rapid onset.

3. Sublingual GTN spray:
   (a) Is an ineffective treatment for acute angina
   (b) Is a potent vasoconstrictor
   (c) Is suitable for hypovolaemic patients
   (d) Can cause vasodilatory side-effects such as headache, flushing and orthostatic hypotension.

4. Patients unable to absorb oral medications, due to gut ileus:
   (a) Should be given their tablets anyway on the off-chance that they may absorb them
   (b) Should receive the equivalent intravenous preparation for all essential medications
   (c) Do not require any further investigation or monitoring
   (d) Should be advised to crush or chew their tablets.

5. Suppositories can be used for what effect?
   (a) Analgesia
   (b) Bowel preparation
   (c) Local treatment, such as haemorrhoids
   (d) All of the above.

6. What is the recommended time interval between eye drops to ensure maximum effect?
   (a) 30 seconds
   (b) 3 minutes
   (c) 5 minutes
   (d) 60 seconds

7. Oral liquid suspensions should be considered for:
   (a) Patients with dysphagia
   (b) Children
   (c) The elderly
   (d) All of the above.

8. Topical beta-blockers:
   (a) Increase intraocular pressure by blockade of sympathetic nerve endings
   (b) Are not absorbed systemically, and therefore there is no potential for cardiovascular effects
   (c) Are indicated for the treatment of glaucoma
   (d) Are generally safe to use in asthmatic patients.

9. Methoxyflurane:
   (a) Is mainly used for immediate, short-term pain relief in the prehospital setting, e.g. by ambulance personnel
   (b) Produces pain relief after 12–20 breaths which continues for several minutes after stopping
   (c) Has high blood solubility
   (d) Has a long duration of action.

10. Which of the following statements is *incorrect*?
   (a) A depot injection deposits a drug in a localised mass, called a depot, from which it is gradually absorbed by surrounding tissue.
   (b) Depot antipsychotics are used as a maintenance treatment for patients with a history of non-adherence with oral antipsychotics.
   (c) Long-acting injectable formulations are intended to have a rapid effect.
   (d) Injections may be used to insert a solid object (or implant) into the body which releases a medication slowly over time.

11. Which of the following statements is *incorrect*?
   (a) Intrathecal administration penetrates the subarachnoid space to allow access of the drug to the cerebrospinal fluid of the spinal cord.
   (b) Intradermal injections are shallow or superficial injections of a drug into the dermis, located below the epidermis.
   (c) A subcutaneous injection is one into the fatty tissues (subcutaneous tissue) between the skin and the muscle.
   (d) Subcutaneous administration is beneficial for drugs that have high oral bioavailability (e.g. insulin).

12. Which of the following statements is *incorrect* regarding dexamethasone?
   (a) Adverse effects are more common with prolonged administration.
   (b) Dexamethasone can be used for severe asthma and COPD exacerbations, suspected croup and severe sepsis.
   (c) Dexamethasone may cause hypoglycaemia.
   (d) Dexamethasone increases the risk and severity of infections.

13. Which of the following statements is *correct*?
   (a) Intramuscular injections are limited to volumes of up to 5 mL.
   (b) An intramuscular injection must be administered at a 45° angle.
   (c) The appropriate degree of entry does not play a role in the successful and comfortable administration of injections.
   (d) The IV route provides delayed onset of action.

14. Which of the following statements is *incorrect*?
   (a) Rectal mucosa is highly vascularised tissue that allows for rapid and effective absorption of medications.
   (b) Buccal administration is achieved by placing the medication between the gums and the inner lining of the cheek.
   (c) Buccal tissue is more permeable than sublingual tissue.
   (d) Peak blood drug levels with sublingual administration are usually achieved 3–10 times faster than via the oral route.

15. Which of the following statements is *incorrect* regarding local drug delivery to the lung?
   (a) Undergoes first-pass metabolism in the liver.
   (b) Delivers high concentration directly to the disease site, minimising risk of systemic side-effects.
   (c) Achieves rapid clinical response.
   (d) Achieves a similar or superior therapeutic effect at a fraction of the systemic dose.

Chapter 7

Adverse drug reactions

Matt Dixon

Aim

The aim of this chapter is to equip the reader with an understanding of what adverse drug reactions are and how they are relevant to clinical practice.

Learning outcomes

After reading this chapter, the reader will be able to:

1. Understand what an adverse drug reaction is and how it is relevant to clinical practice
2. Understand the different types of adverse drug reaction
3. Recognise the signs and symptoms of adverse drug reactions
4. Understand which patient groups are more likely to experience an adverse drug reaction
5. Understand the professional duties around identification and reporting of adverse drug reactions.

Test your knowledge

1. How would you define an adverse drug reaction?
2. Describe how you would recognise an adverse drug reaction.
3. Are adverse drug reactions a common occurrence?
4. Name the patient groups more likely to experience an adverse drug reaction.
5. What actions should be taken when dealing with a suspected adverse drug reaction?

What is an adverse drug reaction?

Originally defined in 1972 by the World Health Organization, and then adopted in the UK by the Medicines and Healthcare products Regulatory Agency, an adverse drug reaction (ADR) is 'any response to a drug which is noxious and unintended and which occurs at doses normally used in man for prophylaxis, diagnosis or therapy'.

This has been expanded upon more recently by the National Institute of Health and Care Excellence (NICE, 2017) which states in addition to the above that an ADR is 'an unwanted or harmful reaction

Fundamentals of Pharmacology for Paramedics, First Edition. Edited by Ian Peate, Suzanne Evans, and Lisa Clegg.
© 2022 John Wiley & Sons Ltd. Published 2022 by John Wiley & Sons Ltd.

which occurs after administration of a drug or drugs, and is suspected or known to be due to the drug'. This definition is important, especially with newer drugs, in including the fact that only suspicion is needed to be able to label a response an ADR.

The National Institute of Health and Care Excellence recommends also that care is taken to distinguish the term 'adverse drug reaction' from 'adverse effect', the latter being preferable to but interchangeable with 'side-effect' and 'toxic effect'. This subtle difference in terminology reflects the fact that a drug can cause an adverse effect, whereas a patient experiences an adverse reaction. The term 'adverse effect' is preferred above others because alongside adverse drug reaction, these terms encompass all unwanted effects. They are unambiguous, make no assumption about mechanism and avoid the risk of misclassification.

111

Classification of adverse drug reactions

Adverse drug reactions are commonly broken down into two categories, Type A and Type B, although there are further subtypes beyond these which provide more accurate classification: Type C, Type D and Type E (MHRA, 2015).

Type A (Augmented) reactions are due to exaggerated but normal pharmacological effects at normal doses. They are dose dependent and therefore readily reversible when reducing the dose or withdrawing the drug. An example of a Type A reaction would be respiratory depression following administration of morphine, which is predictable based on the pharmacology of the drug and would be commonly encountered at higher doses. It would be expected to resolve with cessation or reversal of treatment or reduction in dose. Type A reactions account for approximately 80% of all adverse drug reactions.

Type B (Bizarre) reactions are idiosyncratic and not predictable given the pharmacological nature of the drug. An example of a Type B reaction would be anaphylaxis as a result of penicillin administration. This is uncommon, is not predictable based on the pharmacology of the drug, and will require more intervention to manage beyond moderating the original drug treatment. Type B adverse drug reactions account for approximately the remaining 20% of reactions.

Beyond Type A and B reactions there are the more nuanced C, D and E reactions.

Type C (Continuing) reactions are a subset of Type A and are relatively long-lived. An example of this would be osteonecrosis of the jaw associated with the use of bisphosphonates, which are used to slow the rate of bone turnover in order to help treat certain bony conditions such as osteoporosis (Longmore et al., 2010).

Type D (Delayed) reactions are those which only become apparent some time after the beginning of administration of a drug, and are again a subset of Type A. An example is the onset of leucopenia (reduction in white blood cells) which can be provoked up to 6 weeks after a dose of the anticancer drug lomustine.

Type E (End-of-use) reactions are associated with withdrawal of treatment. Examples include the development of anxiety and fatigue when withdrawing the antidepressant sertraline too quickly. This may be moderated or eliminated by careful tapering of drugs known to cause withdrawal effects.

How prevalent are adverse drug reactions?

Depending on reporting, it may be difficult to accurately quantify the prevalence of ADRs but in the UK a systematic review by Howard et al. (2007) found that 3.73% of all hospital admissions were as a result of ADRs. In a suite of evidence from the UK, NICE (2017) estimates that adverse drug reactions may account for 6–7% of admissions. NICE (2017) goes on to suggest that ADRs occur in 10–20% of hospital inpatients and that 2% of patients admitted with an ADR died. In total, ADRs are believed to contribute to around 1700 deaths and are directly responsible for around 700 potentially avoidable deaths per year in the UK.

Awareness of the prevalence of ADRs is important as the cost burden they place on healthcare systems is considerable. Pirmohamed et al. (2004) calculated that the annual cost to the NHS was £466M, which when adjusted for inflation reflects in 2020 an annual cost of nearly £0.75B. Hidden within this price is considerable morbidity and mortality, an estimated resource burden of 4 in 100 hospital bed-days, as well as costs associated with litigation and insurance coverage. For international context, the estimated cost of medication-related problems was estimated by the Pharmaceutical Society of Australia (2019) to be $AUD 1.4 Billion (~£800M).

The surveillance of ADRs, especially those related to newer medications and those more likely to be experienced by vulnerable groups, is an important area of work for government regulators, given the significant associated costs, both financial and in terms of morbidity and mortality.

The knowledge that around 80% of ADRs are predictable based upon the drug's pharmacology is an important factor in trying to reduce the incidence of adverse reactions. Indeed, the ability to recognise and report adverse reactions is a required element within the College of Paramedics (2018) *Practice Guidance for Paramedics*. This is mirrored in guidance for other professions across the NHS (NICE, 2017).

Who is more likely to experience adverse drug reactions?

Adverse drug reactions are more likely to be experienced amongst certain patient groups (Table 7.1), and when certain classes of medications are involved (Table 7.2).

Table 7.1 Patient characteristics which predispose to adverse drug effects.

Characteristic	Remarks
Age	Patients at the extremes of age are especially susceptible to adverse reactions. Children and neonates in particular are at greater risk of experiencing adverse reactions due to physiological immaturity and variable responses to medications. Extremely small children are at greater risk of calculation errors where drug doses and volumes can be very small. At the upper limit of age patients are once again more vulnerable to adverse reactions due to changes in physiology which affect the ADME processes, as well as potentially lacking physiological reserves to adequately respond to stressors. Absorption may be decreased by slowed gastric transit; the distribution of medications may be affected by increased body fat as well as reduced body water content. A lipid-soluble drug will accumulate in adipose tissue and be less available for metabolism, lengthening its duration of action. Conversely, water-soluble drugs will be found in greater concentrations in the extracellular fluid, including plasma. Drug metabolism can be adversely affected by declining hepatic function and drug and metabolite excretion can be impaired by reduced renal function, both increasing the risk of higher levels of drug and therefore adverse effects. The upper limits of age are also compounded by the increased likelihood of comorbid conditions and polypharmacy
Gender	Physiological and anatomical variations based on gender can affect the pharmacokinetics of many drugs and hence the risk of adverse reactions. Body composition and weight, along with hepatic function, renal function and gastric motility can all vary with gender. Females tend to have a lower body weight and smaller organs, with an increased proportion of adipose tissue, lower glomerular filtration rate and different gastric motility, all of which can leave women at greater risk of adverse reactions. Other gender-related factors such as hormonal and immunological status may contribute to an increased risk of adverse reactions in females
Ethnicity	Ethnic background can have an effect on risk of adverse drug reactions, primarily due to genetic differences. The frequency of some drug reactions can differ greatly between ethnic groups because of variations in the hepatic CYP450 enzymes, for example. One important and notable difference in these metabolising enzymes exists in the gene encoding for the CYP2D6 enzyme which is an important step in the metabolism of codeine to its active metabolite morphine, among many other important metabolic reactions. Some 10% of Caucasian people may have little or no CYP2D6 function, and are classified as poor metabolisers, who are less likely to experience a therapeutic effect from a normal dose of codeine due to slower production of the active metabolite. This variant occurs less frequently in people of Asian and African origin, although there is a greater prevalence of ultra-rapid metabolisers among this population, which increases risk of adverse effects and opiate toxicity (Holmquist, 2009). Another example of this is the antidepressant duloxetine, which is metabolised by the CYP2D6 enzyme from the active form to its inactive metabolites; hence in a poor metaboliser there is increased exposure to the active drug and greater chance of adverse reaction

Table 7.1   (Continued)

Characteristic	Remarks
Environmental factors	Environmental factors can be hard to quantify but some have a well-defined effect on risk of drug reactions. Tobacco smoking is a powerful inducer of the CYP1A2 enzyme (van der Weide et al., 2003) resulting in more rapid metabolism of drugs that are metabolised by this enzyme. Alcohol, diet and other factors may influence the pharmacokinetics of a drug and hence the risk of adverse reaction. A gastric ulcer caused by excessive alcohol intake may impair the absorption of a drug, and a cirrhosed liver due to alcoholism is less capable of the metabolism of drugs
Polypharmacy	Polypharmacy, the term used to describe patients taking multiple drug therapies, is an important factor in assessing for risk of adverse reactions. Those on multiple medications are more likely to experience drug-to-drug reactions when treatments are initiated or changed (Royal Pharmaceutical Society, 2020)
Pregnancy	Pregnancy is a well-known risk factor for increased incidence of adverse drug reactions, as changes in the body, such as increased fluid volume, diluted plasma proteins, cardiac output and renal blood flow increases as well as reduced gastric motility, can all affect a drug's pharmacokinetics. Gastric changes may impair absorption, altered body fluid volumes can affect distribution, and increased renal blood flow will increase the excretion rate. In pregnancy and also in nursing mothers, a potential developmental effect upon the foetus or infant must be considered. While the evidence is limited due to the ethics of such studies, the thalidomide disaster illustrates the potential harm that drugs used by a pregnant mother can cause. More common drugs such as warfarin and ibuprofen are contraindicated in pregnancy due to known concerns about birth defects. Drugs excreted in breast milk can also be passed on the infant, along with the risk of an adverse reaction. The risk of harm to the infant when giving a breast-feeding mother medications must also be carefully considered (McKay et al., 2010)
Host factors	Host disease may predispose to a particular adverse reaction. For example, the antibacterials amoxicillin and ampicillin can cause a rash in patients with glandular fever (infectious mononucleosis)
Patient health and comorbidities	A patient's individual health status can also alter the risk of adverse drug reactions. A patient with chronic kidney disease will excrete medications more slowly, resulting in higher drug levels and potential for accumulation and hence adverse effects. Patients with liver disease may be less able to metabolise drugs and hence unwanted effects may again be more likely. Age, external factors, comorbid conditions and polypharmacy are closely linked, as an older person is more likely to have age-related physiological changes and comorbidities, which increase the likelihood of polypharmacy, all of which compound and increase risk of adverse drug reactions

ADME, absorption, distribution, metabolism and excretion.

Table 7.2   The most common causative medications, ranked by percentage of ADRs.

Drug class	Percentage of ADRs
Non-steroidal anti-inflammatory drugs (e.g. aspirin, ibuprofen)	29.6%
Diuretics (e.g. furosemide)	27.3%
Warfarin	10.5%
Angiotensin-converting enzyme inhibitors (e.g. ramipril)	7.7%
Antidepressants (e.g. sertraline)	7.1%
Beta-blockers (e.g. propranolol)	6.8%
Opiates (e.g. morphine)	6.0%
Digoxin	2.9%
Prednisolone	2.5%
Clopidogrel	2.4%

Source: Adapted with permission from Pirmohamed et al. (2004).

Recognising signs and symptoms of adverse drug reactions

Adverse drug reactions range from life-threatening to functionally benign and the entire spectrum between. The most clinically important adverse drug reaction would be the anaphylactic reaction.

Anaphylaxis

Anaphylaxis is a severe generalised immunological response to a foreign substance; its onset is generally within minutes of exposure to the stimulus and it commonly involves severe and possibly life-threatening symptoms. Anaphylaxis is most commonly caused by drugs such as antibiotics, in particular penicillins, non-steroidal anti-inflammatories, aspirin and some vaccines. It can also be caused by exposure to any allergen and can occur as a result of exposure to bee or wasp stings, latex and foods such as nuts or shellfish in sensitive individuals.

The common symptoms of anaphylaxis are:

- oedema to the lips, tongue, pharynx and epiglottis with associated risk of airway obstruction (Figures 7.1 and 7.2)
- dyspnoea, wheezing, chest tightness, hypoxia and tachypnoea

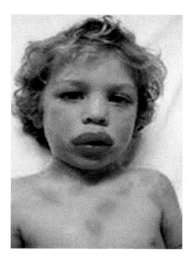

Figure 7.1   Anaphylaxis lips. Source: BBC News.

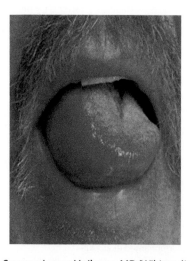

Figure 7.2   Anaphylaxis tongue. Source: James Heilman, MD/Wikimedia Commons.

114

- circulatory collapse (anaphylactic shock) accompanied by tachycardia (as a response to the drop in blood pressure)
- confusion, dizziness, reduced level of consciousness
- erythema, urticaria, angio-oedema
- nausea, vomiting, abdominal pain.

If faced with a patient experiencing an anaphylactic or suspected anaphylactic reaction, it is imperative for the paramedic to act quickly. If known, the stimulus should be removed or its administration stopped. The patient should be treated with high-flow oxygen and airway and ventilation should be supported where needed (noting that in the case of potential airway occlusion, senior help from a hospital emergency department or critical care team will be needed). Pharmacological treatment includes 500 mg intramuscular adrenaline, intravenous steroids such as hydrocortisone (100 mg) and antihistamines, such as chlorphenamine (10 mg) as well as fluid boluses to correct any hypotension. If the patient is experiencing lower airway symptoms such as wheezing or tightness in the chest then bronchodilators may be required, with inhaled salbutamol added to oxygen therapy. The ultimate possible consequence of anaphylaxis could be cardiac arrest, for which treatment is as per standard advanced life support algorithms (Resuscitation Council UK, 2020).

Clinical consideration

Benzylpenicillin is used in paramedic practice to treat suspected meningococcal septicaemia. It is common for patients to report they are allergic to penicillin when in fact they experienced common side-effects only, such as a rash or diarrhoea. In situations where 'allergy' is reported by the patient, the paramedic should establish what the symptoms were, and if they were in fact likely to be side-effects. Unless the patient experienced a true anaphylaxis or a clearly severe allergic reaction, the risk/benefit analysis is likely to be in favour of giving the benzylpenicillin to treat a life-threatening infection, rather than waiting (JRCALC, 2020).

Rashes and skin eruptions

It is common to see a rash as a result of an ADR. This can be an urticarial rash driven by an allergic process or a non-allergic process, such as the erythematous rash often experienced by those taking ampicillin (Figure 7.3).

A fixed drug eruption is another form of cutaneous adverse reaction. This takes the form of well-defined round or oval patches of redness and swelling in the skin, sometimes blistering. In time it will fade to a darker colour and may slough off before healing. The most common sites are hands and feet, lips, eyelids and genitalia. The lesion will predictably appear following administration of the causative agent and fade over time, usually returning upon subsequent dosing (Burge et al., 2016).

Serum sickness

This is a specific type of hypersensitivity reaction to animal proteins in serum and, less commonly, medication. It usually manifests 5–10 days following exposure to the proteins and causes a constellation of symptoms, including rashes (Figure 7.4), itching, small joint arthralgia, fever, malaise, lymphadenopathy and proteinuria. It can be treated on a symptomatic basis if needed but will spontaneously resolve within a week of stopping treatment with the causative agent (Nguyen and Miller, 2017).

Renal disorders

Some classes of drugs are especially prone to causing renal failure, non-steroidal anti-inflammatories (NSAIDs) and angiotensin-converting enzyme inhibitors (ACEi) being two classes that are often implicated in acute renal failure. Acute renal injury can also be produced by antimicrobials such as the penicillins and aminoglycosides (e.g. gentamicin).

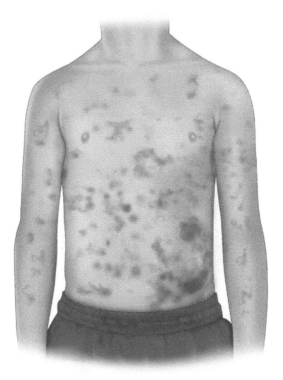

Figure 7.3   Urticarial drug rash.

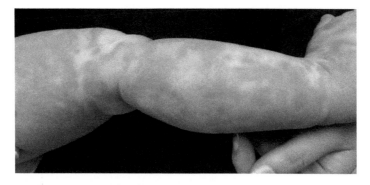

Figure 7.4   Serum sickness rash. *Source:* Brad Sobolewski, MD, MEd.

Geriatric syndrome

Identification of adverse reactions in the elderly can be difficult as these often manifest as symptoms which are already common in this age group. Dizziness, falls and confusion (the geriatric syndrome) may be the only indication of an ADR and should prompt the clinician to consider this possibility as well as looking for other possible causes (Lane et al., 2019).

When suspicious that a patient is experiencing an ADR, it is important for the clinician to either investigate and manage the situation themselves or, if not able to do so, to escalate the concerns to another clinician, such as the patient's general practitioner or hospital doctor, so that further investigation and management can be carried out. It is important to remember that while ADR may present overtly, in the form of anaphylaxis for example, a rash, deterioration in renal function or fall in an elderly patient may be the only indication of a problem. Without considering the potential for an adverse reaction to a medication, it can be easy to miss.

Idiosyncratic reactions

Certain adverse reactions present as idiosyncratic, being unexplainable by the drug's pharmacology. Examples would be Achilles tendinopathy secondary to quinolone antibiotics, aplastic anaemia secondary to the antibiotic chloramphenicol or toxic epidermal necrolysis caused by allopurinol.

Preventing adverse drug reactions

Considering the burden and prevalence of ADRs, the preferable course of action will always be to prevent their occurrence rather than treat and mitigate after they have occurred. The risk of ADRs can be reduced by the use of prescribing strategies which include a comprehensive health and medication history, including use of non-prescription, herbal, alternative and recreational medications. Regular medication reviews, taking into account therapeutic aims, comorbidities and polypharmacy, are important, as is ensuring that the patient is able to take the medication correctly. Cognitive impairment, poor dexterity, poor vision or poorly explained medication regimens can all play a role in incorrect self-administration of medication which may lead to ADRs. Prescribing tools such as the STOPP START tool (Gallagher et al., 2014), which is designed to reduce polypharmacy and optimise prescribed medication use in the elderly, can reduce risk of ADRs.

Once an adverse reaction has occurred and been identified, the next action to take will be to manage it acutely and try to avoid any recurrence.

Questions that can be included in a drug history and when considering starting or changing medication can include the following.

- Have you had this (or similar) medication before and experienced an adverse reaction that you are aware of?
- Did any reaction occur after the drug was started?
- Did anything else happen at the time that might have been contributory? Were you started on another treatment or did your condition change? (Coleman and Pontefract, 2016)

Clinical consideration

When treating a male patient with GTN, the paramedic should ensure they have taken a full medicines history. This is due to a potentially severe interaction between GTN and drugs used to treat erectile dysfunction (Viagra® (sildenafil), Cialis® (tadalafil)). Most erectile dysfunction drugs work by increasing vasodilation in the penis. While this effect is primarily seen locally, there may be more systemic vasodilation and hence hypotension. Thus, if a patient who has recently taken their ED medication is given GTN (which is also a vasodilatory drug), there is a risk of compounding the effects of both and resulting in profound hypotension (JRCALC, 2020).

Managing adverse drug reactions

While every effort should be made to avoid ADRs, given their prevalence it is essential to be able to manage them when they do occur. If the patient is presenting with an anaphylactic reaction then they should be treated as per the protocol on page XX, but if the patient's symptoms are less severe, then less immediate action may be called for. However, once an ADR of any severity is suspected, then it must be investigated and managed appropriately.

Because the signs and symptoms can range from subtle and idiosyncratic to overt, it is essential that the paramedic and indeed all healthcare professionals are aware of the potential for adverse reactions and confident to raise concerns about them where suspected (Montané and Santesmases, 2020).

Presuming that the adverse reaction does not require emergency action or resuscitative measures as these have been covered previously, there are still several measures that should be considered. If possible, administration of the drug suspected of causing the reaction should be ceased.

Clinical consideration

Morphine and other opiates are commonly used in paramedic practice to provide analgesia; a common side-effect of opiate medication, especially by the intravenous route, is hypotension. The paramedic may find that their patient experiences a drop in blood pressure following administration of morphine, and then would need to counter this by stopping the administration of the drug, or in extremis reversing the effect with an opiate antagonist.

Similarly, patients may experience stinging or burning when given intravenous hydrocortisone too rapidly, which may be countered by pausing administration or slowing the rate of administration.

In some situations cessation of treatment may be all that is needed to mitigate the risk and end the adverse reaction, and in all cases appropriate communication with the patient and other healthcare professionals, including their GP, in order to log the adverse reaction, is essential.

Some adverse reactions may need longer-term care and treatment, for example, physiotherapy for quinolone-induced Achilles tendinitis or inpatient care of an acute kidney injury due to NSAID use in a vulnerable patient. In these cases, the paramedic will need to refer the patient on for care by their own GP or an admission to hospital, depending on the circumstances. Advice can be obtained from the patient's GP or senior clinician if unsure.

A useful method for helping to identify ADRs produced by medications which the paramedic administers is to educate the patient on the common adverse effects of any drug given, so they are better placed to recognise a problem and seek help at an earlier stage.

Once any immediate intervention has been made and treatment stopped, the patient should be reviewed with the following considerations.

- Review treatment options. This could include stopping further administration of the suspected causative agent if significant harm has occurred or if the patient requests it.
- If the patient still needs treatment for the underlying condition then an alternative drug should be considered.
- If the drug that caused the adverse reaction is the only one that is suitable then a review of the dose is necessary, for example opiate toxicity in palliative care.
- Temporary cessation of treatment may be adequate, for instance if a patient experienced a kidney injury by taking metformin during a dehydrating illness. This action may be taken retrospectively to treat a kidney injury that has already occurred or prophylactically to reduce the risk of one. The sick day rules provide a useful reference for pre-emptively suspending treatment during minor dehydrating illness (NHS England, 2020).
- Pharmacological management of the adverse reaction may be needed. This could be immediate treatment such as reversal of opioid effects with an opioid antagonist, or it may be the prescribing of a new treatment, although best practice should be to try and avoid prescribing a medication to treat the side-effects of another, given the well-established risks of polypharmacy.
- The adverse reaction should be recorded in the patient's notes such that it is accessible to anyone accessing their shared care record, and should be reported using the Yellow Card system or local incident reporting system if this is not available.

Clinical consideration

Opioid drugs can be used in significant doses in palliative care which may lead to opioid toxicity; the symptoms include confusion, stupor, constricted pupils, nausea, vomiting, constipation, loss of appetite, and in more severe cases circulatory and respiratory depression. While opioid toxicity can be reversed with an opioid antagonist, extreme care should be taken in a palliative care situation, as acute reversal of opiate medication may result in significant pain and distress to the patient and their relatives. The appropriate action is likely to be omission of future doses or dose reduction rather than acute reversal.

Skills in practice: adrenaline dosing in anaphylaxis

A fundamental part of paramedic practice is the ability to manage high-acuity patient presentations, including anaphylaxis. Doses of drugs for emergency use should be memorised, and then checked prior to administration. Table 7.3 presents the adrenaline dosing for anaphylaxis.

Table 7.3   Adrenaline dosing guidance.

Age	Dose	Repeat dose	Dose interval	Maximum dose
12 years and over	500 mg	500 mg	5 minutes	No max. dose
6–11 years	300 mg	300 mg	5 minutes	No max. dose
Birth to 5 years	150 mg	150 mg	5 minutes	No max. dose

Source: JRCALC (2020).

The management of anaphylaxis is likely to involve multiple drug therapies via several administration routes. Adrenaline must only be given by the intramuscular (IM) route when treating anaphylaxis, as rapid administration of concentrated adrenaline intravenously can cause significant side-effects such as chest pain and tachycardia. There is also a risk of local vasoconstriction and tissue necrosis if the IV access is peripheral (McLean-Tooke et al. 2003).

Reporting adverse drug reactions

All healthcare professionals must act in the best interests of their patient, which places a duty of care upon the paramedic to consider the possibility of ADRs as a possible cause of illness when clinically relevant, and to report them without delay (HCPC, 2020).

The reporting of ADRs is an essential part of the process of pharmacovigilance, the scientific method for monitoring, detecting, evaluating and preventing incidences of ADRs and any other medicine-related problem (European Medicines Agency, 2020).

In the UK, ADRs are reported to, and monitored by, the Medicines and Healthcare products Regulatory Agency (MHRA), using the Yellow Card system. Introduced in 1964, following the serious adverse effects identified in the children of pregnant mothers given thalidomide in the 1950s (Coleman and Pontefract, 2016) to identify, monitor and prevent similar situations recurring, this was initially a paper form found in the back of all copies of the *British National Formulary* to be filled out by hand but is now accessible in digital formats and reports can be made physically, by phone or online (MHRA, 2020a). Through the Yellow Card system, the MHRA collects data on all suspected ADRs, including those involving alternative therapies, recreational drugs and medical devices, in adults and children. In Australia, a similar system, known as the Adverse Drug Reactions Advisory Committee (ADRAC) Blue Card system, has been in operation since 1964 (Australian Government, 2021).

The National Institute for Health and Care Excellence (2017) states that a Yellow Card should be submitted to report any suspected or proven adverse reaction in the following circumstances.

- All ADRs in adults and children which are serious, medically significant, or result in harm.
- Any ADR associated with a black triangle product, whether considered harmful or not.

N.B. A black triangle product is a new medicine or vaccine which is under additional monitoring. These medicines are denoted in the BNF, Summaries of Product Characteristics, patient information leaflets and technical literature with an inverted black triangle symbol (▼). Any new medicine, including vaccines, is always monitored more closely, because the clinical trials conducted prior to making a drug available involve a limited number of subjects. Once available to the public, a drug is likely to be used by a much larger and more diverse patient population, so previously unidentified adverse effects may come to light. Sometimes adverse reactions associated with a drug may not become apparent for some time after it has become widely available hence the need for more intensive monitoring when new (MHRA, 2020b).

The MHRA is especially interested in any adverse reactions which:

- occur in children
- occur in anyone aged over 65
- involve biological medicines and vaccines
- involve defective or substandard medicines or devices
- involve fake or counterfeit medicines or devices.
- involve complementary remedies
- produce congenital defects.

Skills in practice: completing a Yellow Card

Reporting of ADRs, either suspected or confirmed, is via the Yellow Card system in the UK (Figure 7.5). It should be carried out as soon as possible once there is suspicion of an adverse reaction. These reports can be made in the following ways.

- Electronically via the MHRA Yellow Card website (https://yellowcard.mhra.gov.uk/).
- Using the yellowcard mobile app.
- By completing the Yellow Card form found in BNFs and posting it to the MHRA.
- By emailing yellowcard@mhra.gsi.gov.uk.
- By calling the national Yellow Card information service (0808 100 3352).]

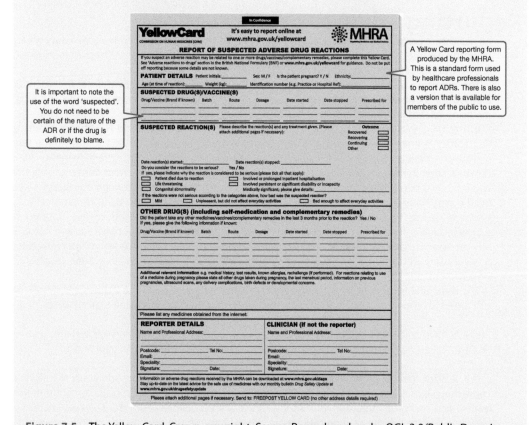

Figure 7.5   The Yellow Card. Crown copyright. *Source:* Reproduced under OGL 3.0/Public Domain.

In addition to reporting an adverse reaction, the clinician must make sure it is documented in the patient's notes and ideally the patient or their carer should be made aware as well.

Once the MHRA has been notified of an adverse reaction, it will assess the date and collate it with any other information in order to produce a report on the medicine, and this will then be published and disseminated widely in order that action to mitigate further potential harm can be taken (Kaufman, 2016).

Actions that may be taken by the MHRA include:

- restricting the use of a medicine or device
- changing the legal status of the medicine or device (from over the counter to prescription only)
- amending the medicine's or device's warning information
- removing the marketing authorisation for the medicine or device and banning its use in the UK.

When reporting an adverse reaction via the Yellow Card system, the following information will be needed (MHRA, 2020a).

- The name and address of the reporter. This can be the clinician who started the treatment suspected of causing the reaction, the clinician who suspected the adverse reaction, or the patient themselves.
- As much information as possible about the patient; this would include initials, sex, age, ethnicity, pregnancy status and an NHS or hospital number.
- Information about the drug suspected of causing the adverse reaction, including, where possible, name, brand, batch, route, dose, start and end dates and the indication it was given for.
- The nature of the suspected reaction, the outcome and severity of the reaction and any treatment given for it.
- Details (if known) of any other drugs the patient was taking within the 3 months prior to the reaction, including over-the-counter and complementary therapies.
- Any other relevant information, which may include medical and drug history, investigation and test results. For example, if the adverse reaction occurred during pregnancy, specific information relating to all other concurrent treatments and clinical information about the pregnancy should be included.

It must be kept in mind that without adequate reporting, the process of pharmacovigilance and the subsequent reduction in incidence and harm caused by adverse reactions will be less effective. While spontaneous notification is the most common method of identifying adverse reactions, its efficacy is significantly limited by under-reporting (Montané and Santesmases, 2020), with some authors suggesting that only around 5% of adverse reactions are actually reported (Coleman and Pontefract, 2016). This should further prompt the clinician to remain alert to the potential for ADRs and to report them whenever they are suspected.

Episode of care

While working as a paramedic on an ambulance, you are called to Harriet, an 85-year-old resident in a nursing home. She is frail, weighs only 53 kg, and has recently been suffering from a bout of gastroenteritis, leaving her dehydrated and feeling dizzy. The dizziness causes her to fall in her room when getting up from her chair. She is found by one of the nurses, who calls an ambulance when Harriet complains of new hip pain.

Upon your arrival, you observe that she is showing signs of pain in the right hip, and the right leg is shorter and rotated externally. You suspect she has fractured the neck of her femur. Harriet is cannulated and given 1 g of paracetamol injection to treat her pain, but this only reduces her pain from 8 to 6 and she is still too uncomfortable to be moved. Following a stepwise approach, you give the patient 5 mg of morphine intravenously which reduces her pain. However, within 5 minutes you note that she has become drowsy, and her previously healthy blood pressure of 140/89 mmHg has dropped to 75/40 mmHg; her respiratory effort remains adequate.

You consider the morphine the likely cause of the drop in blood pressure based on the known actions of morphine and other opioids. You consider reversing the effects of the morphine using naloxone but you are aware this would result in return of the patient's pain. Harriet's blood pressure is stable albeit low and she is still making a good respiratory effort. You decide that giving a fluid bolus to counteract the low blood pressure is an appropriate action which will not affect pain control.

After a bolus of 250 mL 0.9% normal saline (sodium chloride solution), Harriet's blood pressure increases to 135/80 mm Hg and her level of consciousness improves. You discuss what you suspect is an adverse effect of morphine with your clinical supervisor and decide that in future, with frail older patients, a better course of action would be to start with a lower dose of morphine and titrate up gradually. When a similar scenario arises, you are able to mitigate the risk of adverse effects by giving the patient 2.5 mg morphine initially, increasing this gradually, rather than giving a single larger initial dose.

Conclusion

Adverse drug reactions have been discussed in this chapter, including those patient groups more prone to experiencing them, common signs and symptoms, management and reporting. The awareness of ADRs and their consequences is important as the significant prevalence and cost associated with them represent a large burden on the health service.

It is important to understand the types of ADRs and be able to report them but, more importantly, a knowledge of ADRs is essential to underpin medications administration decisions and decisions to treat patients, taking into account their risk factors for adverse reactions. This should assist the paramedic in making informed decisions.

References

Australian Government, Department of Health Therapeutic Goods Administration. (2021). *Blue card adverse reaction reporting form*. www.tga.gov.au/form/blue-card-adverse-reaction-reporting-form

Burge, S., Matin, R. and Wallis, D. (2016). *Oxford Handbook of Medical Dermatology*, 2nd edn. Oxford: Oxford University Press.

Coleman, J.J. and Pontefract, S.K. (2016). Adverse drug reactions. *Clinical Medicine* **16**(5): 48485.

College of Paramedics. (2018). *Practice Guidance for Paramedics for the Administration of Medicines Under Exemptions within the Human Medicines Regulations*. www.collegeofparamedics.co.uk/COP/Professional_development/Medicines_and_Independent_Prescribing/COP/ProfessionalDevelopment/Medicines_and_Independent_Prescribing.aspx?hkey=04486919-f7b8-47bd-8d84-47bfc11d821a

European Medicines Agency. (2020). *Pharmacovigilance: overview*. www.ema.europa.eu/en/human-regulatory/overview/pharmacovigilance-overview

Gallagher, P., Ryan, C., O'Connor, Mm, Byrne, S., O'Sullivan, D. and O'Mahoney, D. (2014). STOPP (Screening tool of older persons prescriptions)/START (Screening tool to alert doctors to right treatment) criteria for potentially inappropriate prescribing in older people version 2. *Age and Ageing* **44**(2): 213–218.

Health and Care Professions Council (HCPC). (2020). *Standards of conduct, performance and ethics*. www.hcpc-uk.org/standards/standards-of-conduct-performance-and-ethics/

Holmquist, G. (2009). Opioid metabolism and effects of cytochrome P450. *Pain Medicine* **10**(s1): S20–S29.

Howard, R., Avery, A. and Slaensburg, S. (2007). Which drugs cause preventable admissions to hospital? A systematic review. *British Journal of Clinical Pharmacology* **63**(2): 136–147.

Joint Royal Colleges Ambulance Liaison Committee (JRCALC). (2020). *Clinical Practice Guidelines*. Bridgwater: Class Professional Publishing.

Kaufman, G. (2016). Adverse drug reactions: classification, susceptibility and reporting. *Nursing Standard* **30**(50): 53–56.

Lane, N., Stukel, T. and Boyd, C. (2019). Long-term care residents geriatric syndromes at admission and disablement over time: an observational cohort study. *Journal of Gerontology* **74**(6): 917–923.

Longmore, M., Wilkinson, I., Davidson, E., Foulkes, A. and Mafi, A. (2010). *Oxford Handbook of Clinical Medicine*, 8th edn. Oxford: Oxford University Press.

McKay, G., Reid, J. and Walters, M. (2010). *Clinical Pharmacology and Therapeutics*, 8th edn. Oxford: Wiley Blackwell.

McLean-Tooke, A., Bethune, C., Fay, A. and Spickett, G. (2003). Adrenaline in the treatment of anaphylaxis: what is the evidence? *BMJ* **327**(7427): 1332–1335.

Medicines and Healthcare products Regulatory Agency (MHRA). (2015). *Guidance on adverse drug reactions*. https://assets.publishing.service.gov.uk/government/uploads/system/uploads/attachment_data/file/949130/Guidance_on_adverse_drug_reactions.pdf

Medicines and Healthcare products Regulatory Agency. (2020a). *About Yellow Card*. https://yellowcard.mhra.gov.uk/the-yellow-card-scheme/

Medicines and Healthcare products Regulatory Agency. (2020b). *Black triangle scheme – new medicines and vaccines subject to EU-wide additional monitoring*. www.gov.uk/guidance/the-yellow-card-scheme-guidance-for-healthcare-professionals#black-triangle-scheme

Montané, E. and Santesmases, J. (2020). *Adverse drug reactions. Medicina Clinica (English Edition)* **154**(5): 178–184.

National Institute for Health and Care Excellence (NICE). (2017). *Adverse drug reactions*. https://cks.nice.org.uk/topics/adverse-drug-reactions/

Nguyen, C. and Miller, D. (2017). Serum sickness-like drug reaction: two cases with a neutrophilic urticarial pattern. *Journal of Cutaneous Pathology* **44**(2): 177–182.

NHS England. (2020). *Sick day rules: how to manage type 2 diabetes if you become unwell with coronavirus and what to do with your medication*. www.england.nhs.uk/london/wp-content/uploads/sites/8/2020/04/3.-Covid-19-Type-2-Sick-Day-Rules-Crib-Sheet-06042020.pdf

Pharmaceutical Society of Australia. (2019). *Medicine Safety Report*. www.psa.org.au/wp-content/uploads/2019/01/PSA-Medicine-Safety-Report.pdf

Pirmohamed, M., James, S., Meakin, S. et al. (2004). Adverse drug reactions as cause of admission to hostpial: prospective analysis of 18820 patients. *BMJ* **329**(7456): 9–15.

Resuscitation Council UK. (2020). *Guidance: anaphylaxis*. www.resus.org.uk/library/additional-guidance/guidance-anaphylaxis

Royal Pharmaceutical Society. (2020). *Polypharmacy: getting our medicines right*. www.rpharms.com/recognition/setting-professional-standards/polypharmacy-getting-our-medicines-right

Van der Weide, J., Steijins, L. and van Weelden, M. (2003). The effect of smoking and cytochrome P450 CYP1A2 genetic polymorphism on clozapine clearance and dose requirement. *Pharmacogenetics* **13**(3): 169–172.

Further reading

Blaber, A., Collen, A. and Ingram, H. (2018). *Independent Prescribing for Paramedics*. Bridgwater: Class Publishing.

Ferner, R. and McGettigan, P. (2018). Adverse drug reactions. *BMJ* **363**: k4051.

Ritter, J., Flower, R., Henderson, G., Loke, Y., MacEwan, D. and Rang, H. (2019). *Rang and Dale's Pharmacology*, 9th edn. St Louis: Elsevier.

United Kingdom Teratology Information Service. (2021). *BUMPS: best use of medicines in pregnancy*. www.medicinesinpregnancy.org/

Multiple-choice questions

1. Which category of adverse drug reaction is most common?
   - (a) D
   - (b) A
   - (c) B
   - (d) E

2. How do you report a suspected adverse drug reaction?
   - (a) MHRA yellowcard scheme
   - (b) Local organisational event reporting system
   - (c) Both

3. What is the approximate percentage of hospital admissions related to adverse drug reactions?
   - (a) 1%
   - (b) 6%
   - (c) 12%
   - (d) 20%

4. What is the estimated cost per year in the UK of adverse drug reactions?
   - (a) £168M
   - (b) £412M
   - (c) £750M
   - (d) £900M

5. Pregnancy is a risk factor for increased chance of an adverse drug reaction.
    (a) True
    (b) False

6. Which of these drugs is most likely to cause a Type E, or end of treatment, reaction?
    (a) Paracetamol
    (b) Sertraline
    (c) Ramipril
    (d) Morphine

7. Anaphylaxis (a Type B reaction) is likely to occur shortly after drug administration.
    (a) True
    (b) False

8. Which of these drugs is least likely to cause an adverse drug reaction?
    (a) Ibuprofen
    (b) Warfarin
    (c) Benzylpenicillin
    (d) Oxygen

9. Who has responsibility for reporting adverse drug reactions?
    (a) Paramedics
    (b) Patients
    (c) Doctors
    (d) All of the above

10. Patients on multiple drugs are at greater risk of adverse drug reactions. What is the term used to describe treatment with multiple drugs?
    (a) Polypharmacy
    (b) Polymyalgia
    (c) Pharmacology
    (d) Pharmacokinetics

11. Adverse drug reactions can be produced by alternative therapies, including herbal remedies.
    (a) True
    (b) False

12. What percentage of adverse drug reactions can be predicted based on the pharmacology of the drug?
    (a) 80%
    (b) 12%
    (c) 55%
    (d) 68%

13. What is the suggested dose of adrenaline to treat anaphylaxis in adults?
    (a) 500 mg
    (b) 1 mg
    (c) 500 µg
    (d) 1 g

14. How many people per 100 000 die as a result of adverse drug reactions per year?
    (a) 0.9
    (b) 2.0
    (c) 2.5
    (d) 3.9

15. Why is reducing adverse drug reactions important?
    (a) To reduce heathcare costs
    (b) To reduce preventable deaths
    (c) To shorten inpatient stays
    (d) All of the above

Chapter 8

Analgesics

Tom Mallinson

Aim

This chapter will provide an introduction and overview to medications commonly used to treat pain, with a focus on those applicable to acute pain in a prehospital setting. Consideration will be given to these medications' pharmacological mechanisms of action and how they can be used synergistically as part of a multimodal approach to analgesia.

Learning outcomes

After reading this chapter the reader will:

1. Understand the mechanism of action of common classes of analgesic drugs
2. Be able to discuss the benefits and limitations of specific drugs or classes of drug
3. Have a greater awareness of the need for a multimodal approach to analgesia
4. Be able to consider appropriate drug choices for a range of conditions.

Pain and analgesia

Assessing pain can be challenging, and discomfort can be experienced due to any number of causes. The provision of analgesia can also be a complex process, requiring a good working knowledge of the pharmacological properties of the medicines being used to facilitate safe and effective polypharmacy. To fully address a patient's pain, we must first understand how and why they are experiencing it and ideally be able to quantify the extent of their discomfort.

Understanding and assessing pain

Pain is a feature of inflammation and injury, these features being *calor* (Heat), *dolor* (Pain), *rubor* (Erythema/Redness), *tumor* (Swelling), *et functio laesa* (Loss of Function), with the functional limitations described possibly also being due to pain.

A widely accepted definition of pain is: *An unpleasant sensory and emotional experience which is associated with actual (or potential) tissue damage, or that is described in terms of such damage.* While this definition is useful, it has some limitations. Most notably, it includes reference to how a sensation is described, yet clearly even if one were unable to articulate a description of pain, that pain would still be experienced. This is especially relevant when we consider the care of those who cannot effectively communicate verbally and any pain assessment tool must take this into consideration.

Fundamentals of Pharmacology for Paramedics, First Edition. Edited by Ian Peate, Suzanne Evans, and Lisa Clegg.
© 2022 John Wiley & Sons Ltd. Published 2022 by John Wiley & Sons Ltd.

Why do we treat pain?

There are many reasons to treat pain, not least because it is unpleasant and from a humanitarian point of view we should seek to reduce suffering whenever possible. Indeed, humanitarian considerations are also a recognised indication for prehospital anaesthesia, where this is felt to be the only option for providing appropriate and safe analgesia. Another core reason to provide appropriate analgesia is to reduce the physiological response to pain which can be detrimental to healing and worsens morbidity (Page, 2013; Tsui et al., 1997) and to mitigate the unwanted psychological sequelae of experiencing a painful event.

Psychology of pain

Experiencing pain is unpleasant. It has both psychological and emotional impact, as well as the physiological response discussed later. Episodes of severe acute pain can precipitate and lead to long-term sequelae such as post-traumatic stress disorder (PTSD), while the presence of PTSD worsens the experience of any subsequent pain. We know that fear and anxiety will heighten psychological arousal and increase the intensity of pain, and many of the non-pharmacological interventions are targeted at reducing such concerns (see Table 8.1).

In relation to chronic pain, pharmacological interventions may be inadequate to offer adequate relief, and as clinicians we may need to look to social or psychological interventions to allow a patient to better manage their pain and facilitate a return to normality. One of the most promising psychological interventions is cognitive behavioural therapy, which is widely used for pain, depression, anxiety and many other conditions. Such interventions require a truly multidisciplinary approach to be successful, and it is important that as clinicians, we understand and respect the beneficial effects of such non-pharmacological interventions (Parkinson, 2015; Russell et al., 2014).

For many patients, psychological distress can severely exacerbate pain, and can make an upsetting experience truly terrifying. This is especially true of those at the extremes of age and other vulnerable groups. In such cases, non-pharmacological interventions to address distress and pain are vitally important. Such non-pharmacological interventions, both psychological and physical, are represented by the TWEED SASH mnemonic (Table 8.1).

Table 8.1   Non-pharmacological interventions to relieve distress and pain (TWEED SASH).

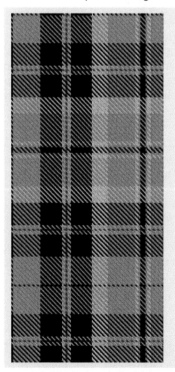

Psychological analgesia:
Therapeutic Touch (e.g. hand-holding)
Warn about any painful interventions
Explain what is happening or about to happen
Establish Eye contact
Defend patient Dignity

Physical interventions:
Stabilise fractures
Apply dressings to burns
Soft surface (*early removal from rigid stretchers*)
Hypothermia avoidance (*hypothermia increases perceived pain intensity*)

Table 8.2 Physiological manifestations of pain.

Body system	Effect of pain
Cardiovascular	• Tachycardia • Hypertension • Vasoconstriction • Increased myocardial oxygen consumption
Respiratory	• Tachypnoea
Neurological	• Mydriasis (pupillary dilation) • Increased sympathetic tone
Endocrine	• Increased serum glucose • Increased serum cortisol
Gastrointestinal	• Reduced gastric emptying • Reduced intestinal motility • Nausea and vomiting • Constipation • Inappetence or anorexia
Urinary	• Sodium retention • Fluid retention
Musculoskeletal	• Hyper-reflexia
General	• Increased oxygen demand • Piloerection • Diaphoresis • Immunosuppression

Physiology of pain

Experiencing pain is not only psychologically unpleasant but can be detrimental to health and healing (Swift, 2018). Pain can cause significant derangement of physiology separately from the illness or injury causing the pain (Table 8.2). This is detrimental for a number of reasons: such deranged physiology may mask or confuse underlying pathology, making diagnosis more challenging, and many of these effects can also lead to further morbidity themselves. Increased myocardial oxygen demand could cause angina, hypertension and tachycardia can contribute to increased blood loss and atelectasis can lead to pneumonia. It is important to remember these detrimental effects of pain when considering the provision of analgesia to our patients, and also when attempting to assess pain in those who cannot clearly communicate with clinicians, such as children, those with significant intellectual disability and anaesthetised patients.

Pain, however, also has an evolutionary benefit, in that it facilitates avoidant and protective behaviours to either stop ongoing injury or tissue damage or promote healing through resting or protecting an injured part of the body. The increase in sympathetic tone seen as a result of pain is also part of the fight or flight mechanism, intended to aid survival.

Pain transmission

In normal physiology, the sensation of pain is perceived when specific nerve impulses reach the brain. The main sensors of painful stimuli are the endings of myelinated A delta and unmyelinated C primary sensory neurons, which detect damaging or potentially damaging (noxious) stimuli. Other sensory receptors and nerve fibres are responsible for touch and proprioception (Table 8.3).

Such stimuli are transmitted through the peripheral (primary) sensory fibres to the spinal cord. Here, they terminate in the dorsal horns and form synapses with secondary neurons which transmit the nerve impulses to the cerebral cortex (this is known as an ascending pathway), where the stimuli are consciously perceived as pain and can trigger avoidant behaviour. Once these nerve impulses reach the brain, they cause activation of multiple regions of the brain including the somatosensory cortices, thalamus, anterior cingulate cortex, motor regions,

Table 8.3 Features of sensory nerve fibres.

Nerve fibre type	Myelin sheath	Conduction speed (metres per second)	Sensory modality
A alpha	Yes	120	Proprioception (muscle length and stretch)
A beta	Yes	75	Stretch, skin touch and pain
A delta	Yes	30	Acute pain, pressure and cold
C	No	2	Pain and warmth

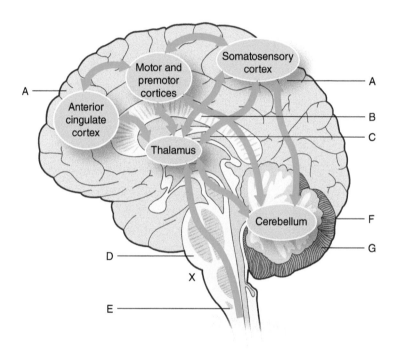

Figure 8.1 The pain matrix.

premotor cortex and cerebellum, collectively known as the 'pain matrix' (Figure 8.1). In response to a stimulus from these ascending pathways, descending modulating pathways will become active.

Pain modulation

A number of theories have been put forward to better understand the modulation of pain. One of the most famous, the gate control theory, suggests that concurrent tactile stimulation of the A beta fibres (for example, by rubbing the skin) near the location of a painful stimulus results in presynaptic inhibition within the spinal cord, thus blocking transmission of pain signals through the slower A delta and C fibres. Another means of pain modulation is the descending modulatory pathways (Figure 8.2). These pathways originate in the midbrain and medulla in areas with high concentrations of opioid receptors and carry impulses from the brain down to the dorsal horn, where they inhibit ascending transmission or pain signals. This interaction within the dorsal horn is regulated by the neurotransmitters serotonin and noradrenaline. In addition to their actions in the midbrain and medulla, endogenous endorphins and enkephalins interact with opioid receptors in the spinal cord to inhibit and modulate pain transmission (Bannister, 2019).

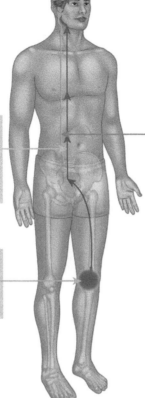

The perception of the pain signals in the somatosensory cortex can be influenced by psychological, physical and social factors.

Primary sensory neurons carry impulses via afferent A-delta and C fibres, which terminate in the dorsal horn of the spinal cord. Secondary neurons carry the signal from the spinal cord to the brain.

Descending efferent pathways send signals to the dorsal horn, activating neurotransmitters to release noradrenaline, serotonin and endorphins which inhibit ascending pain signals.

Stimulation of nociceptors by chemicals (histamine and prostaglandins) released when tissue injury or irritation occurs (i.e. heat, cold, chemicals).

Figure 8.2   The pain pathway.

Clinical consideration

A number of abnormal pain syndromes exist where benign, mild or normally imperceptible stimulation results in increased pain perception. Such conditions can give rise to *allodynia* (pain from light touch), *hyperalgesia* (extreme pain from mild noxious stimuli), *hyperesthesia* (increased sensitivity to mild stimuli) or a host of other abnormal responses.

The condition of phantom limb pain can even cause apparent pain in an arm or leg that has been amputated. These conditions are challenging to manage and require a combination of pharmacological and psychological interventions.

Types of pain

A wide variety of terminology is used when discussing pain and the provision of analgesia. Having an understanding of the types of pain people may experience informs a clinician's choice of analgesia and to some extent may predict which agents may be most effective. Pain sensations can be classified as either nociceptive or neuropathic (or mixed), with these two types responding to different analgesic approaches (Figure 8.3)

The perception of nociceptive pain (from the Latin *nocere* meaning harm) results from damage, or threatened damage, to body tissue. Such insult is signalled by intact and functioning pain nerve fibres which transmit this information to the brain, as opposed to neuropathic pain, discussed below.

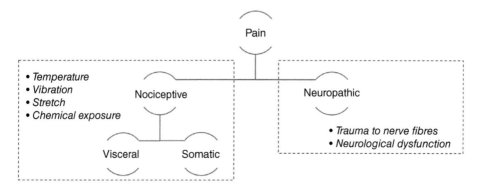

Figure 8.3   Categorisation of pain.

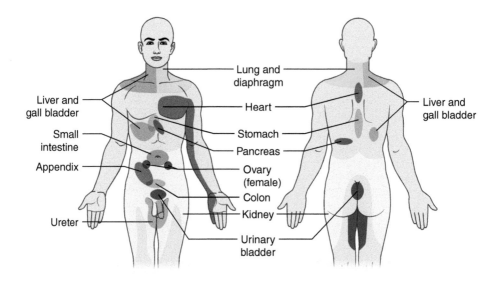

Figure 8.4   Common sites of referred pain.

The sensory fibres involved in this pathway are called nociceptors, and are able to sense and trans-duce a range of noxious stimuli, including extremes of temperature, vibration, stretch and chemical exposure. This includes exposure to inflammatory mediators which both excite and sensitise nociceptors.

Nociceptive pain can be further divided into somatic or visceral pain, depending on where the pain originates. Somatic pain arises from the soma (skin, skeletal muscle and bone) and is often well localised. Visceral pain results from injury or insult to the viscera (internal organs such as the liver, bowel, heart, etc). This is less well localised and may be referred to other adjacent structures (Figure 8.4). Examples include experiencing pain in the shoulder tip as a result of diaphragmatic irri-tation (for example, due to liver pathology), probbly due to a shared innervation of the diaphragm and shoulder tip (C4 nerve root), or pain in the left arm and jaw as a result of myocardial ischaemia or infarction. The causes behind all cases of referred pain are not fully understood, but some are thought to arise from a convergence of nerve fibres from different organs along the pain pathway.

Neuropathic pain, on the other hand, occurs as a result of damage or irritation to the pain fibres themselves. It occurs acutely in traumatic injuries such as amputations or non-freezing cold injuries and can be the cause of significant ongoing morbidity. In many cases, neuropathic pain is harder to diagnose and treat than nociceptive pain.

Clinical considerations

An understanding of nociception and relevant anatomy facilitates accurate testing of specific nerves.
When undertaking cranial nerve testing, for example, cranial nerve I, the olfactory nerve (sense of smell), must be tested with an innocuous/benign scent (e.g. lemon peel/coffee) as any noxious stimuli such as the isopropyl alcohol from a preinjection swab or the ammonia in smelling salts would result in stimulation of intranasal trigeminal pain nerve fibres, thus bypassing a potentially damaged olfactory nerve.

Some injuries create intense pain which appears out of keeping with clinical findings or visible tissue damage. Three important examples are high-voltage electrical burns, high-pressure injection injuries from hydraulic lines and compartment syndrome, all of which require emergency assessment and treatment.

Assessment of pain

It is valuable to be able to quantify the severity of pain, as this allows not only appropriate selection of drug and dosages, but also reassessment of pain levels after interventions have been made (JRCALC, 2019). Commonly used scales include the verbal numerical pain scale/visual analogue scale, the Wong–Baker Scale and the FLACC score, each of which has its benefits and limitations. The verbal numerical pain scale and visual analogue scale are both validated for use in acute pain, can be used to report a quantifiable measure of pain, and are simple to administer with minimal training (Jennings et al., 2009; JRCALC, 2019). The two methods should not be used interchangeably as, despite their commonalities, they are not validated to be used in this way. The Wong–Baker face scale is also validated in acute care, but does require a patient to be able to see the faces on the score chart (Baker and Wong, 1987). It may be a highly useful score to use in children, and it overcomes language differences and perhaps some cultural differences, although the faces may be misconstrued as representing other emotions such as fear, sadness or anxiety. The Wong–Baker scale should be used in black and white, as the inclusion of colour invalidates the tool and may make it less accurate.

The Face, Legs, Activity, Cry and Consolability (FLACC) score has been utilised in paediatric patients (>2 months old) and also in critically ill adults (JRCALC, 2019; Merkel et al., 1997; Voepel-Lewis et al., 2010). It utilises a combined scoring system with five components. Scores range from 0 to 10, with 10 indicating the most intense pain (Table 8.4).

Table 8.4   FLACC Score.

Criterion	Score 0	Score 1	Score 2
Face	No particular expression or smile	Occasional grimace or frown, withdrawn, uninterested	Frequent to constant quivering chin, clenched jaw
Legs	Normal position or relaxed	Uneasy, restless, tense	Kicking, or legs drawn up
Activity	Lying quietly, normal position, moves easily	Squirming, shifting, back and forth, tense	Arched, rigid or jerking
Cry	No cry (awake or asleep)	Moans or whimpers; occasional complaint	Crying steadily, screams or sobs, frequent complaints
Consolability	Content, relaxed	Reassured by occasional touching, hugging or being talked to, distractible	Difficult to console or comfort

Source: Adapted from Merkel et al. (1997) and Voepel-Lewis et al. (2010).

In cases of complex or chronic pain, it is important to remember that pain is a biopsychosocial phenomenon, and a broad history must be obtained to fully understand the patient's experience. The simple mnemonics of SOCRATES or OPQRSTA can sometimes be a useful starting point for understanding a patient's experience of pain (Gregory and Mursell, 2015; JRCALC, 2019). In the OPQRSTA mnemonic, you ask about the Onset of the pain, in relation to when it was first noticed, what they were doing at the time and also the nature of its onset and progression. Next, you ask about any Provoking and relieving factors in relation to the pain; for example, a headache which is exacerbated by a change in posture may be due to raised intracranial pressure. The Quality of the pain is also useful to explore; chest pain described as burning or stinging may indicate a neuropathic cause such as shingles or cord compression, while a dull, heavy or crushing chest pain may point towards ischaemia. Radiation is also important to elicit; for example, lower back pain with pain radiating down both legs (bilateral sciatica) would be considered a red flag, while back pain without such radiation may be benign. An assessment of Severity is useful in both providing an insight into the patient's experience and assessing the efficacy of any treatments given. The tools discussed previously may assist with such quantification. Timing reminds you to clarify the time of pain onset, whether it has occurred at other times, and when the pain subsided, if it is no longer present. Asking about Associated symptoms is also valuable in putting the pain into a wider context, and forming your differential diagnosis. A headache with associated unilateral temporal artery tenderness would prompt you to consider temporal arteritis, while associated amaurosis fugax would make you consider a significant ischaemic insult and associated photophobia with neck stiffness would indicate meningism. In addition, gaining a full social history will provide an insight into complex personal circumstances, and allow you to put the pain symptom into a wider patient context.

Approach to analgesia

Using a combination of pharmacological and non-pharmacological methods can be an effective approach to the provision of effective analgesia (Thies et al., 2018). Multimodal analgesia, the use of multiple pharmacological agents acting via different mechanisms to control pain, is advocated in current clinical guidelines (JRCALC, 2019). In many cases it is most beneficial to give analgesics from various drug families/classes as they will have a synergistic effect and the patient is less likely to experience as great a side-effect burden compared to using a sole agent at higher doses. In Figure 8.5. At a more advanced level, these may be augmented or replaced with different agents or modalities, such as fentanyl, ketamine or regional anaesthesia techniques. The core UK paramedic

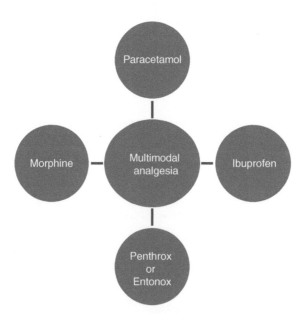

Figure 8.5   Example of multimodal analgesia provision.

analgesic pharmacopoeia will be discussed below (paracetamol, NSAIDs, inhalational analgesia, opioids). These agents can be combined in paramedic practice to provide multimodal analgesia during the prehospital phase. This will be followed by some additional agents which are used by advanced practitioners or doctors.

Find out more

The anatomy, physiology and pharmacology of pain is a huge area, and one which is acutely relevant to paramedic practice. While there are many avenues for further learning, the Faculty of Pain Medicine of the Royal College of Anaesthetists has provided the ePAIN learning platform which is an extremely valuable resource:

   https://fpm.ac.uk/faculty-of-pain-medicine/e-pain

The Royal College of Anaesthetists has also produced a separate suite of e-learning resources covering topics related to analgesia and anaesthesia more broadly, which is a useful source of further reading:

   https://rcoa.ac.uk/e-learning-anaesthesia
   Both of these are available through the e-Learning for Health website:
   https://portal.e-lfh.org.uk/

Paracetamol

Paracetamol (acetaminophen) is an analgesic with a poorly understand and complex mechanism of action. It inhibits prostaglandin synthesis and modulates serotonergic and cannabinoid pathways, acting both centrally and peripherally (Przybyla et al., 2021). Paracetamol can be administered orally, intravenously or rectally. It is a powerful analgesic and should be administered early in a patient's clinical journey for them to gain maximum benefit. It is used internationally in civilian and military prehospital care (Committee on Tactical Combat Casualty Care, 2020). It has a key benefit over the NSAIDs in that it does not cause gastric irritation (Table 8.5).

Paracetamol overdose

The majority of ingested paracetamol (around 90–95%) is conjugated in the liver to a non-toxic metabolite, in a process called glucuronidation, and excreted in the urine. The remaining paracetamol is oxidised by the cytochrome P450 enzyme, producing a hepatotoxic metabolite called *N*-acetyl-*p*-benzoquinone imine (or NAPQI for short), which when taken at therapeutic doses is deactivated through conjugation with glutathione. In overdose, however, the liver's supply of glutathione is exhausted and NAPQI accumulates and can lead to fulminant hepatic failure and death. The antidote to paracetamol overdose, N-acetylcysteine (NAC), replenishes the body's supply of glutathione, allowing metabolism of NAPQI.

Non-steroidal anti-inflammatory drugs

The term non-steroidal anti-inflammatory (NSAID) can be used to describe a wide range of medications (see Table 8.5). They are widely used in healthcare for both chronic and acute pain, but in general ibuprofen is the only one frequently administered by paramedics. These drugs act by inhibition of the cyclo-oxygenase enzymes, resulting in decreased production of inflammatory mediators, specifically the proinflammatory prostaglandins. Their analgesic effect is secondary to inhibition of the inflammatory response. They also have an antiplatelet effect through reducing the synthesis of thromboxane (Figure 8.6).

The NSAIDs may produce an unwanted direct toxic effect on the kidneys, leading to acute kidney injury (AKI) through a combination of acute tubular necrosis and acute interstitial nephritis, and are the cause of around 1 in 8 cases of acute drug-induced renal failure. This risk is exacerbated in the dehydrated or elderly. They can also lead to unwanted gastric irritation due to reduced protection of

Table 8.5   Comparison of common non-opioid analgesics.

	Drug	Maximum 24-hour dose (in adults >70 kg)	Time to peak plasma concentration (h)[a]	Half-life (h)	Gastric irritation
	Paracetamol	4 g	0.5–1	2–4	-
NSAIDs	Aspirin	4 g	1–2	Variable	+++
	Ibuprofen	1.2 g	0.5–1.5	2–3	++
	Naproxen	1 g	1–2	12–17	++++
	Diclofenac	150 mg	1–2	1–2	++++
	Ketorolac	60–90 mg	1	5–6	++
	Meloxicam	15 mg	2	15–20	+
	Celecoxib	400 mg	2–3	10–12	+

[a] When given orally.

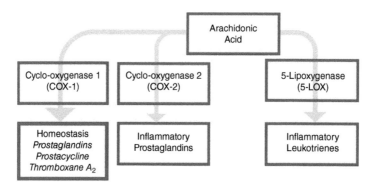

Figure 8.6   Role of the COX and LOX enzymes.

gastro-protective prostaglandins. Such irritation can be mild or may lead to fatal haemorrhage from perforated gastric ulceration. Therefore, concurrent administration of proton pump inhibitors such as omeprazole is often used when a course of NSAIDs is prescribed.

Salicylates

The salicylates include derivatives of acetylsalicylic acid, which gain their name from the white willow tree (*Salix alba*), from the bark of which the active ingredient salicin was identified. Aspirin is the most common example. It acts through irreversible inhibition of the COX-1 enzyme, and thus reduced thromboxane A_2 production with subsequent reduced platelet aggregation, and through modifying the activity of the COX-2 enzyme (see Figure 8.6). Aspirin is metabolised to salicylic acid, itself an active anti-inflammatory. Aspirin is, in general, contraindicated in children due to the occurrence of Reye syndrome, a notable exception being in cases of Kawasaki disease. In overdose, aspirin causes a metabolic acidosis, tinnitus, deafness, dizziness and in severe cases cerebral oedema, hyperpyrexia, seizures and death.

Find out more

Aspirin is also linked to a phenomenon called Samter's triad. This is the association between nasal polyps, asthma and respiratory symptoms triggered by aspirin or NSAIDs.
   You can read more at: www.samterssociety.org/

Propionic acid derivatives

The proprionic acid derivatives include ibuprofen, naproxen and ketoprofen. Ibuprofen is widely used by the topical and oral routes, and is available to many paramedics as part of their approach to multimodal analgesia. These medications are extremely useful for musculoskeletal pain, but have an associated risk of gastric irritation and if administered long term may worsen renal function. Naproxen is often preferred due to its twice-daily dosing but it confers a greater risk of gastric irritation.

Acetic acid derivatives

This class of NSAID includes diclofenac and ketorolac. Diclofenac is a commonly used analgesic agent available over the counter. It is often used as a topical gel or in tablet form. Diclofenac is also believed to inhibit both the COX and LOX enzymes, giving a dual anti-inflammatory effect (see Figure 8.6).

135

Ketorolac is an injectable NSAID used worldwide both in and out of hospital for numerous causes of pain. It can be delivered by the intravenous or intramuscular routes, making it a useful adjunct in acute pain for patients who are 'nil by mouth'.

Enolic acid derivatives

This group of NSAIDs, also known as the oxicams, contains the drugs piroxicam and meloxicam, and a number of others. Meloxicam is a favoured analgesic in military or remote settings due to its effectiveness, reduced platelet inhibition, low gastrointestinal risk and once-daily administration due to its long half-life (Committee on Tactical Combat Casualty Care, 2020; Wedmore and Butler, 2017). Many enolic acid derivatives are non-selective COX-1 and COX-2 inhibitors, but meloxicam is selective for COX-2.

Selective COX-2 inhibitors

These drugs, also known as the coxibs, selectively inhibit the COX-2 enzyme (see Figure 8.6). They have the benefit over many other NSAIDs that they only require once- or twice-daily dosing, due to their long duration of action. The risk of gastrointestinal bleeding and platelet dysfunction with COX-2 inhibitors is also less than many other NSAIDs. However, concerns have been raised about their cardiovascular safety profile, as their use seems to correlate with an increased risk of ischaemic cardiac events (Antman et al., 2007). Newer drugs are being developed which are dual COX-2 and 5-LOX inhibitors, which it is hoped will provide additional benefit by reducing leukotriene synthesis. 5-LOX inhibitors are found in small amounts in a number of plants, including St John's wort, used to treat depression.

Find out more

It is challenging to clearly delineate which of the non-opioids is better or stronger or more effective, and there is certainly significant individual variation between patients. The closest resource we have to answer this is probably the Oxford league table of analgesics. This is based on the drug's number needed to treat (NNT) in order to achieve a 50% reduction in pain when compared to a placebo. The lower the NNT number, the greater the efficacy of the analgesic in question.

While various similar tables are available in the literature, the table provided by the Bandolier team on its Oxford Pain Site is a useful place to start:

www.bandolier.org.uk/booth/painpag/Acutrev/Analgesics/Leagtab.html

Episode of care

Forty-year-old Emily calls an ambulance for severe back pain and pain down the back of one thigh. She relates a history of lower back pain for around 2 weeks, after lifting a lot of boxes when she moved house.

She has none of the red flags for serious pathologies, but is in enough pain to severely limit her ability to move. The attending crew feel she could safely be discharged on scene, but want to provide appropriate analgesia. They administer 1 g of oral paracetamol and 400 mg of oral ibuprofen and discuss non-pharmacological interventions like gentle stretching and mobilisation. They also provide safety netting advice, especially discussing the red flags for back pain.

Before they leave, the crew contact Emily's GP to enquire about other analgesic options. The duty doctor phones Emily back later that day and undertakes a telephone consultation. They then prescribe amitriptyline and opt to continue the ibuprofen but add in regular omeprazole for gastric protection. They provide further safety netting advice and will phone the patient back in a week's time.

Inhalational analgesia

Nitrous oxide

There are two main inhalation anaesthetics which are known to have analgesic properties along with their anaesthetic actions, and these are in frequent prehospital use at subanaesthetic doses, for analgesia. The first is nitrous oxide, which is administered in a mixture with 50% oxygen (JRCALC, 2019). The use of such a nitrous oxide:oxygen mixture has a number of drawbacks.

First, the two gases will separate at low temperatures (anything below around 5–10 °C), resulting in the administration of a high concentration of oxygen or an increasingly hypoxic concentration of nitrous oxide. Therefore, cold cylinders should be rewarmed and then inverted a number of times before use. Second, nitrous oxide diffuses into any gas-filled cavity within the body, potentially distending that space. Therefore, it should be avoided in conditions where this may cause significant harm, such as bowel obstruction, pneumocephaly, bullous emphysema or for patients who have recently been diving. Entonox use also raises intracranial pressure by increasing cerebral blood flow and should be avoided in head injuries.

Prolonged or repeated use of nitrous oxide can lead to the symptoms of vitamin B12 deficiency, due to its ability to oxidise and inactivate cobalamin (B12). These symptoms include sensory neuropathy, myopathy and encephalopathy, and it would be prudent to avoid its use in patients with known B12 deficiency or peripheral neuropathies. It is also unsuitable in a number of concurrent conditions and it is vital to be familiar with its specific contraindications (Box 8.1).

Methoxyflurane

The second most widely used inhalational agent is methoxyflurane (Penthrox®) which is a fluorinated hydrocarbon anaesthetic agent. When used for acute pain, however, it is being used at analgesic, rather than anaesthetic doses.

Methoxyflurane's analgesic effects occur through action in both the brain and spinal cord. It has this effect through interaction with various receptors including GABA receptors, potassium channels, glutamate and glycine receptors. It also interacts directly with components of second messenger systems.

Box 8.1   Contraindications to nitrous oxide:oxygen (50:50 mix) administration

- Decompression sickness[a]
- Head injuries
- Impaired consciousness
- Pneumothorax[a]
- Pneumocephalus[a]
- Pneumoperitoneum[a]
- Violent psychiatric patients
- Intraocular gas injection in preceding 8 weeks[a]
- Suspected bowel obstruction[a]

[a]Related to its diffusion into and distension of gas-filled spaces.

These functions lead to reduced transmission across synapses and conduction within neurons. Unlike some other analgesics, it produces little in the way of euphoria and does not appear to have an effect on the circulating levels of dopamine, serotonin or endogenous opioids. In prehospital care, it is inhaled as a vapour using the Green Whistle device, and produces an analgesic effect within 6–10 breaths, with one dose (3 mL) providing around 30 minutes of analgesia. It has been used successfully to provide analgesia for painful procedures and as a prehospital analgesic (Forrest et al., 2019).

Methoxyflurane does, however, have a number of contraindications and limitations related to its chemical nature and metabolism. The most significant of these is its contraindication in patients with a history of malignant hyperthermia from any cause, including other anaesthetic vapours, as it can trigger this condition (Box 8.2).

Box 8.2   Contraindications to methoxyflurane administration

- Malignant hyperthermia (in patient or family)
- Allergy/adverse reaction to anaesthetic vapours
- Impaired consciousness
- Significant head injuries
- Cardiovascular instability
- Renal impairment
- Ventilatory compromise

Skills in practice: Penthrox preparation and administration

1. Insert the activated charcoal chamber into the dilutor hole on the top of the green whistle.
2. Open the bottle of methoxyflurane, either by hand or using the base of the green whistle to loosen it.
3. Hold the green whistle at a 45° angle and pour the contents of the bottle into the base of the whistle.
4. Allow the patient to hold the device, and coach them to inhale through the mouthpiece.
5. Advise the patient to take a few small breaths initially to get used to the taste and smell.
6. Encourage the patient to inhale through the green whistle, which allows the activated charcoal chamber to absorb exhaled methoxyflurane.
7. Intermittent periods of inhalation through the device may be enough to provide analgesia, but continuous use of the device is also possible.
8. If a higher concentration of inhaled methoxyflurane is required, the hole on top of the activated charcoal chamber can be occluded, which reduces the entrainment of extra diluting air.
9. Once treatment is completed, dispose of the green whistle and methoxyflurane bottle in accordance with local policy.
10. If required, a second green whistle can be used for the same patient.

Opioids
Agonists
The opiates and opioids are drugs with active contents related to the chemicals found in the opium poppy (*Papaver somniferum*). Opiates are those medications which are directly related to the natural compounds found in such poppies, while opioids are synthetic compounds which have similar action to the natural opiates.

Opioid medications exert their action through binding with opioid receptors, which are predominantly located in the central nervous system but are also present in peripheral sites, such as the intestines. In this regard, the opioids we administer are activating intrinsic modulatory pathways which utilise endorphins and enkephalins. Unfortunately, one of these central locations is the chemoreceptor trigger zone on the surface of the medulla oblongata, which contains mu opioid receptors, resulting in nausea and vomiting with opioids.

The different subtypes of opioid receptors lead to different clinical effects when bound by an agonist (Table 8.6). Opioid agonists also share a common group of side-effects (Figure 8.7), with each individual drug having a slightly different side-effect profile. Some opioids, notably codeine and morphine, have a direct effect upon mast cells, leading to their degranulation and histamine release. Such an effect may mimic an allergic reaction, causing erythema, pruritus and flushing.

Table 8.6 Terminology for opioid receptors.

Preferred terminology	Alternative terminology	Clinical effect of agonist binding
δ, delta, DOP	OP1	• Respiratory depression • Cough suppression • Reduced gastric motility • Spinal analgesia
κ, kappa, KOP	OP2	• Spinal analgesia • Dysphoria • Hallucinations
μ, mu, MOP	OP3	• Spinal and supraspinal analgesia • Respiratory depression • Reduced gastrointestinal motility • Bradycardia • Euphoria • Nausea and vomiting
NOP[a], nociceptin receptor	OP4	• Anxiety • Possible role in opioid tolerance and dependence

[a] NOP receptors bind nociceptin (an antianalgesic) but not naloxone; it has little affinity to opioid drugs.

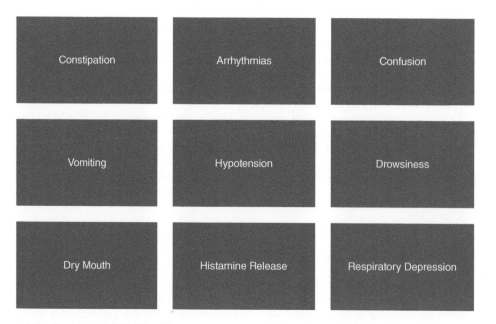

Figure 8.7 Common opioid side-effects

Morphine

Morphine is often considered the standard and archetypal opiate and other drugs in this class are often compared to it, in terms of their individual strengths or limitations. Clinically, morphine is a versatile drug and can be administered by various routes. Most commonly, in prehospital practice it is administered intravenously or intramuscularly, but the intranasal and intraosseous routes are also used. Nebulised morphine is also being researched as an option for acute pain, although findings are mixed at this time (Grissa et al., 2015; Mofidi et al., 2020). The metabolites of morphine are shown in Figure 8.8.

Codeine

Codeine is a weak agonist at the mu opioid receptor (MOP), but the majority of its analgesic effects are produced by its active metabolite – morphine (Figure 8.9). There is significant genetic variation in terms of gene expression of the hepatic enzymes responsible for the metabolism, meaning the rate of metabolism and therefore clinical effect of codeine vary significantly between patients. Due to this genetic difference, those of Asian or African descent may experience significantly less analgesic effect from codeine than someone whose genetic heritage is northern European. Some people even appear to gain no analgesic benefit from codeine at all, and this variability of effect is a significant drawback of codeine.

Diamorphine (heroin)

Diamorphine is a highly lipid-soluble opioid, which facilitates a rapid onset of action and also rapid movement across the blood–brain barrier. Its analgesic actions, which result from its active metabolites (Figure 8.10), are accompanied by a significant level of euphoria, making it a widely used drug of abuse (Scarth and Smith, 2016).

Diamorphine is increasingly being utilised in prehospital care in the UK by both the intravascular and intranasal routes of administration. It is available as a white powder in ampoules for reconstitution with water and a fairly large dose can be reconstituted into a small volume, making it ideal for intranasal or subcutaneous administration. It is commonly used in children by the intranasal route.

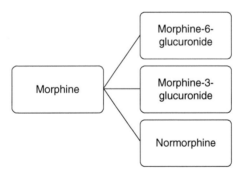

Figure 8.8   Morphine metabolism.

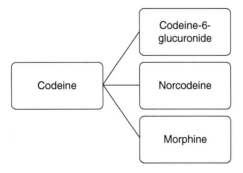

Figure 8.9   Codeine metabolism.

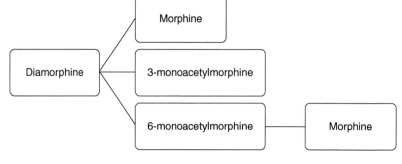

Figure 8.10   Diamorphine metabolism.

Fentanyl

Fentanyl is a versatile synthetic opioid, suitable for use in trauma, with a more rapid onset of action and greater analgesic potency than morphine. It also produces less cardiovascular depression than morphine and lacks the unwanted histamine release seen with codeine and morphine, potentially making it a better choice for use in the prehospital setting. It can be administered by multiple routes, including intravenously, intranasally and orally as a lozenge. It has been widely adopted in civilian and military prehospital practice as a first-line analgesic for acute severe pain (Committee on Tactical Combat Casualty Care, 2020; Ellerton et al., 2013; Thies et al., 2018; Wedmore and Butler, 2017). Its metabolites are shown in Figure 8.11.

Other fentanyl-related compounds include alfentanil, sufentanil and remifentanil, which are both more potent and more lipophilic. They all respond to naloxone.

A comparison of the pharmacokinetic properties of the common opioids is shown in Table 8.7.

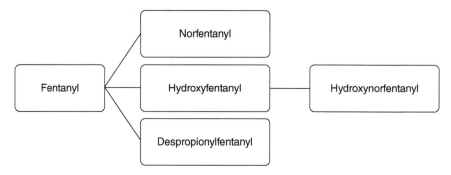

Figure 8.11   Fentanyl metabolism.

Table 8.7   Pharmacokinetics of common opioids.

	Pharmacologically active metabolites	Excretion	Duration of action (h)	Half-life
Morphine	Yes	90% excreted in urine. 10% excreted as conjugated morphine in faeces	3–6	1.5–4.5 h
Codeine	Yes	17% unchanged in urine. Other metabolites mostly excreted in urine	4–6	2.8 h
Diamorphine	Yes	60% excreted in urine as metabolites. 0.1% excreted unchanged in urine	4–5	3 minutes[a]
Fentanyl	No	5–20% excreted unchanged in urine. 9% in faeces	0.5–1	2.3–14 h

[a] Rapidly converted to morphine.

Episode of care

Tenzing was riding his motorbike on an autumnal afternoon when he lost control on a sharp corner and was thrown from the bike. He received injuries to the left side of his thorax and his left femur, with pain in his neck and back. Prior to this incident he was a fit and well 28-year-old man.

He is initially attended to by a paramedic and an ambulance technician on a double-crewed ambulance. They apply a traction splint to his broken leg, gain intravenous access and administer 10^mg of morphine and an antiemetic. Tenzing is still in severe pain and they request further assistance. Entonox is avoided due to the suspicion of a pneumothorax. While waiting, they prepare their immobilisation equipment and attempt to keep him warm.

An advanced paramedic arrives to assist the crew, and administers a left-sided femoral nerve block to provide complete analgesia for the fractured femur. They also administer an analgesic dose of ketamine and a gram of paracetamol intravenously. Being mindful that they want to accurately titrate Tenzing's analgesia but avoid unwanted side-effects, they opt for further aliquots of ketamine while en route to the hospital rather than further morphine.

On arrival at hospital, Tenzing is found to have multiple fractured ribs and the anaesthetic team provide him with a thoracic epidural after his femoral fixation surgery in order to facilitate deep breathing and reduce the risk of subsequent pneumonia. Ongoing multimodal analgesia is provided with morphine, paracetamol and the epidural.

Find out more

Fentanyl has been used for many years by mountain rescue teams in the UK and such patients often receive onward transfer from the ambulance service. To facilitate excellence in multiagency working and high-quality patient care, it may be useful to review the analgesic agents used by other prehospital care providers working in your area.

An overview of the usage of analgesic agents by mountain rescue team members is presented in Ellerton's 2013 paper.

Ellerton, J.A., Greene, M. and Paal, P. (2013). The use of analgesia in mountain rescue casualties with moderate or severe pain. *Emergency Medicine Journal* **30**(6): 501–505.

Skills in practice: intranasal diamorphine administration

1. Consult a dosage table for the concentration required for patient by age or weight.
2. Add the specific volume of 0.9% saline to a 10 mg ampoule of diamorphine powder.
3. A volume of 0.2 mL of this solution is drawn up into a syringe (or more if accounting for device-specific dead space).
4. Attach the nasal atomiser/aerosol device to the syringe via a Luer-Lock connector.
5. Tilt the patient's head backwards and place the tip of the atomisation device just inside the nostril.
6. Aim slightly outwards towards the ipsilateral ear.
7. Compress the syringe plunger rapidly, delivering half of the medication into the nostril.
8. Move the device to the other nostril and repeat steps 5–7 to deliver the remaining medication.

Antagonists

There are two key antagonists of the opioid receptors: naloxone and naltrexone. Naloxone is commonly available in prehospital medicine to facilitate reversal of opioid overdose (e.g. heroin overdose or iatrogenic overdose) where this has caused unwanted decreased consciousness and

Reflection

If you were assessing a patient with significant chronic pain, who was experiencing respiratory depression as a result of an accidental morphine overdose (or drug accumulation from long-term therapy or concurrent renal failure), how would you adjust your naloxone dosing?

What is the risk of administering a large bolus dose of naloxone to such a patient?

cardiorespiratory depression. Administration of naloxone is not risk free, however, as it can elicit hyperalgesia, rapid opioid withdrawal, pulmonary oedema and significant dysrhythmias. Naltrexone is used in alcohol and opioid dependence, but not in the acute setting. It has a very similar chemical structure to naloxone. Naloxone should be available whenever opioids are being administered for acute pain.

The duration of action of naloxone depends on both administration route and dose but it is often a lot shorter than the effects of the opioid it is counteracting. This is one of the reasons why an intramuscular loading dose is sometimes advocated, and why significant opioid overdoses should be observed for a number of hours (JRCALC, 2019).

Atypical analgesics

Ketamine

Ketamine is a dissociative anaesthetic (1–2 mg/kg) and, in smaller doses (0.2–0.75 mg/kg), an analgesic agent. These effects are due to its actions as a glutamate N-methyl-D-aspartate (NMDA) receptor antagonist with additional capabilities to reduce the presynaptic release of glutamate. Some of its analgesic effects may be due to interaction with opioid receptors, adding to its analgesic properties, although its effects cannot be reversed with naloxone. Ketamine additionally has antagonistic effects on various other neurotransmitters, probably explaining its anticholinergic symptoms. It is also a bronchodilator and indirectly increases sympathetic tone, resulting in increased heart rate, blood pressure and cardiac output. It also has a direct negative inotropic effect on the myocardium, which is usually masked by the indirect positive effects, but the negative inotropic effect may become clinically apparent in patients who are critically ill and catecholamine depleted.

As a result of ketamine's positive inotropic and chronotropic effects, it is not a suitable agent for patients with ischaemic cardiac chest pain. In such patients, increasing their myocardial oxygen demand may worsen ischaemia and pain.

Ketamine is fast acting with an onset of action of around 30 seconds when given intravenously. It is a safe and effective prehospital analgesic, particularly suited to situations where maintenance of airway reflexes, respiratory rate and cardiovascular stability is vital, such as during technical rescue or when providing Care Under Fire (Committee on Tactical Combat Casualty Care, 2020; Metcalfe, 2018; Russell et al., 2014; Wedmore and Butler, 2017). It is especially important to carefully dose ketamine, as while it is an effective analgesic at lower doses, with higher doses it acts as a general anaesthetic, inducing loss of consciousness, and in overdose can easily prove fatal. This is particularly important when more than one concentration of ketamine is available to the clinician, where a 10-fold overdose could easily occur. At the lower analgesic doses, unwanted dissociation and agitation may occur, requiring concurrent administration of a sedative agent.

Find out more

Providing analgesia in remote and hostile environments is challenging. The Wilderness Medicine Society has provided a clinical practice guideline discussing this issue entitled 'Wilderness Medical Society practice guidelines for the treatment of acute pain in remote environments: 2014 update' available from: https://wms.org/research/guidelines

Antidepressants and antiepileptics

A number of drugs originally developed as either psychiatric medications or antiepileptics are now used to treat neuropathic pain. Drugs from the family of selective serotonin reuptake inhibitors (SSRIs), traditionally used for anxiety and depression, are often used to treat neuropathic pain in the primary care setting, but have limited to no value during the acute phase.

Amitriptyline is often considered the first-line treatment option for neuropathic pain. It is a tricyclic antidepressant (TCA) medication, now used widely in primary and secondary care to treat pain. Other TCAs such as nortriptyline and desipramine are also increasingly being used in pain medicine and may provide a more favourable side-effect profile. While not yet common practice internationally, there have been positive experiences in using amitriptyline for acute pain associated with cold injuries, traumatic injuries and postoperatively (Joslin et al., 2014; Wong et al., 2014), and its use could become more common in civilian urban and rural practice.

Anticonvulsants such as pregabalin and gabapentin are also used to treat pain (Reed and Schurr, 2020). They have been used successfully to treat neuropathic pain of various aetiologies. Unfortunately, they have also both become drugs of abuse due to their perceived euphoric effects. There is some evidence to support the use of pregabalin acutely for painful burns, but other than this their use is usually limited to chronic and postoperative pain.

Nefopam

Nefopam is an analgesic agent often used in primary care for a wide variety of pathologies. It acts centrally as a serotonin, norepinephrine and dopamine reuptake inhibitor. It also exerts an action on sodium and calcium channels to inhibit glutamatergic transmission. Nefopam also has an anticholinergic effect and many of its side-effects are related to this mode of action. It can be administered by the oral route, or by intravenous or intramuscular injection. It is unsuitable for use in patients with a history of seizures, for those taking other serotonergic medications or for ischaemic cardiac pain.

Adjuncts to analgesia

Magnesium sulfate

Magnesium sulfate ($MgSO_4$) has been discussed for some time as an adjunct to other analgesic agents. This is probably due to its membrane-stabilising activity, but magnesium is also a cofactor in ATP production and appears to antagonise calcium release, inhibit catecholamine release, antagonise NMDA receptors, and have an anti-inflammatory effect, reducing interleukin-6 and TNF-alpha plasma levels, all of which may contribute to its analgesic properties. It has been shown to be effective in reducing pain in a postoperative setting (de Oliveira et al., 2013; Mussrat et al., 2019) and for patients with acute pain (Hutchins and Rockett, 2019). However, a dosing regimen for its use specifically for analgesia is still unclear and its use in the treatment of pain in the prehospital setting is not standard clinical practice.

Local anaesthetics

Lidocaine, which has been used for many years as an antidysrhythmic due to its sodium channel-blocking actions, has also been used as an adjunct to analgesia. Significant work has been undertaken to explore intravenous infusion of lidocaine as an analgesic, most commonly to enhance intra- and postoperative analgesia, but also for chronic pain. It is also increasingly being used in the management of acute pain (Hutchins and Rockett, 2019; Meaney et al., 2020); however, this is not without risks and is not currently standard practice. Lidocaine is also used as a transdermal patch (Figure 8.12), by local infiltration and also when used to deliver regional anaesthesia. Local anaesthetic toxicity is treated with lipid emulsion infusion, and this should be available to clinicians undertaking regional anaesthesia with local anaesthetic agents.

While lidocaine can be carefully administered intravenously, other local anaesthetics, such as bupivacaine, when given intravenously may cause catastrophic cardiovascular collapse, neurotoxicity and death.

143

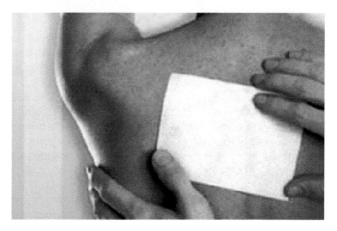

144

Figure 8.12   Lidocaine patch being applied.

Local anaesthetic agents can be effectively utilised in the prehospital setting when undertaking regional anaesthesia techniques, such as fascia iliaca compartment block or ring blocks, which can provide excellent analgesia and reduce the need for opioid administration and the attendant side-effects (Simpson et al., 2012; Williams and Laws, 2019). For some techniques, longer acting local anaesthetics such as levobupivacaine may be used to provide a longer duration of analgesia/anaesthesia for the patient.

Conclusion

The assessment of pain can be challenging, and a biopsychosocial approach may be required to truly understand a patient's lived experience. There are multiple effective analgesics available to the paramedic and there is often benefit in utilising multiple agents acting synergistically (multimodal analgesia), to achieve relief from pain and also to minimize dose-related side-effects from any one class of drug. With paramedics increasingly working in diverse and advanced roles, a broad knowledge of analgesics is essential to allow clinicians to select the best treatments and minimise pain and distress for their patients.

Reflection choice of analgesia

Condition	Your notes
Ischaemic cardiac chest pain (angina)	
Inflammatory cardiac chest pain (pericarditis)	
Polytrauma with cardiovascular instability	
A brief painful procedure	
Field amputation of a lower limb	

Reflection: consider how the physical and pharmacological properties of these commonly used prehospital analgesics compare with those of an ideal (imaginary) analgesic drug

Analgesic	Pharmacological and physical properties
Ideal (imaginary) analgesic	Pharmacological Physical
Morphine sulfate	Pharmacological Physical
Paracetamol	Pharmacological Physical
Nitrous oxide/oxygen (Entonox)	Pharmacological Physical

Glossary

ATP	Adenosine triphosphate
DOP	Delta opioid receptor
ECG	Electrocardiogram
Glutamate	An excitatory neurotransmitter
Interleukin-6	A proinflammatory cytokine and anti-inflammatory myokine
JRCALC	Joint Royal Colleges Ambulance Liaison Committee
KOP	Kappa opioid receptor
TNF-alpha	Tumour necrosis factor alpha, an endogenous pyrogen which regulates immune cells
MOP	Mu opioid receptor
Narcan®	Trade name for naloxone
NOP	Nociceptin opioid receptor
NSAID	Non-steroidal anti-inflammatory
Opiate	A substance derived from opium poppy
Opioid	Any substance (natural or synthetic) which binds to opioid receptors
Penthrox	Trade name for methoxyflurane administered via the Penthrox inhaler
TCA	Tricyclic antidepressant

References

Antman, E.M., Bennett, J.S., Daugherty, A., Furberg, C., Roberts, H. and Taubert, K.A. (2007). Use of nonsteroidal antiinflammatory drugs: an update for clinicians: a scientific statement from the American Heart Association. *Circulation* **115**(12): 1634–1642.

Baker, C. and Wong, D. (1987). Q.U.E.S.T.: a process of pain assessment in children. *Orthopaedic Nursing* **6**(1): 11–21.

Bannister, K. (2019). Descending pain modulation: influence and impact. *Current Opinion in Physiology* **11**(1): 62–66.

Committee on Tactical Combat Casualty Care. (2020). *Tactical Combat Casualty Care (TCCC) Guidelines for Medical Personnel*. Washington, DC: US Department of Defense: Defense Health Agency (DHA): Joint Trauma System.

de Oliveira, G.S., Castro-Alves, L.J., Khan, J.H. and McCarthy, R.J. (2013). Perioperative systemic magnesium to minimize postoperative pain: a meta-analysis of randomized controlled trials. *Anesthesiology* **119**(1): 178–190.

Ellerton, J.A., Greene, M. and Paal, P. (2013). The use of analgesia in mountain rescue casualties with moderate or severe pain. *Emergency Medicine Journal* **30**(6): 501–505.

Forrest, M., Porter, K. and van der Velde, J. (2019). Methoxyflurane (Penthrox®) – a case series of use in the prehospital setting. *Journal of Paramedic Practice* **11**(2): 54–60.

Gregory, P. and Mursell, I. (2015). *Manual of Clinical Paramedic Procedures*. Hoboken: John Wiley & Sons.

Grissa, M.H., Boubaker, H., Zorgati, A. et al. (2015). Efficacy and safety of nebulized morphine given at 2 different doses compared to IV titrated morphine in trauma pain. *American Journal of Emergency Medicine* **33**(11): 1557–1561.

Hutchins, D. and Rockett, M. (2019). The use of atypical analgesics by intravenous infusion for acute pain: evidence base for lidocaine, ketamine and magnesium. *Anaesthesia and Intensive Care Medicine* **20**(8): 415–418.

Jennings, P.A., Cameron, P. and Bernard, S. (2009). Measuring acute pain in the prehospital setting. *Emergency Medicine Journal* **26**(8): 552–555.

Joint Royal Colleges Ambulance Liaison Committee (JRCALC). (2019). *Clinical Practice Guidelines 2019*. Bridgwater: Class Professional Publishing.

Joslin, J., Worthing, R., Ladbrook, M. and Mularella, J. (2014). Amitriptyline use for acute pain in remote environments. *Wilderness and Environmental Medicine* **25**(4): 488–489.

Meaney, E.D., Reid, L. and Srivastava, D. (2020). A survey on the use of intravenous lidocaine infusion for acute pain in Scottish hospitals. *British Journal of Pain* **14**(2): 98–103.

Merkel, S.I., Voepel-Lewis, T., Shayevitz, J.R. and Malviya, S. (1997). The FLACC: a behavioral scale for scoring postoperative pain in young children. *Pediatric Nursing* **23**(3): 293–297.

Metcalfe, M. (2018). Ketamine administration by HART paramedics: a clinical audit review. *Journal of Paramedic Practice* **10**(10): 430–437.

Mofidi, M., Dashti, A., Rezai, M., Ghodrati, N., Ameli, H. and Amiri, H. (2020). Comparing the efficacy of nebulized morphine with intravenous morphine in traumatic musculoskeletal pain management. *Journal of Research in Clinical Medicine* **8**: 21.

Mussrat, R., Zahoor, A., Khan, M.A. and Ahmad, S. (2019). Comparison of perioperative magnesium sulphate infusion with placebo for postoperative analgesia. *Professional Medical Journal* **26**(11): 1937–1941.

Page, G.G. (2013). *The immune-suppressive effects of pain. Madame Curie Bioscience Database*. Austin: Landes Bioscience.

Parkinson, M. (2015). Pain: understanding the biopsychosocial model and the paramedic's role within the multidisciplinary team. *Journal of Paramedic Practice* **7**(5): 250–255.

Przybyła, G.W., Szychowski, K.A. and Gmiński, J. (2021). Paracetamol – an old drug with new mechanisms of action. *Clinical and Experimental Pharmacology and Physiology* **48**(1): 3–19.

Reed, R.N. and Schurr, M.J. (2020). Acute pain in the trauma patient. *Current Trauma Reports* **6**: 1–7.

Russell, K., Scaife, C., Weber, D. et al. (2014) Wilderness Medical Society Practice Guidelines for the Treatment of Acute Pain in Remote Environments: 2014 Update. *Wilderness and Environmental Medicine* **25**(4): S96–S104.

Scarth, E. and Smith, S. (2016). *Drugs in Anaesthesia and Intensive Care*, 5th edn. Oxford: Oxford University Press.

Simpson, P.M., McCabe, B., Bendall, J.C., Cone, D.C. and Middleton, P.M. (2012). Paramedic-performed digital nerve block to facilitate field reduction of a dislocated finger. *Prehospital Emergency Care* **16**(3): 415–417.

Swift, A. (2018). Understanding pain and the human body's response to it. *Nursing Times* **114**(3): 22–26.

Thies, K-C., Mountain, A. and Goode. P. (eds). (2018). *European Trauma Course: The Team Approach*, 4th edn. Market Drayton: European Trauma Course Organisation.

Tsui, S.L., Law, S., Fok, M. et al. (1997). Postoperative analgesia reduces mortality and morbidity after esophagectomy. *American Journal of Surgery* **173**(6): 472–478.

Voepel-Lewis, T., Zanotti, J., Dammeyer, J.A. and Merkel, S. (2010). Reliability and validity of the face, legs, activity, cry, consolability behavioral tool in assessing acute pain in critically ill patients. *American Journal of Critical Care* **19**(1): 55–61.

146

Wedmore, I.S. and Butler, F.K. (2017). Battlefield analgesia in tactical combat casualty care. *Wilderness and Environmental Medicine* **28**(2): S109–S116.

Williams, J. and Laws, S. (2019). Fascia iliaca compartment block versus IV morphine for femoral fracture pain. *Journal of Paramedic Practice* **11**(4): 156–164.

Wong, K., Phelan, R., Kalso, E. et al. (2014). Antidepressant drugs for prevention of acute and chronic postsurgical pain: early evidence and recommended future directions. *Anesthesiology* **121**(3): 591–608.

Further reading

AnaesthesiaUK. www.frca.co.uk/default.aspx
Online learning resource covering anatomy, physiology and pharmacology, as well as overviews of some of the medical equipment used in clinical anaesthesia.

British Pain Society Publications. www.britishpainsociety.org/british-pain-society-publications/
A comprehensive suite of resource for both professionals and patients.

Dickman, A. (2012). *Drugs in Palliative Care*, 2nd edn. Oxford: Oxford University Press.
A useful pocket reference for the pharmacopoeia of palliative medicine.

Watson, M., Ward, S., Vallath, N., Wells, J. and Campbell, R. (2019). *Oxford Handbook of Palliative Care*. Oxford: Oxford University Press.
A comprehensive reference for the field of palliative care, and a valuable resource for both pharmacological and non-pharmacological symptom management.

Multiple-choice questions

1. Ketamine is often used in military and austere environments. Why is this?
   - (a) Lower risk of hypotension compared to opioids
   - (b) It is easy to spell
   - (c) It has no restrictions in terms of import and export laws internationally
   - (d) You cannot be allergic to ketamine
2. Ketorolac belongs to which class of medication?
   - (a) Inhalational analgesic
   - (b) NMDA Antagonist
   - (c) Opioid
   - (d) NSAID
3. At which of the following receptors does morphine *not* have an effect?
   - (a) δ
   - (b) ψ
   - (c) μ
   - (d) κ
4. In terms of opioid mechanism of action, what does MOP stand for?
   - (a) Morphine-receptors occurring peripherally
   - (b) Morphine-related opiate
   - (c) Morphine phosphate
   - (d) Mu opiate receptor
5. Paracetamol in overdose causes which organ to fail?
   - (a) Heart
   - (b) Spleen
   - (c) Skin
   - (d) Liver
6. In comparison to morphine, fentanyl is:
   - (a) Slower acting
   - (b) 100 times less potent
   - (c) Approximately 20 times less likely to cause side effects
   - (d) More lipophilic

7. Methoxyflurane is what type of chemical?
   (a) A noble gas
   (b) A fluorinated hydrocarbon
   (c) An inert nitrous oxide donor
   (d) A sympathomimetic
8. Which other medication is often prescribed alongside a course of ibuprofen?
   (a) A Class I anti-dysrhythmic
   (b) Amlodipine
   (c) A beta-2 adrenoreceptor
   (d) A proton pump inhibitor
9. Which of these statements is true regarding magnesium sulfate ($MgSO_4$)?
   (a) Should be administered as a rapid IV bolus
   (b) Reduces pain in the postoperative period
   (c) Is the British Army's first-line analgesic
   (d) Is usually administered intranasally
10. Aspirin is linked to what undesirable outcome in paediatric patients?
    (a) Patau syndrome
    (b) Reye syndrome
    (c) Kawasaki disease
    (d) Lennox-Gestaut syndrome
11. A common side-effect of morphine is:
    (a) Leukonychia
    (b) Respiratory depression
    (c) Asterixis
    (d) Inverted T-waves on ECG
12. Which of the following is incorrect in relation to diamorphine?
    (a) It can be administered intranasally
    (b) Morphine is a metabolite
    (c) It is highly lipophilic
    (d) It cannot be given to paediatric patients
13. Which of these statements is true about naloxone?
    (a) Naloxone is a beta opioid antagonist
    (b) Naloxone administration causes no side-effects
    (c) The effects of fentanyl can be reversed by naloxone
    (d) The effects of ketamine will be increased by naloxone
14. An overdose of aspirin may cause each of these, apart from:
    (a) Blindness
    (b) Tinnitus
    (c) Metabolic acidosis
    (d) Hyperpyrexia
15. COX inhibitors exert their analgesic effect by:
    (a) Upregulating the noradrenaline and serotonin receptors
    (b) Reducing GABA receptor activity
    (c) Stimulating interleukin-3 release
    (d) Reducing prostaglandin synthesis

Chapter 9

Antibacterials

Dean Whiting, Deborah Flynn and Dawn Ball

Aim

The aim of this chapter is to encourage the reader to develop an understanding and appreciation of the differences in antibacterial use.

Learning outcomes

1. To understand how pathogens cause infections and the use of terminology associated with this category of medication.
2. To understand the different antibacterial classes and be able to explain their actions and associated side-effects.
3. To be able to explain the prehospital considerations for the use of each antibacterial class.
4. To understand the paramedic's health-promoting role in antibacterial therapy and antimicrobial stewardship.

Test your knowledge

1. What is the difference between bacteriostatic and bactericidal treatments?
2. Describe the professional responsibilities of registered healthcare professionals in relation to antimicrobial stewardship.
3. What are the pharmacokinetics of aminoglycosides?
4. What considerations should be taken into account when administering benzylpenicillin?
5. What does the term 'teratogenic' mean?

Introduction

This chapter explores antibacterials. These are the miracle drugs of the last two centuries, as their use reduced mortality rates in previously life-threatening conditions such as bacterial pneumonia, sepsis and tuberculosis. This trend has started to reverse due to the development of resistance to currently available antibacterials combined with a lack of research into the development of new antimicrobial treatments (World Health Organization, 2020), which include antibiotics, antivirals and antifungals. A

Fundamentals of Pharmacology for Paramedics, First Edition. Edited by Ian Peate, Suzanne Evans, and Lisa Clegg.
© 2022 John Wiley & Sons Ltd. Published 2022 by John Wiley & Sons Ltd.

research briefing on trends in infectious disease produced by the United Kingdom Parliamentary Office of Science and Technology (2017) suggests that infectious disease creates a significant burden to the UK's health and economic systems, causing 7% of all deaths and being responsible for a large proportion of sick days.

Micro-organisms are ubiquitous in the world but can only be seen under microscopic examination. They include bacteria, viruses, fungi and protozoa. Micro-organisms live on and inside us, often being more beneficial than harmful. The normal body flora, for example, consists of colonies of mostly bacterial micro-organisms acquired through contact with the outside world. These micro-organisms can be further classified as aerobic bacteria, which require the presence of oxygen for survival, and anaerobic bacteria, which do not require oxygen for survival.

The presence of normal flora prevents colonisation by disease-causing micro-organisms, known as pathogens. The capacity to cause disease depends on the micro-organism, its characteristics and location. It is known that many strains of bacteria such as *E.coli* live harmlessly in the alimentary tract, but can cause infection if they spread to other body compartments, such as the urinary tract. Some strains of *E. coli* can also cause severe diarrhoea when they enter the intestines of a healthy human. Normally harmless micro-organisms can also cause disease when the host is particularly vulnerable, for example during suppression of the immune system.

Language and terminology

The terms *antimicrobial*, *antibacterial* and *antibiotic* are often used interchangeably, but each term has its own specific meaning. An antimicrobial is active against bacteria and/or other micro-organisms including viruses, fungi and protozoa. An antibacterial is active against bacteria. An antibiotic is a drug that is produced by one type of micro-organism to protect itself from another micro-organism, and is therefore from natural sources. The more general terms antimicrobial and antibacterial can refer to drugs that are both natural and synthetic in origin.

Selective toxicity is the ability of an antimicrobial to harm microbes without injuring human cells. Antimicrobials do this by a range of different mechanisms, many of which exploit differences of structure or function between microbial and human cells. However, when these differences are small, antimicrobial actions can cross over to human cell function and cause cell damage.

The goal of antibacterial therapy is to either eliminate a bacterial infection or reduce the number of bacteria to a level which the immune system can effectively deal with. Antibacterial drugs can either be *bactericidal*, meaning they directly kill bacteria (e.g. penicillins and aminoglycosides), or *bacteriostatic*, meaning they inhibit bacterial growth and rely on the immune system to kill the bacteria (e.g. tetracyclines). Some drugs are partly bactericidal and partly bacteriostatic, depending on the dosage and plasma concentration of the drug, the number of bacteria, the time from the start of treatment and the health of the person. Antibacterials with a relatively narrow therapeutic index, such as aminoglycosides, require monitoring of the serum concentration to ensure it lies within therapeutic range, to prevent underdosing or drug toxicity.

Based on the spectrum of their activity, antibacterials are categorised as broad spectrum or narrow spectrum. Table 9.1 details the main differences.

Antibacterial mechanisms of action

There are four main antibacterial mechanisms of action.

Table 9.1　Broad- and narrow-spectrum antibiotics.

Broad-spectrum antibiotics	Narrow-spectrum antibiotics
Effective against gram-positive and gram-negative bacteria Kills a variety of organisms Used when cause of infection is unknown. **Examples:** erythromycin, ciprofloxacin, doxycycline	Effective against gram-positive bacteria only Used when causative organisms are known **Examples:** macrolides, older penicillins (although others can be broad spectrum, e.g. amoxicillin, ampicillin), vancomycin

Disruption of bacterial cell wall synthesis: beta-lactams

Most bacterial cells have an outer, relatively rigid wall made up of a substance unique to bacteria, called peptidoglycan. The cell wall supports the inner cell membrane and prevents it from rupturing due to the high intracellular osmotic pressure. Penicillins, cephalosporins and carbapenems, known collectively as beta-lactams because they all contain a beta-lactam ring in their chemical structures, disrupt bacterial cell wall synthesis by binding with penicillin-binding proteins, the enzymes responsible for bacterial cell wall synthesis, and preventing the formation and maintenance of the cell wall. The weakened cell wall causes the bacteria to swell and burst due to the osmotic pressure.

Interference in folate metabolism: sulfonamides, trimethoprim

Bacteria, unlike human cells, must produce their own folic acid, which is necessary for synthesis of DNA and RNA for growth and reproduction. The sulfonamides contain a chemical group which is similar to para-aminobenzoic acid (PABA), a vital step in the production of folic acid. Sulfonamides compete with PABA in this metabolic step, interrupting folic acid synthesis. Trimethoprim inhibits a later step in folic acid production. Sulfonamides and trimethoprim are often used in combination, as their actions may be synergistic.

151

Inhibition of bacterial DNA synthesis: quinolones

Bacterial cells have a single chromosome which consists of a supercoiled DNA molecule within the bacterial cytoplasm. The quinolones inhibit the action of an enzyme, DNA gyrase, that is essential for the replication of bacterial DNA and the survival of the bacterial cell.

Inhibition of bacterial protein synthesis: tetracyclines, aminoglycosides, macrolides, chloramphenicol, lincosamides

Ribosomes are required for bacterial protein synthesis, as in human cells, but the ribosomal subunits in bacteria are slightly different from those in human cells. Drugs such as aminoglycosides bind irreversibly to the bacterial ribosomal subunit 30S, disrupting the initiation of the synthetic process, the reading of the genetic code or the completion of protein synthesis

Choosing the right treatment

'The right drug for the right bug' (Burchum and Rosenthal, 2019, p.1042).

Antimicrobials should only be prescribed and administered when infection has been recognised or there is a high degree of suspicion of infection and when there is likely to be clear benefit to the patient. The Joint Formulary Committee (NICE 2021) suggests that the key factor in choosing the right treatment is establishing the causative micro-organism. Antimicrobial protocols are developed through surveillance of common causative micro-organisms and trends in antimicrobial resistance. In the prehospital environment, identification of the causative micro-organism is unlikely and therefore prompt empirical prescribing of the appropriate antibiotic to patients with signs and symptoms suggestive of serious infection, such as sepsis or meningitis, is recommended. There may also be a role for prehospital antimicrobial use in complex wound and open fracture management but further research is required to inform and change future practice (Lack et al., 2019; Smit and Boyle, 2014).

Prior to prescribing or administering antibiotics, the paramedic must take note of the patient's allergies, medical and drug history, liver and kidney function, susceptibility to disease, route tolerance (for example, ability to swallow), severity of illness, age and whether pregnant, breast feeding or taking oral contraceptives. Race may need to be considered, as genetics can influence the metabolism of some antibacterials (Tsai et al., 2015).

Antimicrobial resistance

The World Health Organization (2020) defines antimicrobial resistance (AMR) as 'the ability of microorganisms (like bacteria, viruses and some parasites) to stop an antimicrobial (such as antibiotics, antivirals and antimalarials) from working against it. As a result, standard treatments become ineffective, infections persist and may spread to others'. Globally, addressing the problem of AMR is now considered a public health priority, as resistance to antimicrobials is making infections harder and more costly to treat. For example, the occurrence of bacteria resistant to penicillins, tetracyclines, cephalosporins, carbapenems, macrolides and quinolones is rising (World Health Organization, 2020).

Preventing antimicrobial resistance

The main method of preventing antimicrobial resistance is to preserve and prolong the effectiveness of current antibacterials and prevent the occurrence and transmission of infections. The World Health Organization (2020) sets out action points for individuals, healthcare professionals, health policy makers and the healthcare industry.

The individual's responsibility centres around managing expectations regarding the prescribing of antibiotics and concordance with medication regimens, in addition to preventing the transmission of infection.

The focus of the paramedic in preventing antimicrobial resistance is patient education. Patients may need some explanation about the actions of antibacterials to clarify that these drugs cannot be prescribed simply to provide symptom relief. The paramedic should explain to those who are prescribed antibacterials the importance of completing the entire course, even if they feel better, as incomplete treatment of a bacterial infection encourages resistance. Patients should similarly be warned against keeping antibacterials for future use or sharing them with friends with similar symptoms. The importance of taking the medication as prescribed should also be reinforced, to maintain an adequate plasma level of drug and prevent the development of resistant micro-organisms. The paramedic also plays a vital role in promoting behaviour which prevents the spread of infection and development of antibacterial resistance through measures such as hand washing, covering nose and mouth when sneezing, vaccination, practising safe sex, maintaining awareness of current public health campaigns, reducing unnecessary or inappropriate prescribing of antibacterials and supporting rapid diagnostics (World Health Organization, 2020).

The role of policymakers is to ensure there are robust systems for infection prevention and control as well as surveillance of antimicrobial resistance.

Clinical consideration: Summary of the paramedic's role in the principles of good assessment, combating microbial resistance and prescribing practice considerations

- Establish if the person has a history of hepatic and/or renal impairment and allergies, is pregnant or breast feeding and assess for any contraindications or cautions present in their history specific to antibacterial groups.
- Prescribe and administer antibiotics in accordance with official guidelines and protocols.
- See best evidence, local guidelines or manufacturer's guidance for specialist instructions regarding dilution/reconstitution, route and rate of administration and concentration and scheduling of administration.
- In treatment failure, the identity of the causative micro-organism should be established through a microscopy, culture and sensitivity (MC&S) test.
- Assess the severity of the current illness.
- Determine previous antibacterial therapy.
- Ask about previous adverse/allergic reactions.
- Evaluate the therapeutic effect, for example improved wellbeing.
- Consider concurrent medications and be aware of interaction risk and monitor for potential effects.
- Encourage the person to adopt health-promoting behaviours towards the prevention of infection spreading and maintain principles of antimicrobial stewardship.

Antimicrobial stewardship (AMS)

According to the British Society for Antimicrobial Chemotherapy (2017), the definition of AMS is 'the right antibiotic, for the right indication (diagnosis), in the right patient, at the right time, with the right dose and route, causing the least harm to the patient and future patients'. Furthermore, it argues that there is a need to tackle the multifactorial drivers of antibiotic use through adoption of cautious prescribing guidelines driven by AMS overarching goals. These goals include improving patient outcomes, reducing collateral damage and impact costs. National Institute for Health and Care Excellence (NICE) guidelines (2018) agree that this is about changing prescribing practice to slow development of AMR and prolong the effectiveness of currently available antibacterials.

Antibacterials by clinical use

The conditions most frequently treated with antimicrobials in the primary care setting are respiratory and urinary tract infections, with penicillin accounting for 50% of all prescriptions, followed by macrolides (13%), tetracyclines (12%) and trimethoprim (11%) (Dolk et al., 2017).

The next section details the pharmacokinetics of each group of antibiotics, their actions, contraindications and cautions, adverse effects, drug interactions and clinical considerations. However, some antimicrobials mentioned will not be discussed in detail in this chapter, namely sulfonamides and quinolones.

Beta-lactams

Penicillins

Examples of this group, used to treat mild to moderate infections, are benzylpenicillin, flucloxacillin, ampicillin and piperacillin (with tazobactam). The spectrum of activity of the various penicillins ranges from narrow to extended and they are bactericidal. The main differences between the penicillins are their spectrum of activity, stability in stomach acid and duration of action.

Benzylpenicillin sodium (Pen G) and flucloxacillin are known narrow-spectrum penicillins, whereas ampicillin and piperacillin (when combined with tazobactam) are broad spectrum. The pharmacokinetics of the penicillins differ. Benzylpenicillin sodium is the example used below. The variations of Pen G are available in four salts which differ in route of administration and time course of action. Table 9.2 describes the general pharmacokinetics of Pen G.

Contraindication, cautions and adverse effects

The penicillins are largely free from serious adverse effects. Hypersensitivity is the most common adverse effect and can range from skin rash to anaphylaxis. Allergy to any penicillin may mean an allergy to other penicillins and beta-lactam drugs, so a previous allergic reaction to any member of the class is a contraindication to the use of any beta-lactam, as is a history of atopic allergy (asthma, eczema and hay fever).

Diarrhoea is a common adverse effect, especially in oral treatment with broad-spectrum penicillins, potentially leading to pseudomembranous enterocolitis (also known as antibiotic-associated colitis). Superinfections (the opportunistic overgrowth of another microbe, such as yeast, after antibacterial treatment) are commonly associated with the killing of the normal intestinal flora by broad-spectrum agents.

Table 9.2 Pharmacokinetics of benzylpenicillin sodium.

Action	
Absorption	Poorly absorbed from the gastrointestinal tract. Best administered by intramuscular or intravenous routes. Intrathecal injection of benzylpenicillin is not recommended
Distribution	Distributes well to most tissues and fluids except cerebrospinal fluid (if no inflammation present), joints and eyes
Metabolism	Minimal metabolism
Excretion	Renal – excreted largely unchanged

Drug interactions

This is not an exhaustive list, so further reading in NICE (2021) is recommended. This group has interactions with anticoagulants (alters effect) and methotrexate (increases risk of toxicity). Risk of hepatotoxicity increases when flucloxacillin is combined with alcohol or paracetamol. Concurrent administration of ampicillin and allopurinol increases the risk of a skin rash. Piperacilllin with tazobactam increases the effect of suxamethonium and similar drugs if used in combination.

Considerations in the administration of penicillins

- Promote principles of good patient assessment, prescribing practice and antimicrobial stewardship through patient education.
- Oral doses of penicillin should be taken with a full glass of water 1 hour before or 2 hours after meals (antibiotic specific). Some food/drink (fruit juice, soft drinks, milk) may reduce the absorption of some oral penicillins.
- Gastrointestinal discomfort is a common effect of penicillins. Patients should be advised how to maintain adequate nutrition and hydration.
- Monitor renal function, by assessing fluid intake and output, to prevent injury, particularly in older people, those with renal impairment, acutely ill or very young.
- Monitor patients following administration for signs of allergy.
- Advise patients with a known penicillin allergy to wear/carry appropriate identification.
- Advise patient to report any signs of an allergic reaction (skin rash, fever, itching, hives, wheezing or swollen joints).
- If concomitant medications include anticoagulants, INR (how long it takes blood to form a clot) should be monitored and dose adjusted as required.
- Consider concurrent medication and be aware of interaction risk.
- High-dose penicillins and aminoglycosides should not be administered in the same intravenous solution, as aminoglycosides are inactivated.
- Monitor parenteral injection site as pain and inflammation can occur

Episode of care

You are dispatched to the home of Jaysal, a 24-year-old web designer, who has been unwell for about 2 days with coryzal symptoms. His partner is very concerned as Jaysal has deteriorated over the last 2 hours and seems to be confused with headache, stiff neck, aversion to bright lights, rapid breathing, pale skin, and cold hands and feet. His partner informs you that Jaysal has no significant past medical history, but she thinks that he had a mild reaction to penicillin as a child. He looks unwell and you suspect that he may have meningitis. You consider administering benzylpenicillin 1.2 g IV and plan to urgently transfer Jaysal to the hospital.

Cephalosporins

These have a broad antibacterial spectrum and are mostly bactericidal. There are five generations of cephalosporins, and each successive generation has a broader spectrum of activity, greater resistance to beta-lactamases and greater ability to penetrate the cerebrospinal fluid. The pharmacokinetics for the generational group of cephalosporins are similar and are presented in Table 9.3.

Contraindications, cautions and adverse effects

Gastrointestinal disturbances are the most common adverse effects, with the risk of pseudomembranous enterocolitis. Allergy and hypersensitivity risks are present with all beta-lactams. Cautious use is recommended in people with renal impairment due to risk of toxicity. Common neurological effects include, dizziness, headache, and lethargy.

Generally, this antibacterial group is well tolerated. Blood disorders can occur; for example, ceftriaxone can cause bleeding tendencies by interfering with the metabolism of vitamin K. Thrombophlebitis can occur at the IV injection site or an abscess at the site of an intramuscular injection.

Table 9.3 Pharmacokinetics of cephalosporins.

Action	
Absorption	Only three (cefaclor, cephalexin and cefuroxime) are well absorbed after oral administration. The rest are administered intramuscularly or intravenously
Distribution	Widely distributed in tissues. Later generation agents (e.g. cefotaxime) cross the blood–brain barrier more easily. They are known to cross the placental barrier and enter breast milk
Metabolism	Primarily hepatic
Excretion	Mainly renal but some (e.g. cefoperazone) in bile

Drug interactions

There is an increased risk of nephrotoxicity when cephalosporins are combined with some medications, including aminoglycosides Additionally, certain cephalosporins (ceftriaxone) can increase the risk of bleeding if taken concurrently with drugs such as anticoagulants, thrombolytics, non-steroidal anti-inflammatory drugs and other antiplatelet drugs

A disulfiram-like reaction (flushing, sweating, palpitations, dyspnoea, syncope, vertigo, blurred vision, hypotension, throbbing headache, chest pain, nausea and vomiting, potentially leading to convulsions, cardiovascular collapse and death), although rare, may occur if cephalosporins (particularly cefazolin) are combined with alcohol, even after treatment has been completed.

Considerations in the administration of cephalosporins

- Promote principles of good patient assessment, prescribing practice and antimicrobial stewardship through patient education.
- Advise the patient to take with food if gastric discomfort occurs.
- Advise the patient about the signs and symptoms of an allergic reaction – urticaria, rash, itching, hypotension, dyspnoea and hives.
- If given intramuscularly or intravenously, monitor injection sites for signs of irritation (abscess or phlebitis). Inform the person of potentially painful intramuscular injection.
- Advise the patient to refrain from alcohol for up to 72 hours after treatment to prevent a disulfiram-like reaction.
- Monitor renal function if patient is taking cephalosporins and another drug with potential nephrotoxicity.
- Monitor patients at risk of potential blood loss (bleeding gums, easy bruising) especially if taking anticoagulant drugs (or similar). If prescribed ceftriaxone, observe for and instigate measures to reduce haemorrhage risk. Prothrombin time and/or bleeding time should be monitored, and if significant bleeding is present. administer parenteral vitamin K and transfer to hospital.
- If diarrhoea is experienced, advise the patient about replacing fluids and maintaining hydration.
- Inform the patient about treatment schedule and adverse effects and monitor them for signs of superinfection.
- If CNS effects occur, refer to primary care practitioner or transfer to hospital.

Episode of care

Isini, a 36-year-old woman, is 12 weeks pregnant, and was seen by the nurse practitioner 2 days ago for a lower urinary tract infection. Isini was prescribed cefalexin 500 mg BD for 3 days and was advised to seek further assistance if the symptoms did not improve or if symptoms of upper urinary tract infection developed. You arrive at her home and recognise that she looks quite unwell and is complaining of vomiting, rigors, fever, lethargy and loin pain. Her past medical history is diabetes mellitus, and she has had three urine infections over the last 6 months.

Table 9.4   Pharmacokinetics of imipenem.

Action	
Absorption	Is not absorbed by the GI tract therefore intravenous administration only
Distribution	Distributes well to body fluids and tissues and penetrates the CSF. It is known to pass into the breast milk but it is unclear if it passes the placental barrier
Metabolism	Renal
Excretion	Renal

CSF, cerebrospinal fluid; GI, gastrointestinal.

Carbapenems

Agents within this group include imipenem (with cilastatin), meropenem and ertapenem. They have the widest spectrum of activity and are bactericidal in action. Carbapenems should be used sparingly, which will delay development of resistance to them. Table 9.4 presents the pharmacokinetics of imipenem.

Contraindications, cautions and adverse effects

Caution is advised in central nervous system disorders and epilepsy and in patients with renal impairment.

Thrombophlebitis is a potential common side-effect. Commonly, GI tract effects can occur; however, rarely, pseudomembranous colitis, superinfections, seizures or hypersensitivity reactions ensue.

Drug interactions

These drugs increase the risk of seizures when given with the antivirals ganciclovir or valganciclovir. They also decrease the concentration of the anticonvulsant valproate, increasing the risk of breakthrough seizures

Considerations in the administration of carbapenems

- Promote principles of good patient assessment, prescribing practice and antimicrobial stewardship through patient education.
- Assess for possible cautions or contraindications: known history of renal impairment or allergy to carbapenem and/or other beta-lactam antibiotic or seizure disorder, pregnancy, lactational state or inflammatory bowel disorders.
- If essential administration of imipenem is required alongside valproate, consider additional anticonvulsant therapy to prevent the occurrence of breakthrough seizures.
- Regular urine function testing is advised, due to the metabolism and excretion route.
- Advise the patient to report any altered bowel patterns or superinfection symptoms.
- Advise on the need to take appropriate safety precautions, such as ensuring patient is accompanied if CNS effects such as dizziness occur.
- Advise patient about signs of hypersensitivity.

Clinical consideration: medication consideration during adulthood

Poor antimicrobial stewardship: management for antibiotic demand through patient education regarding indications for use, completing the course, non-stockpiling for future use or sharing of antibiotics with symptomatic people

Awareness of drug allergies and emergence of resistant strains

Consider use of contraceptive measures in women of reproductive age, if the prescribed antibiotic is known to be teratogenic, and provide relevant patient education

Cautions for use in pregnancy: dosage adjustment due to increased maternal hepatic metabolism and glomerular infiltration rate; balance benefits of treatment against risk of foetal harm, due to drugs crossing the placental barrier, for example sulfonamides

Caution in lactation as most drugs cross into the breast milk; for example, may cause tooth deformities and staining of teeth

Interference with hormone-based contraceptives

Awareness of renal or hepatic impairment in patient history or associated conditions

Table 9.5   Pharmacokinetics of tetracycline.

Action	
Absorption	Absorption from the gastrointestinal tract, as predominantly administered orally. Absorption is reduced by the presence of food, drink or medications containing calcium, iron, aluminium or magnesium in the stomach, as the drugs bind readily to these ions
Distribution	Distributed to most body fluid and tissues but there is poor penetration to the cerebrospinal fluid. Is known to cross the placental barrier and enter breast milk
Metabolism	Concentrates in the liver
Excretion	Urine

Tetracyclines

These include tetracycline, doxycycline, minocycline and demeclocycline. They have bacteriostatic properties. Table 9.5 details the pharmacokinetics of tetracycline.

Contraindications, cautions and adverse effects

Contraindications include allergies, renal or hepatic impairment, pregnancy and lactation. Tetracyclines are not recommended for administration to children under 12 years as they can cause teeth discolouration in the younger child. If taken during pregnancy, the milk (deciduous) teeth of the baby can be discoloured. These effects are due to the tendency of tetracyclines to bind to calcium ions, resulting in their incorporation in teeth and bones.

Gastrointestinal adverse effects include direct irritation to the gastrointestinal tract causing oesophageal irritation or ulceration, epigastric burning, nausea, vomiting, cramps and diarrhoea. Fungal superinfection can result in vaginal or anal itching, sore mouth and black, furry tongue.

Dermatological effects include photosensitivity (increased skin sensitivity to ultraviolet light) as a common adverse effect. Skin rashes and hypersensitivity reactions (urticaria to anaphylaxis) are less common.

Intravenous high-dose tetracyclines can be hepatotoxic, especially in pregnant and postpartum women who also have renal disease

Drug interactions

The most clinically significant interaction is between tetracyclines and antacids and mineral supplements and is due to the tendency of tetracycline to bind to metal ions such as calcium, iron and magnesium, reducing the absorption of the drug. Tetracyclines are also known to interact with digoxin (monitor levels), anticoagulants (increases their action due to reduced gut flora producing less vitamin K), retinoids (vitamin A drugs) (increased risk of benign intracranial hypertension) and finally antacids and milk (interferes with absorption of tetracycline and may reduce effectiveness). Hepatotoxicity is a further risk when tetracycline is taken with, for example, atorvastatin, valproate, paracetamol or methotrexate. There is some evidence that tetracyclines may reduce the levels of oral contraceptives, but whether this effect is clinically significant is not established. Additional birth control precautions are, however, recommended for patients taking oral contraceptives with a tetracycline.

Considerations in the administration of tetracyclines

- Promote principles of good patient assessment, prescribing practice and antimicrobial stewardship through patient education.
- Take a whole tablet on an empty stomach 1 hour before or 2–3 hours after medication or meals.
- Do not take with dairy products, iron preparations, calcium supplements, magnesium- containing laxatives or antacids. If required, there should be a minimum of 2 hours between ingestion of tetracycline and these medications.
- Stand/sit upright and drink a full glass of water with each dose; this can prevent oesophageal irritation/ulceration. Do not take immediately before going to bed.

Advise the patient:

- if the drugs produce GI disturbances on administration (epigastric burning, cramps, nausea), tetracyclines should be taken with meals but this may affect the degree of absorption of the drug. The meal should not include dairy products
- to seek medical advice for any hypersensitivity reaction
- to report any diarrhoea, due to superinfection risk
- to consult prescriber if any adverse effects occur, such as other infections, changes in faeces/urine colour or pattern, severe abdominal cramps, difficulty in breathing, light sensitivity, rash/itching, jaundice, headache or visual disturbances
- to avoid prolonged exposure to sunlight, wear protective clothing and use sunscreen (SPF 30 and above) and avoid using sunbeds
- if drug was administered by injection, to report any signs of thrombophlebitis, such as swelling, redness, tenderness and heat at the injection site.

Chloramphenicol

This is a broad-spectrum antibiotic with both bacteriostatic and bactericidal effects, dependent on the sensitivity of individual bacteria. However, it should be reserved for life-threatening infections when used systemically. See Table 9.6 for the pharmacokinetics of chloramphenicol.

Contraindications, cautions and adverse effects

A common side-effect of chloramphenicol is bone marrow failure, leading to blood cell abnormalities. Because of this, chloramphenicol is only used to treat life-threatening infections. Acute porphyria is therefore a contraindication for its systemic use. Repeated or prolonged courses of oral or intravenous treatment should be avoided, as this would increase the risk of blood disorders, and even prolonged use of otic preparations of chloramphenicol should be avoided. Sore throat, fever and unusual tiredness could indicate signs of blood abnormalities.

Intravenous and oral administration of chloramphenicol is best avoided in patients with severe renal impairment but can be used (with caution) in patients with hepatic impairment, as there is an increased risk of bone marrow depression. Intravenous and oral administration should be avoided in pregnancy, as neonatal grey baby syndrome may occur, especially if used in the third trimester. This syndrome presents with abdominal distension, diarrhoea, vasomotor collapse, hypothermia, flaccidity, pallid cyanosis, abnormal respiratory rate and ashen skin colour. Chloramphenicol should also be avoided for breast-feeding mothers, as it may cause bone marrow toxicity in the infant. Pregnant and

Table 9.6   Pharmacokinetics of chloramphenicol.

Action	
Absorption	It can be administered via oral, intravenous and topical routes. Rate of absorption varies with route
Distribution	Distributes well through the body, including into cerebrospinal fluid, across the placenta and into breast milk
Metabolism	Hepatic
Excretion	Renal

lactating women should only receive chloramphenicol in optic preparations, if necessary, as it carries a theoretical risk of bone marrow toxicity.

Other adverse effects, including eye and ear irritation, aplastic anaemia, headache and depression after parenteral administration, ototoxicity, nausea and vomiting or circulatory collapse after oral administration, are less common.

Drug interactions

Chloramphenicol is known to increase the levels of oral anticoagulants, antihyperglycaemics, immunosuppressants (tacrolimus) and the anticonvulsant phenytoin. Phenobarbital or rifampicin may reduce the effect of chloramphenicol.

Considerations in the administration of chloramphenicol

- Promote principles of good patient assessment, prescribing practice and antimicrobial stewardship through patient education.
- Monitor plasma concentration after intravenous and oral administration in older persons or patients under 4 years of age or with hepatic or renal impairment.
- Monitor blood cell counts for abnormalities prior to and during a course of treatment.
- Avoid using ear buds in the external ear canal during treatment.
- Potentially transient eye irritation occurs, so provide advice about avoiding driving and hazardous work during initial stage of treatment. Periodic eye tests are advisable.
- When administered in combination with antihyperglycaemic drugs, monitor capillary blood glucose.
- When administered in combination with anticoagulants, monitor INR.

When administered in combination with phenytoin, monitor seizure pattern. Aminoglycosides

These include gentamicin, streptomycin, neomycin, tobramycin and amikacin. They have a broad spectrum of activity and are bactericidal. The pharmacokinetics are similar for all aminoglycosides (Table 9.7).

Contraindications, cautions and adverse effects

A known allergy to aminoglycosides is a contraindication for these drugs as well as myasthenia gravis.

They should be used with caution in the older person, in dehydration, with renal impairment, hearing or vestibular disorders, or in neuromuscular conditions such as Parkinson disease, as they can cause muscle weakness and respiratory depression.

Aminoglyosides can produce ototoxicity (mostly irreversible), resulting in deafness and/or vestibular (balance) disruption. These effects are dose dependent, and existing hearing impairment, tinnitus or vertigo may increase the risk of ototoxicity, as will use of aminoglycosides in combination with other ototoxic drugs. Because the drugs are cleared entirely by the kidneys, their use in renally impaired patients increases their toxicity, as they are likely to achieve higher plasma levels.

Table 9.7 Pharmacokinetics of aminoglycosides.

Action	
Absorption	Not absorbed from the gastrointestinal tract. Gentamicin is mainly administered parenterally but is also available as eye and ear preparations. Other aminoglycosides are available in topical preparations
Distribution	Distribution tends to be limited to the extracellular fluid and does not reach sufficient concentration in the cerebrospinal fluid unless given intrathecally
Metabolism	Not metabolised
Excretion	Renal

Nephrotoxic (usually reversible) effects can occur, and are more likely with existing renal impairment or when combined with other nephrotoxic drugs.

These drugs should be used with caution in pregnancy as there is a risk of auditory or vestibular damage in the foetus, especially if used in the second or third trimester – the benefits of the drug must outweigh the risk to the foetus.

Drug interactions

Ototoxicity and nephrotoxicity generally occur when there is concurrent administration of other agents with ototoxic or nephrotoxic effects.

Concurrent administration with neuromuscular blocking drugs, e.g. pancuronium, increases the risk of respiratory arrest, as aminoglycosides intensify the neuromuscular blockade.

Aminoglycosides are synergistic when used with penicillins, increasing bactericidal efficiency.

Considerations in the administration of aminoglycosides

- Promote principles of good patient assessment, prescribing practice and antimicrobial stewardship through patient education.
- Limit parenteral use of aminoglycosides to 7 days to reduce risk of toxicity.
- Initial dosing should be individualised due to variations in serum levels achieved with the same dose. Factors affecting serum levels include weight, renal function, age, percentage body fat, presence of fever, oedema and dehydration.
- Monitoring of both peak and trough plasma levels should be carried out to ensure both are within therapeutic range.
- Correct dehydration before commencement of aminoglycosides.
- With intramuscular or intravenous gentamicin administration, doses for obese patients should be calculated using ideal body weight to avoid excessive dosage.
- Serum concentration monitoring in parenteral administration of aminoglycosides must be determined in older people, obese people, people with cystic fibrosis, those with renal impairment (lengthen dose interval or reduce dose) and if high doses are being given. It should be monitored in all persons receiving parenteral aminoglycosides. This is extended to when being used in pregnancy.
- Encourage the patient to report signs and symptoms of ototoxicity (tinnitus, persistent headache, high-frequency hearing loss, nausea, unsteadiness, dizziness, vertigo), and monitor for signs of inner ear problems.
- Monitor for signs of nephrotoxicity (proteinuria, urinary casts, dilute urine production, increased serum creatinine and blood urea nitrogen). If oliguria or anuria develops, report to medical team.
- Flush IV line if the patient has multiple antibiotic administrations.
- Observe patients with myasthenia gravis and those receiving muscle relaxants or general anaesthetics with aminoglycosides due to the risk of respiratory depression resulting from neuromuscular blockade.

Clinical consideration: medication administration in the older adult

Signs and symptoms of infections can differ in this group

Culture and sensitivity are important to establish causative micro-organism

This group reacts more sensitively and with individual variability to the treatment regimens than younger adults

Pharmacokinetic changes due to age-related decline of body systems require attention to sites of metabolism (liver/kidney) and excretion (kidney) – may require dose adjustment

Rate of drug absorption is slower

More likely to have liver (prolongs drug effect) or renal (non-excretion of drug) impairment

More likely to experience adverse drug reaction due to body system impairment, polypharmacy, severe illness and pre-existing illness and drug regimens consisting of high-risk drug–drug interactions

More susceptible to adverse effects of antimicrobials. Give consideration to hydration and nutritional status alongside safety measures if CNS side-effects are noted

Consider dose adjustment and lengthen dose intervals in clients with liver or renal impairment, those who depend on alcohol or take concomitant nephrotoxic or hepatoxic drugs

Unintentional non-concordance due to forgetfulness, inability to follow instructions, complicated drug regimens, appearance of side-effects, inaccessibility to medication due to poor packaging or health inequalities (distance to pharmacy or cost)

Intentional non-concordance due to complicated drug regimen, poor patient education, client feels the drug is not necessary, increased side-effects, dosage is too high or poor client–practitioner relationship.

Macrolides

Macrolides, which include erythromycin, azithromycin and clarithromycin, have a similar antibacterial spectrum to penicillin. Erythromycin has both bacteriostatic and bactericidal properties. It is considered one of the safest antibiotics available. Table 9.8 describes the pharmacokinetics of erythromycin.

Contraindications, cautions and adverse effects

Contraindications include known allergy to any member of the group, as cross-sensitivity occurs. Cautious use in hepatic impairment as metabolism may be reduced and in renal impairment due to effects on excretion.

The most common adverse effects are gastrointestinal, these being decreased appetite, anorexia, nausea, vomiting and diarrhoea. Antibiotic-associated colitis and superinfections are rare effects. There is a risk that the drugs may cause QT prolongation (with oral and intravenous administration) and they may exacerbate myasthenia gravis. CNS effects such as hallucinations or seizures occur rarely.

Drug interactions

Erythromycin in combination with aminophylline increases the risk of hypokalaemia. Plasma levels of carbamazepine, digoxin and some immunosuppressants can increase in the presence of macrolides, increasing the risk of toxicity. Combination with warfarin leads to increased risk of bleeding. There is a risk of increased adverse effects of ergotamine (antimigraine) and erythromycin. Concomitant use of mizolastine (non-sedating antihistamine) and erythromycin increases the risk of adverse effects on the heart, and concomitant use of erythromycin and statins increases the risk of muscle pains. The potential for cardiotoxicity is increased when erythromycin is given with medications such as amiodarone which increase the QT interval.

Table 9.8 Pharmacokinetics of erythromycin.

Action	
Absorption	Absorption from GI tract is generally poor as erythromycin is destroyed by gastric acid. Acid-resistant formulations are better absorbed. It can be administered IV but not IM as deemed too painful
Distribution	Distributes well to most tissues but penetration to CSF is poor. Crosses the placental barrier and enters breast milk
Metabolism	Hepatic
Excretion	Bile (faeces) and urine (small amounts)

CSF, cerebrospinal fluid; GI, gastrointestinal; IM, intramuscular; IV, intravenous.

Erythromycin should not be used with chloramphenicol or clindamycin, as they antagonise each other's antibacterial actions. Verapamil (calcium channel blocker), azole antifungal drugs (ketoconazole) and HIV protease inhibitors such as ritonavir inhibit the metabolism of erythromycin.

Considerations in the administration of macrolides

- Promote principles of good patient assessment, prescribing practice and antimicrobial stewardship through patient education.
- Limit oral course to a maximum of 14 days to limit the risk of liver damage.
- Advise patient to take the medication on an empty stomach, with a full glass of water, 1 hour before meals or 2 hours afterwards.
- Advise that gastrointestinal adverse effects can be reduced by taking erythromycin (variant dependent) with meals, if necessary.
- Monitor for signs of toxicity if patient is also taking aminophylline (monitor potassium levels), carbamazepine or warfarin (monitor INR).
- Advise patient about reporting any adverse effects experienced, especially severe GI disturbances due to potential for antibiotic-associated (pseudomembranous) colitis.
- Monitor hepatic and renal function.
- Monitor IV site for pain, swelling and redness.

Lincosamides

Although similar, lincosamides, which include clindamycin and lincomycin, are considered more toxic than macrolides. Clindamycin is a bacteriostatic but it can assume bactericidal properties. Table 9.9 presents the pharmacokinetics of clindamycin.

Contraindications, cautions and adverse effects

Contraindications include diarrhoeal illness, as diarrhoea associated with *Clostridium difficile* infection is a risk with these drugs. This can develop up to 6 weeks after completing a course of a lincosamide. This is known to occur more frequently with clindamycin than other types of antibiotics. These drugs should be used with caution in older people due to this risk.

Use should be avoided in patients with acute porphyria as it could induce an acute crisis. Caution is advised in patients with renal or hepatic impairment.

Caution is advised in the first trimester of pregnancy and in breast-feeding women due to a risk of infantile diarrhoea, as the drugs enter breast milk.

Clindamycin cream damages latex condoms and diaphragms, so additional birth control measures are required.

Adverse effects include skin reactions, which are common, abdominal pain (with parenteral and topical administration) and vulvovaginal infection (with parenteral, oral and vaginal administration).

Electrocardiogram changes, hypotension or cardiac arrest may occur with rapid intravenous administration.

Table 9.9 Pharmacokinetics of clindamycin.

Action	
Absorption	Absorbed from the gastrointestinal tract so can be administered orally. Intravenous, intramuscular and topical administration also possible
Distribution	Distributes well to most tissues and body fluids, including bone and synovial fluid, but does not penetrate the cerebrospinal fluid or cross the blood–brain barrier
Metabolism	Hepatic
Excretion	Urine and bile

Drug interactions

Clindamycin increases the effects of neuromuscular blockers (used in anaesthetic induction and surgery) such as atracurium, cisatracurium and suxamethonium.

Considerations in the administration of lincosamides

- Promote principles of good patient assessment, prescribing practice and antimicrobial stewardship through patient education.
- Advise patient to report any bouts of diarrhoea to their healthcare professional and discontinue treatment immediately if prolonged, severe or bloody diarrhoea occurs.
- Oral capsules should be swallowed whole, with a glass of water.
- Advise using additional contraceptive measures if using vaginal preparations.
- If patient is breast feeding, advise monitoring the child for diarrhoea, bloody stools or candidiasis.
- In treatment (systemic) regimens of 10 days or more, monitor hepatic and renal function.
- Monitor hepatic and renal function in neonates and infants (by systemic use).

163

Conclusion

This chapter has provided the reader with an overview of the use of antibacterial medication. The role of the paramedic is key in ensuring the principles of effective antimicrobial stewardship are maintained to ensure their sustained usability to protect from emerging resistant pathogens. The HCP's role is paramount, primarily by offering advice and information to those who use health and social care services regarding expectations of antimicrobial therapies.

The following is a list of conditions associated with the use of antibiotics. Take some time and write notes about each of the conditions. Think about the medications that may be used in order to treat these conditions and be specific about the pharmacokinetics and pharmacodynamics. Remember to include aspects of patient care. If you are making notes about people you have offered care and support to, you must ensure that you have adhered to the rules of confidentiality.

The condition	Your notes
Nausea and vomiting	
Pseudomembranous colitis	
Anaphylaxis	

References

British Society for Antimicrobial Chemotherapy. (2017). *Antimicrobial Stewardship. From Principles to Practice.* www.bsac.org.uk/antimicrobialstewardshipebook/BSAC-AntimicrobialStewardship-From PrinciplestoPractice-eBook.pdf

Burchum, J.R.. and Rosenthal, L.D. (2019). *Lehne's Pharmacology for Nursing Care.* St Louis: Elsevier.

Dolk, F.C., Pouwels, K., Smith, D. et al., (2018). Antibiotics in primary care in England: which antibiotics are prescribed and for which conditions? *Journal of Antimicrobial Chemotherapy* **73**(2): ii2–ii10.

Lack, W., Seymour, R., Bickers, A., Studnek, J. and Karunakar, M. (2019). Prehospital antibiotic prophylaxis for open fractures: practicality and safety. *Prehospital Emergency Care* **23**(3): 385–388.

National Institute for Health and Care Excellence. (2018). *Antimicrobial stewardship.* www.nice.org.uk/guidance/ng15

National Institute for Health and Care Excellence. (2021). *British National Formulary.* https://bnf.nice.org.uk/

Parliamentary Office of Science and Technology. (2017). *UK Trends in Infectious Disease.* https://researchbriefings.files.parliament.uk/documents/POST-PN-0545/POST-PN-0545.pdf

Smit, L and Boyle, M. (2014). Antibiotic prophylaxis in pre-hospital trauma care: a review of the literature. *Australasian Journal of Paramedicine* **11**(5).

Tsai, D., Jamal, J.A., Davis, J.S. et al. (2015). Interethnic differences in pharmacokinetics of antibacterials. *Clinical Pharmacokinetics* **54**(3): 243–260.

World Health Organization. (2020). *Antibiotic resistance.* www.who.int/en/news-room/fact-sheets/detail/antibiotic-resistance

Further reading

Ashelford, S., Raynsford, J. and Taylor, V. (2016). *Pathophysiology and Pharmacology for Nursing Students*. London: Sage Publications.

British Medical Association. (2018). *New Guide to Medicines and Drugs*, 10th edn. London: Dorling Kindersley.

Barber, P. and Robertson, D. (2020). *Essential Pharmacology for Nurses*, 4th edn. Buckingham: Open University Press.

Cattini, P. Kiernam, M. (2020). Infection prevention and control. In: *The Royal Marsden manual of Clinical Nursing Procedures*, 10th edn (eds S. Lister, J. Hofland and H. Grafton). Chichester: Wiley-Blackwell Publishing.

Coppoc, G.L. (1996). *Chloramphenicol*. www.cyto.purdue.edu/cdroms/cyto2/17/chmrx/cap.htm

Department of Health and Social Care. (2019). *Antimicrobial resistance (AMR)*. www.gov.uk/government/collections/antimicrobial-resistance-amr-information-and-resources

Ha, D., Forte, M., Olans, R. et al. (2019). A multidisciplinary approach to incorporate bedside nurses into antimicrobial stewardship and infection prevention. *Joint Commission Journal on Quality and Patient Safety* **45**(5): 600–605.

Karch, A.M. (2017). *Focusing on Nursing Pharmacology*, 7th edn. Philadelphia: Wolters Kluwer Publishing.

Moffa, M. and Brook, I. (2015). Tetracyclines, glycylcyclines and chloramphenicol. In: *Mandell, Douglas and Bennett's Principles and Practice of Infectious Diseases*, 8th edn (eds J.E. Bennett, R. Dolin and M. Balser). St Louis: Elsevier.

Olans, R.N., Olans, R.D. and DeMaria Jr, A. (2018). The critical role of the staff nurse in antimicrobial stewardship – unrecognised, but already there. *Clinical Infectious Diseases* **62**: 84–88.

Pearce, L. (2019). Antimicrobial resistance: how you can make a difference, *Nursing Standard* **34**(5): 53–54.

Peate. I. (2015). Antimicrobial resistance: the nurse's essential role. *British Journal of Nursing* **24**(1): 5.

Wilson, A. (2019). Antimicrobial resistance: what can nurses do? *British Journal of Nursing* **28**(1): 16–17.

World Health Organization. (2016). *Global action plan on antimicrobial resistance*. www.who.int/publications/i/item/9789241509763

Xiu, P. and Datta, S. (2019). *Pharmacology*, 5th edn. London: Elsevier.

Multiple-choice questions

1. What does the term 'bactericidal' mean?
   (a) Inhibits bacterial growth
   (b) Destroys bacteria
   (c) Aids bacterial growth
   (d) Aids bacterial cell replication
2. Which group of antibacterials does imipenem belong to?
   (a) Sulfonamides
   (b) Quinolones
   (c) Aminoglycosides
   (d) Beta-lactams
3. Neonatal grey baby syndrome is associated with which antibiotic?
   (a) Cefalexin
   (b) Chloramphenicol
   (c) Ciprofloxacin
   (d) Co-trimoxazole
4. The action of clindamycin is:
   (a) Folate interference
   (b) Bacterial DNA inhibition
   (c) Protein synthesis interference
   (d) Disruption of the cell wall
5. Erythromycin is known to increase the levels of which drug?
   (a) Warfarin
   (b) Paracetamol
   (c) Ferrous sulfate
   (d) Gabapentin

6. Tetracycline is contraindicated in:
   (a) Pregnant women
   (b) Breast-feeding mothers
   (c) People with renal impairment
   (d) All of the above

7. In which group of antibiotics is there a possibility of disulfiram-like reaction occurring if alcohol is consumed alongside the treatment?
   (a) Penicillin
   (b) Aminoglycosides
   (c) Sulfonamides
   (d) Cephalosporins

8. Antibacterials can have _____ adverse effects.
   (a) Hepatotoxic
   (b) Nephrotoxic
   (c) Ototoxic
   (d) All of the above

9. Ototoxicity is a known adverse effect of which antibacterial group?
   (a) Aminoglycosides
   (b) Tetracyclines
   (c) Cephalosporins
   (d) Penicillins

10. Concomitant administration of erythromycin and which medication can induce hypokalaemia?
    (a) Theophylline
    (b) Ferrous sulfate
    (c) Warfarin
    (d) Iburofen

11. Which antibiotic group disrupts the bacterial cell wall?
    (a) Carbapenems
    (b) Lincosamides
    (c) Chloramphenicol
    (d) Aminoglycosides

12. The term *antibacterial* is used interchangeably with which other term?
    (a) Antihypertensive
    (b) Antibiotic
    (c) Antiemetic
    (d) Anticoagulant

13. Which factors can affect the pharmacokinetics of antibiotics?
    (a) Age
    (b) Renal function
    (c) Hepatic function
    (d) All of the above

14. Photosensitivity is a potential adverse effect of which antibiotic group?
    (a) Cephalosporins
    (b) Penicllins
    (c) Carbapenems
    (d) Tetracyclines

15. A main priority of good antimicrobial stewardship is:
    (a) Monitor for tendon damage
    (b) Identify the causative organism
    (c) Monitor hepatic function
    (d) Monitor renal function

16. Breakthrough seizures are a possibility when imipenem is concurrently administered with which drug?

   (a) Paracetamol

   (b) Levothyroxine

   (c) Valproate

   (d) Ferrous sulfate

Chapter 10

Medications used in the cardiovascular system

Lisa Clegg and Fraser D. Russell

Aim

This chapter aims to provide the student paramedic with an understanding of the pharmacological agents used to treat patients with cardiovascular disease.

Learning outcomes

After reading this chapter, the reader will be able to:

1. Define lifestyle choices that mitigate future development of cardiovascular disease
2. Understand the key role that the renin-angiotensin-aldosterone system (RAAS) plays in regulation of blood volume and systemic vascular resistance and as a target for management of patients with hypertension and heart failure
3. Compare pharmacological therapies for their potential to improve health outcomes (e.g. potential to reduce hospitalisation for heart failure, reduce risk of stroke, reduce rate of mortality)
4. Recognise the pharmacological therapies that may be associated with unwanted effects, even at therapeutic doses (e.g. hypotension, cough, hyperkalaemia).

Cardiovascular diseases

Paramedics have a critical role in the assessment and management of patients presenting with cardiovascular disease (CVD). About 7.4 million people in the UK and 1.2 million people in Australia live with CVD (Australian Bureau of Statistics, 2018; British Heart Foundation, 2021). With an estimated 17.9 million deaths per year, CVD is the leading cause of death worldwide (World Health Organization, 2021).

Coronary artery disease involves the impairment of blood flow through the coronary arteries, commonly caused by atheromatous plaques and thrombosis formation. Risk factors for CVD described as modifiable include hypertension, dyslipidaemias (hypercholesterolaemia) and physical inactivity, while non-modifiable factors include family history and advanced age. Given the prevalence of CVDs in the community, patients with CVD presentations such as hypertension, heart failure and acute coronary syndrome are common in paramedic-led care.

Fundamentals of Pharmacology for Paramedics, First Edition. Edited by Ian Peate, Suzanne Evans, and Lisa Clegg.
© 2022 John Wiley & Sons Ltd. Published 2022 by John Wiley & Sons Ltd.

Hypertension and heart failure

Hypertension is a leading cause of cardiovascular morbidity and mortality. Hypertension is diagnosed when office or clinic systolic blood pressure (SBP) is ≥140 mmHg (≥135 mmHg for home measurements) and/or diastolic blood pressure (DBP) is ≥90 mmHg (≥85 mmHg for home measurements) (Unger et al., 2020).

Chronic hypertension leads to structural changes within the ventricles such as ventricular hypertrophy, resulting in ventricular dysfunction. High blood pressure increases afterload (the pressure the ventricle works against to open the pulmonary or aortic valves to eject the blood). This eventually leads to heart failure as the ventricle loses its ability to pump adequately, resulting in increased blood volume and pressure at the end of diastole (end-diastolic volume and end-diastolic pressure) (Oh and Cho, 2020).

Hypertension is a modifiable risk factor not only for heart failure, but also for renal failure and stroke and patients lower their risk through lifestyle changes and pharmacotherapies that include the use of blood pressure-lowering medications.

Heart failure is defined as 'a complex clinical syndrome with typical symptoms and signs that generally occur on exertion but can also occur at rest. It is secondary to an abnormality of cardiac structure or function that impairs the ability of the heart to fill with blood at normal pressure or eject blood sufficient to fulfil the needs of the metabolising organs' (Atherton et al., 2018).

This definition describes two processes that cause heart failure: the inability of the heart to adequately fill (diastolic failure) and the inability of the heart to eject enough blood to meet metabolic needs (systolic failure) (Figure 10.1).

The left ventricular ejection fraction (LVEF), the fraction of the left ventricular volume in systole divided by the end-diastolic volume, expressed as a percentage, is commonly used in the classification of heart failure. Normal LVEF is 50–70%; heart failure with reduced ejection fraction (HFrEF) is <40%; heart failure with midrange ejection fraction (HFmEF) is 40–49% and heart failure with preserved ejection fraction (HFpEF) is ≥50% (Kemp and Conte, 2012).

Heart failure with reduced ejection fraction is commonly caused by ischaemic heart disease that results in negative inotropy (decreased force of cardiac contraction). This leads to an increase in left ventricular end-diastolic pressure (LVEDP) and left ventricular end-diastolic volume (LVEDV). Right ventricular failure, primarily caused by an increase in afterload due to the high pressure in the pulmonary system resulting from left ventricular failure (Arrigo et al., 2019), is reported to occur in at least 60% of patients with HFrEF (Bosch et al., 2017).

Heart failure with preserved ejection fraction results from a failure of the left ventricle to adequately relax and typically denotes a stiffer ventricular wall. The 'stiffness' and decreased compliance of the ventricular wall cause an increase in ventricular end-diastolic pressure. Right ventricular failure occurs in 30–40% of patients with this form of heart failure (Bosch et al., 2017).

Management of hypertension and heart failure

Lifestyle modification is the cornerstone for reducing risk of hypertension and heart failure and is achieved through smoking cessation, increased physical activity, weight loss, improved diet (including increased consumption of fish, legumes, poultry, fruits, vegetables, whole grains and low-fat dairy products), reduced sodium intake, enhanced dietary intake of potassium and moderation in alcohol intake for individuals who drink alcohol (Arnett et al., 2019; Grundy et al., 2019; Unger et al., 2020).

First-line pharmacological therapies for hypertension and heart failure include angiotensin-converting enzyme (ACE) inhibitors, angiotensin receptor blockers (ARBs), angiotensin receptor-neprilysin inhibitor (ARNI), beta-blockers and aldosterone receptor antagonists (Yancy et al., 2013, 2016, 2017; Unger et al., 2020). For patients with hypertension without comorbid heart failure, blood pressure-lowering medication can reduce the incidence of heart failure (Table 10.1). First-line treatment for a hypertensive emergency requiring immediate reduction in blood pressure (e.g. hypertensive encephalopathy; acute ischaemic stroke with SBP >220 mmHg or DBP >120 mmHg; acute haemorrhagic stroke and SBP >180 mmHg) includes a beta-blocker such as labetalol and a dihydropyridine calcium channel blocker such as nicardipine (Unger et al., 2020).

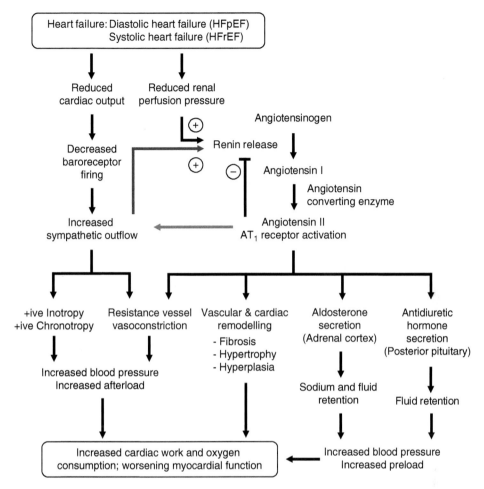

Figure 10.1 Overview of pathways that lead to worsening myocardial function in heart failure patients. Note the interplay between the sympathetic nervous system (blue arrow) and the renin-angiotensin-aldosterone system (RAAS; orange arrow). HFpEF, heart failure with preserved ejection fraction (diastolic heart failure); HFrEF, heart failure with reduced ejection fraction (systolic heart failure).

Beta-adrenoceptor antagonists (beta-blockers)

The administration of beta-blockers to patients with HFrEF is seemingly paradoxical given the suppressive effect that these drugs have on myocardial contractility. While initial treatment may cause a small reduction in ejection fraction, chronic administration of beta-blockers to patients with HFrEF reduces mortality. The clue to success of this therapy resides in the underlying pathophysiology of heart failure. During HFrEF, the reduced cardiac output is detected as a reduction in arterial pressure, resulting in a compensatory increase in sympathetic outflow, to restore arterial pressure by increasing cardiac rate and contractility (see Figure 10.1). Since arterial pressure is not the problem in these patients, chronically elevated sympathetic drive is a cause of pathogenic myocardial remodelling and increased risk for ventricular arrhythmias. Increased release of noradrenaline at JG beta-1 adrenoceptors also stimulates renin secretion. Chronic use of beta-blockers interrupts these effects, improving haemodynamic performance of the heart. In patients with HFrEF who are treated with beta-blocker therapy, rate of hospitalisation associated with cardiac causes decreases, as does risk of sudden cardiac death and total mortality rate (Packer et al., 1996).

- Beta-blockers can cause worsening of heart failure. The risk for this is curtailed by administration of low doses that are slowly titrated upwards.
- Beta-blockers can compromise airflow by interfering with the binding of adrenaline to airway beta-2 adrenoceptors and are therefore contraindicated in patients with asthma.

Table 10.1   Drug therapies for management of patients with hypertension or heart failure.

Aetiology	Treatment	References
Hypertension • Reduce the incidence of HF	Black populations: thiazide-like diuretic with DHP-CCB, or DHP-CCB with an ARB. A diuretic and aldosterone receptor antagonist may be added Non-black populations: ACE inhibitor or ARB with DHP-CCB. A thiazide or thiazide-like diuretic and aldosterone receptor antagonist may be added	[1]
HFrEF • Reduce morbidity and mortality • Reduce HF hospitalisations (ivabradine)	ACE inhibitor, or ARBs, or ARNI with evidence-based beta-blockers and aldosterone antagonists. For patients (NYHA Class II or III) who can tolerate ACE inhibitors or ARBs, ARNI is the therapy of choice. ARNI is contraindicated in patients who have a history of angio-oedema and should not be used in conjunction with ACE inhibitors or within 36 h of the last dose of ACE inhibitor. ARBs are used in preference to ACE inhibitors if ACE inhibitors cause cough or angio-oedema. Ivabradine is used to lower heart rate	[2-4]
Atrial fibrillation (patient with HFrEF) • Reduce hospitalisations for HF • Reduce risk of stroke (oral anticoagulants)	Heart rate control: beta-blocker and/or digoxin (low dose – 0.125–0.25 mg/day)	[2,5,6]
HFmEF • Reduce cardiovascular events • Reduce hospitalisations for HF	ACE inhibitors, ARBs, beta-blockers and aldosterone receptor antagonists. Diuretics to manage volume overload	[7,8]
Atrial fibrillation (patients with HFmEF)	Heart rate control: beta-blockers, non-dihydropyridine calcium channel blockers (verapamil, diltiazem)	[6]
HFpEF • Reduce hospitalisations for HF	Diuretics to manage volume overload. Beta-blockers, ACE inhibitors, ARBs to reduce SBP and DBP (coronary revascularisation for patients with coronary artery disease)	[2,4,8]
Atrial fibrillation (patients with HFpEF)	Heart rate control: beta-blockers, non-DHP-CCB (verapamil, diltiazem)	[5,6,9,10]

ACE, angiotensin-converting enzyme; ARBs, angiotensin receptor blockers; ARNI, angiotensin receptor-neprilysin inhibitor; DBP, diastolic blood pressure; DHP-CCB, dihydropyridine calcium channel blocker; HFmEF, heart failure with midrange ejection fraction (40–49%); HFpEF, heart failure with preserved ejection fraction (≥50%); HFrEF, heart failure with reduced ejection fraction (<40%); SBP, systolic blood pressure.

[1] Unger et al., 2020; [2] Yancy et al., 2013; [3] Yancy et al., 2016; [4] Yancy et al., 2017; [5] January et al., 2019; [6] Hindricks et al., 2021; [7] Margonato et al., 2020; [8] Ponikowski et al., 2016; [9] Gard et al., 2020; [10] Mullens et al., 2019.

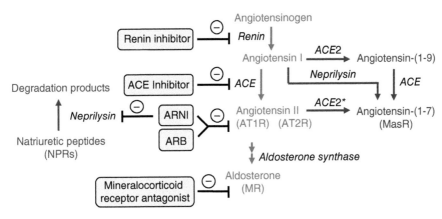

Figure 10.2 Classes of drug that target the renin-angiotensin-aldosterone-system (RAAS) and neprilysin for the management of patients who have hypertension or heart failure. The diagram illustrates classic (orange) and alternative RAAS pathways (purple), and the metabolism of natriuretic peptides by neprilysin (blue). ACE, angiotensin-converting enzyme; ACE2, angiotensin-converting enzyme 2; ARB, angiotensin receptor blocker; ARNI, angiotensin receptor-neprilysin inhibitor; AT1R, angiotensin 1 receptor; AT2R, angiotensin 2 receptor; MasR, mitochondrial assembly receptor; MR, mineralocorticoid receptor; NPRs, natriuretic peptide receptors. *ACE2 is the main enzyme in the kidneys responsible for converting angiotensin II to angiotensin-(1-7), while prolyloligopeptidase is important in the circulation and lungs.

Renin-angiotensin-aldosterone-system

The renin-angiotensin-aldosterone system (RAAS) has a critical role in the maintenance of physiological blood volume and electrolyte balance. Angiotensin II, the primary effector of RAAS, mediates its effects through activation of angiotensin II type 1 (AT_1) and type 2 (AT_2) receptors. Angiotensin II is produced by sequential processing of the precursor molecules angiotensinogen and angiotensin I. JG cells secrete renin into the blood in response to (i) low renal perfusion pressure, (ii) sympathetic outflow that leads to JG cell beta-1 adrenoceptor activation, and (iii) low distal tubule sodium chloride concentration (Friis et al., 2013). Renin converts angiotensinogen to angiotensin I, which is in turn converted to angiotensin II by ACE that is expressed in vascular endothelial cells and epithelial cells of the lungs and kidneys (Figure 10.2).

While important for normal regulation of blood pressure and fluid and electrolyte balance, a dys-regulated RAAS can contribute to detrimental pathophysiological remodelling of the cardiovascular system. Angiotensin II mediates a plethora of effects that contribute to the development of hypertension and heart failure, for example vasoconstriction, vascular smooth muscle cell and cardiomyocyte hypertrophy and cardiac and renal fibrosis (AlQudah et al., 2020; Shafiq et al., 2008). The RAAS represents an important target for drug treatment of patients with hypertension and/or heart failure (see Figure 10.2).

Angiotensin-converting enzyme (ACE) inhibitors

Angiotensin-converting enzyme inhibitors (quinapril, enalapril, fosinopril, lisinopril, perindopril, ramipril, captopril, trandolapril) are used to treat patients with heart failure and/or hypertension. In patients with HFrEF, ACE inhibitors are reported to decrease all-cause mortality (risk ratio 0.72; $p < 0.01$ at 6 months) and cardiovascular mortality (risk ratio 0.83; $p < 0.001$ at 6–42 months) and lead to fewer admissions to hospital for heart failure (risk ratio 0.71; $p < 0.01$) or for cardiovascular complications (risk ratio 0.94; $p < 0.01$) (Boeuf-Gibot et al., 2021).

Angiotensin receptor blockers (ARBs)

The ARBs (irbesartan, candesartan, valsartan, olmesartan, telmisartan, losartan, eprosartan) are AT1 receptor-selective antagonists. Angiotensin II mediates opposing cardiovascular effects through activation of AT1 and AT2 receptors, and chronic activation of AT1 receptors can contribute to the pathogenesis of hypertension and heart failure through effects such as vasoconstriction, vascular inflammation, cardiomyocyte hypertrophy, fibroblast hyperplasia and oxidative stress. A series of large-scale clinical trials have shown a significant reduction in cardiovascular death and all-cause mortality in HFrEF patients treated with candesartan (Pfeffer et al., 2003; Young et al., 2004). The effects of angiotensin II at AT2 receptors may be cardioprotective. Activation of AT2 receptors leads to vasodilation and suppression of myocardial fibrosis (Sumners et al., 2019; Wang et al., 2017).

Angiotensin receptor-neprilysin inhibitor (ARNI)

Natriuretic peptides modulate electrolyte–fluid balance by causing diuresis and have a critical role in cardiovascular homeostasis since their actions tend to reduce fluid overload in the venous circulation. The primary forms of natriuretic peptide are atrial natriuretic peptide, B-type natriuretic peptide and C-type natriuretic peptide. The effects of the natriuretic peptides are terminated by the activity of neprilysin, a membrane-bound endopeptidase (Bayes-Genis et al., 2016). ARNI, a combination of sacubitril (a neprilysin inhibitor) and valsartan (an ARB), prolongs the beneficial effects of the natriuretic peptides by inhibiting their enzymatic breakdown and blocks the cardiovascular effects of angiotensin II (see Figure 10.2). Sacubitril, in combination with the ARB valsartan, has been found to be superior to the ACE inhibitor enalapril for reducing cardiovascular mortality and hospitalisations for heart failure (McMurray et al., 2014). Based on these findings, ARNI is now recommended for patients who can tolerate ACE inhibitors or ARBs and who have HFrEF (see Table 10.1).

Mineralocorticoid receptor antagonists

The mineralocorticoid aldosterone causes the reabsorption of sodium ions from renal tubules back into the blood, thereby maintaining plasma sodium and blood volume. In heart failure, this action worsens fluid overload. Mineralocorticoid receptor antagonists reduce blood volume and provide cardioprotective effects as a result.

- Troublesome cough is experienced in ~20% of patients who are treated with an ACE inhibitor and this is attributed to reduced metabolism, and hence accumulation of bradykinin. For these patients, ACE inhibitors can be replaced with an ARB.
- Combined use of ACE inhibitors and ARBs provides no survival benefit when compared to monotherapy with an ACE inhibitor or ARB and may cause a hypotensive response. For these reasons, combined use of ACE inhibitors and ARBs is generally avoided.
- Angiotensin II is critical for normal renal development. Administration of ACE inhibitors and ARBs is contraindicated in pregnancy because of the risk for fetopathy, including neonatal renal impairment and pulmonary hypoplasia.
- Aldosterone contributes to potassium excretion. By blocking the effects of aldosterone, mineralocorticoid receptor antagonists can cause hyperkalaemia. Potassium levels >5.1 mmol/L have been associated with increased mortality (Krogager et al., 2017).

Calcium channel blockers (CCBs)

Calcium channel blockers produce relaxation of vascular smooth muscle and negative chronotropic and ionotropic effects in the heart. Dihydropyridine CCBs (DHP-CCBs) such as nifedipine and amlodipine have greater selectivity for vascular smooth muscle over cardiac muscle compared to non-dihydropyridine CCBs (NDHP-CCBs) such as diltiazem and verapamil and are therefore less likely to produce cardiac effects. Both types of CCB are used to treat patients with hypertension and angina pectoris. NDHP-CCBs are also used to manage patients with supraventricular tachyarrhythmias (they are known as Class IV antiarrhythmic agents). NDHP-CCBs should be avoided in patients who are being treated with beta-blockers and those who have HFrEF, because of the potential to cause excessive myocardial depression. There is insufficient evidence of a benefit of CCBs to support their use in patients with HFpEF.

Diuretics

Diuretics are a first-line therapy for patients with uncomplicated hypertension (see Table 10.1). Diuretics can also assist in alleviating the congestion in patients with congestive heart failure by removing excess sodium and water and are therefore recommended for patients with HFrEF and HFpEF (Ponikowski et al., 2016). Loop, thiazide and thiazide-like diuretics can cause potassium wasting, a situation that is avoided by coadministration of a potassium-sparing diuretic. Readers are referred to Chapter 11 for the pharmacology and clinical utility of diuretic agents in patients with hypertension and heart failure.

Positive inotropes for patients with decompensated heart failure

A primary concern of low cardiac output is hypoxia caused by hypoperfusion of tissues that can lead to end-organ dysfunction. Positive inotropes provide haemodynamic support in instances of low cardiac output (e.g. in acute decompensated heart failure, cardiogenic shock, prior to heart transplantation and following cardiac surgery). Most positive inotropes increase myocardial contraction by increasing intracellular calcium concentration. Unfortunately, the use of positive inotropes in patients with chronic heart failure has often failed to produce long-term clinical benefit and may have increased the risk for death (see review by Ahmad et al., 2019).

Calcium sensitisers are agents that provide inotropic support without increasing cyclic AMP or intracellular calcium concentration. Omecamtiv mecarbil increases myocyte contractility by increasing sarcomere duration of contraction without causing appreciable effects on calcium transients. The Global Approach to Lowering Adverse Cardiac outcomes Through Improving Contractility in Heart Failure (GALACTIC-HF) clinical trial has been established to examine the safety and efficacy of omecamtiv mecarbil in patient with HFrEF (Teerlink et al., 2020).

173

Acute coronary Syndrome (ACS)

Acute coronary syndrome includes unstable angina and myocardial infarction (MI). Patients with ACS often experience pain or discomfort in the chest, commonly known as angina. The main cause is an ulcerated atheromatous plaque with thrombus that occludes the coronary artery, resulting in myocardial ischaemia which can lead to myocardial cell death if coronary artery blood flow is not restored through coronary reperfusion.

Coronary reperfusion is required in patients diagnosed with ST-segment elevation myocardial infarction (STEMI), with primary percutaneous coronary intervention (primary PCI) being the first-line therapy. In PCI, a balloon catheter is inserted into the blocked coronary artery, opening the artery to restore blood flow to the myocardium. A stent (mesh tube) may also be inserted to maintain coronary artery patency.

A fibrinolytic agent is used if the patient cannot receive PCI intervention within 2 hours of STEMI diagnosis (Fazel et al., 2020; Ibanez et al., 2018). Major bleeding is a risk when fibrinolysis is coupled with PCI (Fazel et al., 2020).

Management of acute coronary syndrome

Fibrinolytic therapy

Thrombin (coagulation factor IIa) catalyses the conversion of soluble fibrinogen to insoluble fibrin. While fibrin is a critical factor in haemostasis to prevent blood loss following injury, it may also contribute to thrombosis, resulting in reduced blood flow. The thrombus is dissolved by plasmin, a naturally occurring fibrinolytic modulator derived from plasminogen. Plasminogen is converted to plasmin by endothelial-derived tissue plasminogen activator (t-PA). Alteplase, produced using recombinant technologies, is identical in structure to t-PA, with a half-life in plasma of less than 5 minutes. Reteplase and tenecteplase mimic the effects of t-PA, but with plasma half-lives of 15 and 20 minutes, respectively. Reteplase and tenecteplase have similar efficacy and safety profiles and are used clinically in patients who have had a recent acute myocardial infarction (Zia-Behbahani et al., 2019). Fibrinolytic agents are contraindicated in patients who have severe hypertension, recent surgery or stroke, because of the risk of haemorrhage. The effect of fibrinolytic agents can be reversed using tranexamic acid, a drug that inhibits plasminogen activation.

Common clinical manifestations of ACS include the following:

- prolonged chest pain described as crushing, squeezing or stabbing
- anxiety or fear of death
- nausea and vomiting
- breathlessness.

Paramedics should also be aware that these clinical manifestations are not always present, and patients may present pain free. Paramedics should not discount cardiac causes for atypical presentations.

Aspirin and dual antiplatelet therapy

Prior to PCI, patients are treated with dual antiplatelet therapy (DAPT) comprising a combination of aspirin and an adenosine 5′-diphosphate (ADP) $P2Y_{12}$ receptor inhibitor such as prasugrel or ticagrelor. Aspirin inhibits cyclo-oxygenase, which is responsible for the production of thromboxane A_2 and the prostaglandins, resulting in attenuated platelet aggregation. DAPT is indicated in patients with acute coronary syndrome, particularly if undergoing PCI, and in patients who have had stent implantation for coronary artery disease (Valgimigli et al., 2018). Benefits ascribed to DAPT include reduced rate of myocardial infarction and stent thrombosis, aiding maintenance of arterial patency. Risk scores are used to determine the duration of DAPT, with the aim of maximising cardiovascular benefits and minimising bleeding risk.

$P2Y_{12}$ receptor inhibitor monotherapy has been evaluated for efficacy and safety. Recent clinical trials suggest that ticagrelor monotherapy produces similar cardiovascular risk reductions as DAPT, but with a lower incidence of bleeding (Mehran et al., 2019).

Glyceryl trinitrate (nitroglycerin)

Glyceryl trinitrate (GTN) is used for rapid alleviation of angina pectoris and for treatment of patients with acute heart failure and myocardial infarction. GTN causes dilation of venules (reducing preload) and arterioles (reducing afterload). Where atherosclerotic plaques limit delivery of blood to tissues, GTN dilates collateral blood vessels to facilitate improved tissue perfusion. It also dilates coronary arteries to improve delivery of blood to the myocardium. The mechanism involves the liberation of nitric oxide, which is a potent vasodilator.

Glyceryl trinitrate is administered sublingually as a spray or tablet, or intravenously, as the drug undergoes extensive first-pass metabolism when ingested orally. Chronic exposure to GTN causes tolerance (reduced responsiveness), via an as yet unidentified mechanism (Bilska-Wilkosz et al., 2019). Intermittent use of the GTN patch (e.g. removal of the patch at night with reapplication in the morning) helps to circumvent the loss of responsiveness to the drug. GTN is contraindicated in patients who have a hypersensitivity to the drug, following use of phosphodiesterase type 5 inhibitors, such as sildenafil, and in patients with severe anaemia.

Lipid-lowering therapies

Lipid-lowering therapies provide significant survival benefits in patients who are at elevated risk of an adverse cardiovascular event. Statins are the first-line therapy for reducing blood cholesterol levels. Therapy is tailored to patient clinical profile, with high-, moderate- and low-intensity statin therapies used to reduce serum LDL concentration by $\geq50\%$, 30–49% and <30%, respectively (Grundy et al., 2019). Other lipid-lowering drugs can be combined with statins if target LDL-C concentrations are not achieved.

HMG-CoA reductase inhibitors (statins)

Acetyl-coenzyme A is a precursor in a sequence of biochemical reactions that culminate in the formation of cholesterol in liver cells. In an early step in this pathway, 3-hydroxy-3-methylglutaryl-coenzyme A (HMG-CoA) is converted to mevalonic acid by the enzyme HMG-CoA reductase. By inhibiting this enzyme, statins interfere with cholesterol synthesis. The response to this reduction in cholesterol synthesis is an increase in LDL receptor number, which leads to increased clearance of LDL from the blood. Statins approved for clinical use include atorvastatin, rosuvastatin, simvastatin, pravastatin, lovastatin and fluvastatin.

Statin therapy has been reported to reduce the risk of a first major vascular event by 21%, the risk of a major coronary event by 24%, and risk of vascular mortality by 12% when calculated as effect per 1.0 mmol/L reduction in LDL-C (Cholesterol Treatment Trialists' Collaboration, 2016). Increasing age was associated with smaller risk reductions in major vascular events and vascular deaths. Statin therapy is typically well tolerated and safe. Side-effects include myalgia, with rare cases of myopathy and rhabdomyolysis (Grundy et al., 2019). A systematic review of side-effects of the statins has found that muscle symptoms are often reported at a similar rate in patients taking a placebo as those taking the statin (Ganga et al., 2014).

175

Ezetimibe

This drug acts to reduce the uptake of cholesterol from the small intestine by inhibiting Niemann-Pick C1-like 1 (NPC1L1), a transport protein that carries cholesterol from the intestinal lumen into the intestinal cells, from where it is transported into the lymphatic vessels in the form of chylomicrons. This drug would usually only be considered as monotherapy if a patient could not tolerate statins, as there is no evidence that it reduces cardiovascular risk when used on its own. It is also used in combination with a statin if the statin alone does not produce a sufficient reduction in LDL.

PCSK9 inhibitors

Proprotein convertase subtilisin/kexin type-9 (PCSK9) targets LDL receptors in cells for destruction rather than recycling, reducing their capacity to remove LDL from the circulation. By binding to PCSK9, monoclonal antibodies such as evolocumab and alirocumab inhibit the enzyme, enabling LDL recycling and continued sequestration of LDL from the blood.

Episode of care: chest pain

A paramedic crew has been called to attend Max Simons, a 76-year-old patient with chest pain and breathing difficulties. The time of day is 0530 hours and it is a Friday morning in November.

On arrival the crew find the patient sitting on the couch, clutching at his chest. The patient is pale, diaphoretic and grimacing.

Presenting medical history

Max tells the crew that he woke with severe chest discomfort which he described as central crushing pain and a dull ache in the left arm (radiating pain).

Past medical history

Max states that he had a heart attack 5 years previously which resulted in stenting of two arteries. Occasionally when exercising, he develops angina and he has also had high blood pressure (hypertension) for many years. Max also says that he has high cholesterol (hypercholesterolaemia).

Medications

Max is prescribed atorvastatin for high cholesterol, aspirin to prevent platelet aggregation, GTN for episodes of angina and irbesartan for hypertension.

Assessments and clinical manifestations

After gaining patient consent, the crew undertake the following assessments with a **12-lead ECG** as a priority.

- Perfusion assessment:
  - Skin: pale, cool, diaphoretic
  - Oxygen saturations: 93%
  - Pulse rate: 91
  - BP: 155/95

- Respiratory assessment:
  - Respiratory rate: 24
  - Speech: sentences
  - Ventilatory effort: slight increase
  - Breath sounds: clear
  - Conscious state: orientated to time and place.
- Other findings:
  - 12-lead ECG: sinus rhythm with ST elevation in V2, V3, V4 indicating an anterior wall myocardial infarction (AWMI)
  - Pain score: 7/10
  - Temperature: 37.0
  - Blood glucose level: 4.4 mmol

Management

Based on the patient's history and clinical manifestations, a provisional diagnosis of AWMI is made. Max is treated with the following.

- Positioning: upright to improve ventilatory function
- Oxygen: high flow to increase the fraction of inspired oxygen (FiO_2)
- Glyceryl trinitrate (GTN): causes vasodilation of veins and arteries resulting in decreased preload and afterload. This reduces the workload of the heart, thereby reducing myocardial oxygen demand
- Aspirin to prevent the development of thrombosis and the extension of any current thrombi that may have caused the coronary artery occlusion
- Analgesia such as fentanyl to help reduce pain
- Continual 12-lead ECG monitoring
- Transport to hospital

Risk factors and considerations

Max has a history of hypertension and hypercholesterolaemia which are risk factors for atherosclerosis, a common cause of cardiovascular disease which can cause myocardial infarction.

Reflection

Take some time to consider if time of day is an important factor in patients presenting with chest pain. If so, why do you think this is?

Skills in practice: electrode placement for a 12-lead ECG

Explain the procedure and gain patient consent.
Always ensure the patient's privacy is maintained.
Patient's skin may need to be cleaned to ensure attachment of the ECG electrodes.
Chest hair may need to be removed.

Limb lead placement
- Right arm lead – inner wrist
- Left arm lead – inner wrist
- Right leg lead – inner ankle
- Left leg lead – inner ankle

Chest lead placement
- V1: fourth intercostal space, just right of the sternum
- V2: fourth intercostal space, just left of the sternum
- V3: in between V2 and V4
- V4: fifth intercostal space, midclavicular line
- V5: adjacent to V4, anterior axillar line
- V6: adjacent to V5, midaxillar line

In practice, it may not always be possible to access the patient's limbs, for example a patient who has been in a car crash where their legs are pinned under the dashboard. Modification can be made to the limb leads using the patient's torso.
- Right shoulder
- Left shoulder
- Right lower quadrant (lateral)
- Left lower quadrant (lateral)

Conclusion

Cardiovascular disease is the leading cause of death worldwide. Given this, calls to ambulance services from patients presenting with cardiovascular disease are common and therefore it is essential that paramedics have a sound understanding of cardiovascular disease pathophysiology, clinical manifestations patients may present with and treatment regimes. It is important that paramedics understand the pharmacology of drugs used in the clinical management of patients who have cardiovascular disease.

The following is a list of conditions that are associated with the cardiovascular system. Take some time and write notes about each of the conditions. Think about the medications that may be used in order to treat these conditions and be specific about the pharmacokinetics and pharmacodynamics. Remember to include aspects of patient care. If you are making notes about people you have offered care and support to, you must ensure that you have adhered to the rules of confidentiality.

The condition	Your notes
Hypertension	
Heart failure	
Hypercholesterolaemia	
Arrhythmias	
Myocardial infarction	

Glossary

ACS	Acute coronary syndrome
CVD	Cardiovascular disease
HFmEF	Heart failure with midrange ejection fraction
HFpEF	Heart failure with preserved ejection fraction

HFrEF	Heart failure with reduced ejection fraction
LVEDP	Left ventricular end-diastolic pressure
LVEF	Left ventricular ejection fraction
MI	Myocardial infarction
PPCI	Primary percutaneous coronary intervention
STEMI	ST-elevation myocardial infarction

References

Ahmad, T., Miller, P.E., McCullough, M. et al. (2019). Why has positive inotropy failed in chronic heart failure? Lessons from prior inotrope trials. *European Journal of Heart Failure* **21**(9): 1064–1078.

AlQudah, M., Hale, T.M. and Czubryt, M.P. (2020). Targeting the renin-angiotensin-aldosterone system in fibrosis. *Matrix Biology* **91-92**: 92–108.

Arnett, D.K., Blumenthal, R.S., Albert, M.A. et al. (2019). 2019 ACC/AHA guideline on the primary prevention of cardiovascular disease: a report of the American College of Cardiology/American Heart Association Task Force on Clinical Practice Guidelines. *Circulation* **140**(11): e596–e646.

Arrigo, M., Huber, L.C., Winnik, S. et al. (2019). Right ventricular failure: pathophysiology, diagnosis and treatment. *Cardiac Failure Review* **5**(3): 140–146.

Atherton, J.J., Sindone, A., De Pasquale, C.G. et al. (2018) National Heart Foundation of Australia and Cardiac Society of Australia and New Zealand: Guidelines for the prevention, detection, and management of heart failure in Australia 2018. *Heart, Lung and Circulation* **27**(10): 1123–1208.

Australian Bureau of Statistics. (2018). *National Health Survey: first results.* www.abs.gov.au/statistics/health/health-conditions-and-risks/national-health-survey-first-results/latest-release#chronic-conditions

Bayes-Genis, A., Barallat, J. and Richards, A.M. (2016). A test in context: neprilysin. Function, inhibition and bio-marker. *Journal of the American College of Cardiology* **68**(6): 639–653.

Bilska-Wilkosz, A., Kotańska, M. Górny, M. et al. (2019). Is the mechanism of nitroglycerin tolerance associated with aldehyde dehydrogenase activity? A contribution to the ongoing discussion. *Acta Biochimica Polonica* **66**(4): 627–632.

Boeuf-Gibot, S., Pereira, B., Imbert, J. et al. (2021). Benefits and adverse effects of ACE inhibitors in patients with heart failure with reduced ejection fraction: a systematic review and meta-analysis. *European Journal of Clinical Pharmacology* **77**(3): 321–329.

Bosch, L., Lam, C.S.P., Gong, L. et al. (2017). Right ventricular dysfunction in left-sided heart failure with preserved versus reduced ejection fraction. *European Journal of Heart Failure* **19**(12): 1664–1671.

British Heart Foundation UK. (2012). *CVD Factsheet.* bhf-cvd-statistics-uk-factsheet%20(1).pdf

Cholesterol Treatment Trialists' (CTT) Collaboration. (2016). Impact of renal function on the effects of LDL cholesterol lowering with statin-based regimens: a meta-analysis of individual participant data from 28 randomised trials. *Lancet* **4**(10): 829–839.

Fazel, R., Joseph, T.I., Sankardasa, M.A. et al. (2020). Comparison of reperfusion strategies for ST-segment-elevation myocardial infarction: a multivariate network meta-analysis. *Journal of the American Heart Association* **9**(12): e015186.

Friis, U.G., Madsen, K., Stubbe, J. et al. (2013). Regulation of renin secretion by renal juxtaglomerular cells. *Pflügers Archives – European Journal of Physiology* **465**: 25–37.

Ganga, H.V., Slim, H.B. and Thompson, P.D. (2014). A systematic review of statin-induced muscle problems in clinical trials. *American Heart Journal* **168**(1): 6–15.

Gard, E., Nanayakkara, S., Kaye, D. et al. (2020). Management of heart failure with preserved ejection fraction. *Australian Prescriber* **43**(1): 12–17.

Grundy, S.M., Stone, N.J., Bailey, A.L. et al. (2019) 2018 AHA/ACC/AACVPR/AAPA/ABC/ACPM/ADA/AGS/APhA/ASPC/NLA/PCNA Guideline on the management of blood cholesterol: a report of the American College of Cardiology/American Heart Association Task Force on Clinical Practice Guidelines. *Circulation* **139**(25): e1082–e1143.

Hindricks, G., Potpara, T., Dagres, N. et al. (2021). 2020 ESC guidelines for the diagnosis and management of atrial fibrillation developed in collaboration with the European Association of Cardio-Thoracic Surgery (EACTS). *European Heart Journal* **42**(5): 373–498.

Ibanez, B., James, S., Agewall, S. et al. (2018). 2017 ESC Guidelines for the management of acute myocardial infarction in patients presenting with ST-segment elevation. *European Heart Journal* **39**(2): 119–177.

January, C.T., Wann, L.S., Calkins, H. et al. (2019). 2019 AHA/ACC/HRS focused update of the 2014 guideline for management of patients with atrial fibrillation: a report of the American College of Cardiology/American Heart Association task force on clinical practice guidelines and the heart rhythm society. *Journal of the American College of Cardiology* **74**(1): 104–132.

Kemp, C.D. and Conte, J.V. (2012). The pathophysiology of heart failure. *Cardiovascular Pathology* **21**(5): 365–371.

Krogager, M.L., Torp-Pedersen, C., Mortensen, R.N. et al. (2017). Short-term mortality risk of serum potassium levels in hypertension: a retrospective analysis of nationwide registry data. *European Heart Journal* **38**(2): 104–112.

Margonato, D., Mazzetti, S., de Maria, R. et al. (2020). Heart failure with mid-range or recovered ejection fraction: differential determinants of transition. *Cardiac Failure Review* **6**: e28.

McMurray, J.J.V., Packer, M., Desai, A.S. et al. (2014). Angiotensin-neprilysin inhibition versus enalapril in heart failure. *New England Journal of Medicine* **371**(11): 993–1004.

Mehran, R., Baber, U., Sharma, S.K. et al. (2019). Ticagrelor with or without aspirin in high-risk patients with PCI. *New England Journal of Medicine* **381**(21): 2032–2042.

Mullens, W., Damman, K., Harjola, V.-P. et al. (2019). The use of diuretics in heart failure with congestion – a position statement from the Heart Failure Association of the European Society of Cardiology. *European Journal of Heart Failure* **21**(2): 137–155.

Oh, G.C. and Cho, H-J. (2020). Blood pressure and heart failure. *Clinical Hypertension* **26**: 1.

Packer, M., Bristow, M.R., Cohn, J.N. et al. (1996). The effect of carvedilol on morbidity and mortality in patients with chronic heart failure. U.S. Carvedilol Heart Failure Study Group. *New England Journal of Medicine* **334**(21): 1349–1355.

Pfeffer, M.A., Swedberg, K., Granger, C.B. et al. (2003). Effects of candesartan on mortality and morbidity in patients with chronic heart failure: the CHARM-Overall programme. *Lancet* **362**(9386): 759–766.

Ponikowski, P., Voors, A.A., Anker, S.D. et al. (2016). 2016 ESC Guidelines for the diagnosis and treatment of acute and chronic heart failure. *European Heart Journal* **37**(27): 2129–2200.

Shafiq, M.M., Menon, D.V. and Victor, R.G. (2008). Oral direct renin inhibition: premise, promise, and potential limitations of a new class of antihypertensive drug. *American Journal of Medicine* **121**(4): 265–271.

Sumners, C., Peluso, A.A., Haugaard, A.H. et al. (2019). Anti-fibrotic mechanisms of angiotensin AT_2-receptor stimulation. *Acta Physiologica* **227**(1): e13280.

Teerlink, J.R., Diaz, R., Felker, G.M. et al. (2020). Omecamtiv mecarbil in chronic heart failure with reduced ejection fraction: GALACTIC-HF baseline characteristics and comparison with contemporary clinical trials. *European Journal of Heart Failure* **22**: 2160–2171.

Unger, T., Borghi, C., Charchar, F. et al. (2020). 2020 International Society of Hypertension Global Hypertension Practice Guidelines. *Hypertension* **75**(6): 1334–1357.

Valgimigli, M., Bueno, H., Byrne, R.A. et al. (2018). 2017 ESC focused update on dual antiplatelet therapy in coronary artery disease developed in collaboration with EACTS. *European Heart Journal* **39**(3): 213–254.

Wang, Y., Del Borgo, M., Lee, H.W. et al. (2017). Anti-fibrotic potential of AT_2 receptor agonists. *Frontiers in Pharmacology* **8**: 564.

World Health Organization. (2021). *Cardiovascular Diseases Fact Sheet*. www.who.int/en/news-room/fact-sheets/detail/cardiovascular-diseases-(cvds)

Yancy, C.W., Jessup, M., Bozkurt, B. et al. (2013). 2013 ACCF/AHA Guideline for the management of heart failure: a report of the American College of Cardiology Foundation/American Heart Association Task Force on Practice Guidelines. *Circulation* **128**(16): e240–e327.

Yancy, C.W., Jessup, M., Bozkurt, B. et al. (2016). 2016 ACC/AHA/HFSA focused update on new pharmacological therapy for heart failure: an update of the 2013 ACCF/AHA Guideline for the management of heart failure: a report of the American College of Cardiology/American Heart Association Task Force on Clinical Practice Guidelines and the Heart Failure Society of America. *Circulation* **134**(13): e282–e293.

Yancy, C.W., Jessup, M., Bozkurt, B. et al. (2017). ACC/AHA/HFSA focused update of the 2013 ACCF/AHA guideline for the management of heart failure: a report of the American College of Cardiology/American Heart Association Task Force on Practice Guidelines and the Heart Failure Society of America. *Journal of Cardiac Failure* **23**(8): 628–651.

Young, J.B., Dunlap, M.E., Pfeffer, M.A. et al. (2004). Mortality and morbidity reduction with Candesartan in patients with chronic heart failure and left ventricular systolic dysfunction: results of the CHARM low-left ventricular ejection fraction trials. *Circulation* **110**(17): 2618–2626.

Zia-Behbahani, M., Hossein, H., Kojuri, J. et al. (2019). Tenecteplase versus reteplase in acute myocardial infarction: a network meta-analysis of randomized clinical trials. *Iranian Journal of Pharmaceutical Research* **18**(3): 1622–1631.

Further reading

Australian Paramedic Clinical Practice Guidelines. www.clinicalguidelines.gov.au/

Joint Royal Colleges Ambulance Liaison Committee (JRCALC). (2019). *Clinical Practice Guidelines 2019*. Bridgwater: Class Professional Publishing.

Ward, J., Connolly, M. and Aaronson, P. (2020). *The Cardiovascular System at a Glance*, 5th edn. Oxford: Wiley Blackwell.

Multiple-choice questions

1. Drugs used to interfere with the renin-angiotensin system for control of blood pressure include:
   (a) Verapamil and digoxin
   (b) Digoxin and endothelin-1
   (c) Captopril and candesartan
   (d) Salbutamol and salmeterol

2. Renin is released from juxtaglomerular cells in response to:
   (a) An elevation in renal perfusion pressure
   (b) Release of prostacylin (PGI_2) from the macula densa
   (c) An increase in Na^+ concentration in the distal tubule
   (d) Stimulation of receptors in the juxtaglomerular cell by angiotensin II

3. The enzyme chymase converts angiotensin I to angiotensin II. This type of processing may also be achieved by the activity of:
   (a) Angiotensin-converting enzyme (ACE)
   (b) Bradykinin
   (c) Endothelin-converting enzyme (ECE)
   (d) Renin

4. A patient undergoes catheter-based radiofrequency ablation of the sympathetic nerves that are located adjacent to the renal arteries to treat their hypertension. A *direct* effect of renal denervation would be:
   (a) Decreased release of adrenaline from the adrenal medulla
   (b) Decreased renin secretion from the juxtaglomerular cells
   (c) Decreased released prostacyclin from the macula densa
   (d) Decreased reabsorption of chloride ions from the distal tubule

5. Why is the beta-1 adrenoceptor-selective antagonist, atenolol, contraindicated in patients who have asthma?
   (a) Beta-1 adrenoceptor-selective antagonists cause receptor supersensitivity
   (b) At therapeutic doses, some airway beta-2 adrenoceptors will be blocked
   (c) Beta-1 adrenoceptors are the predominant receptor subtype on bronchial smooth muscle cells
   (d) At therapeutic doses, renin release is inhibited

6. Dobutamine is a beta-1 adrenoceptor agonist and is used therapeutically in the:
   (a) Management of patients who have asthma
   (b) Chronic management of patients who have moderate heart failure
   (c) Acute inotropic support of patients who have end-stage heart failure
   (d) Treatment of patients who have ventricular arrhythmias

7. Treatment of a patient with myocardial infarction could include:
   (a) The use of antiplatelet agents such as clopidogrel and aspirin
   (b) A fibrinolytic drug such as tenecteplase
   (c) Primary percutaneous coronary intervention
   (d) Any of the above

8. The fibrinolytic agent tenecteplase:
   (a) Combines with antithrombin III to inhibit factor Xa
   (b) Stimulates conversion of plasminogen to plasmin
   (c) Is inactivated by plasmin inhibitors such as PAI-1
   (d) Inhibits the conversion of prothrombin to thrombin

9. Which of the following positive inotropes increases force of myocardial contraction without increasing intracellular calcium concentration or sensitising troponin-C to calcium?

(a) Digoxin
(b) Dobutamine
(c) Omecamtiv mecarbil
(d) Endothelin-1

10. The mechanism by which glyceryl trinitrate reduces cardiovascular preload is:
    (a) Venodilation, resulting in reduced venous return
    (b) Diuresis resulting in reduced intravascular volume
    (c) Reduction in venous compliance
    (d) Increase in ventricular compliance

11. Why is glyceryl trinitrate (GTN) used intermittently?
    (a) To avoid tolerance that is associated with extended use of the drug
    (b) To minimise toxicity that is associated with long-term use of GTN
    (c) To minimise extensive metabolism of GTN by enzymes present in the
    (d) To reduce the probability of development of a hypersensitivity reaction that is

12. Which of the following would be the primary indication for angiotensin receptor-neprilysin inhibitor (ARNI), sacubitril/valsartan?
    (a) A patient who has heart failure with reduced ejection fraction, and who can tolerate ACE inhibitors or ARBs
    (b) A patient who has low cardiac output and requires haemodynamic support
    (c) A patient requiring treatment for familial hypercholesterolaemia
    (d) A patient who has chest pain associated with coronary artery disease

13. Administration of ACE inhibitors and ARBs is contraindicated in someone who:
    (a) Has diabetes
    (b) Has elevated systolic blood pressure
    (c) Is pregnant
    (d) Has elevated diastolic blood pressure

14. Which of the following agents could be used to reduce the blood concentration of low-density lipoprotein (LDL)?
    (a) Alirocumab, a proprotein convertase subtilisin/kexin type-9 (PCSK9) inhibitor
    (b) Atorvastatin, an HMG-CoA reductase inhibitor
    (c) Both a) and b)
    (d) None of the above

15. Which of the following is a potential cause of hypokalaemia?
    (a) Lisinopril (angiotensin-converting enzyme inhibitor)
    (b) Candesartan (angiotensin AT1 receptor blocker)
    (c) Spironolactone (aldosterone receptor antagonist)
    (d) Furosemide (loop diuretic)

Chapter 11

Medications used in the renal system

Anthony Kitchener

Aim

The aim of this chapter is to orientate the reader to the renal system, explore some of the common pathologies encountered by healthcare professionals and consider the pharmacological interventions used in the management of these conditions.

Learning outcomes

After reading this chapter, the reader will:

1. Have gained an understanding of acute kidney injury and chronic kidney disease, including pharmacology that can contribute to renal demise
2. Know how common renal-conditions can be treated or managed by pharmacological intervention
3. Be able to describe the different drug classifications used in renal medicine
4. Be able to differentiate and understand the side-effects of common renal pharmacotherapy and how this knowledge can contribute to effective patient counselling for prescribed medications.

Test your knowledge

1. Identify the difference between acute kidney injury and chronic kidney disease.
2. Name four common renal conditions.
3. Discuss the potential risks associated with reduced renal function.
4. List the common types of drugs used to treat renal disorders.
5. Discuss the role and function of the National Institute of Health and Care Excellence (NICE) in the management of renal disorders.

Fundamentals of Pharmacology for Paramedics, First Edition. Edited by Ian Peate, Suzanne Evans, and Lisa Clegg.
© 2022 John Wiley & Sons Ltd. Published 2022 by John Wiley & Sons Ltd.

Introduction

The study of renal medicine is termed 'nephrology' and includes several conditions, both acute and chronic, that can cause injury to the kidney. Acute kidney injury (AKI) is a sudden drop in renal function that can be caused by a reduction in blood flow to the kidney, produced by severe dehydration, for example, or by certain groups of medicines that are toxic to the kidneys. Chronic kidney disease (CKD) reflects a long-term disease process or stress on the kidney, which gradually reduces renal function. Chronic, severe reduction in renal function is end-stage renal disease (ESRD), at which point treatment options are limited to renal dialysis or renal transplant surgery.

Around 3 million people in the UK have CKD around 700 million globally and the largest contributors to this are uncontrolled diabetes and hypertension. Due to comorbid states and the finite resources associated with dialysis and transplant, the options for treatment are sometimes limited or include a lengthy wait. Haemodialysis and peritoneal dialysis are methods used to replace the work of the kidneys until a renal transplant can be performed (if the patient is eligible). Patients in ESRD will have disordered fluid and electrolyte balance, and are particularly at risk of cardiac arrhythmia due to abnormally high extracellular potassium levels (hyperkalaemia) which can lead to sudden cardiac death. There are approximately 30 000 people in the UK on dialysis at any one time, several million worldwide. For every five people that need a renal transplant in the UK each year, there are only three kidney donors. Eight of 10 patients on the donor organ waiting list are waiting for donor kidneys.

A discussion of the complex physiology of the renal system is outside the scope of this chapter, but because of the multiple physiological roles played by the kidneys, the loss of renal function can be expected to produce a range of disorders, as illustrated in Figure 11.1.

Renal diseases can be classified into pre-renal, intrarenal and postrenal, reflecting the causes of the disease, which are reduced blood flow to the kidney (pre-renal), intrinsic damage to the kidneys themselves (intrarenal) or damage due to obstructed outflow from the kidney (postrenal), as shown in Table 11.1.

Acute kidney injury

Acute kidney injury can be caused by pre-renal, intrarenal and postrenal pathophysiology. The clinical presentation may be oliguria (reduced urine output) or complete anuria (no urine output). There is a resultant abnormally high level of nitrogenous products in the blood (azotaemia) due to failure to excrete them and this may present clinically as being tired all the time (TATT), peripheral oedema, muscle cramps, insomnia and itching. There may be a history of infection or other insult preceding the clinical presentation or the diagnosis. Certain medications (see Box 11.1) are thought to be a

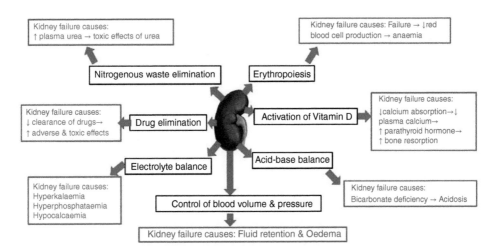

Figure 11.1 The major physiological functions of the kidneys (black boxes) and the sequelae of renal failure (red boxes).

Table 11.1   Pre-renal, intrarenal and postrenal disease characteristics.

	Pre-renal disease	Intrarenal disease	Postrenal disease
Mechanism	Reduced blood flow to kidney	Direct damage by drugs or toxins.	Obstruction of renal pelvis, ureters, bladder or urethra
Aetiology	• Prolonged hypotension • Cardiac failure • Anaphylaxis • Pulmonary embolism • Sepsis • Renal artery stenosis • Blood loss • Hyperemesis • Vascular occlusion • Medication • Hepatorenal syndrome (seen in alcohol use disorders)	• CKD progression • Autoimmune disease • Glomerulonephritis • Localised infection • Bacterial infections (haemolytic uraemia) • Acute tubular necrosis	• Obstruction from calculi • Retained clots • Enlarged prostate • Bladder tumour • Physical injury • Cervical cancer • Urethral stricture • Meatal stenosis • Meatal phimosis
Plasma urea levels	Increased	Increased	Increased
Plasma creatinine levels	Increased	Increased	Increased
Estimated glomerular filtration rate (eGFR)	Reduced	Reduced	Reduced
Urine output	Reduced	Reduced	Reduced

CKD, chronic kidney disease.

Box 11.1   Drugs known to be nephrotoxic.

- Some antibiotics (e.g. aminoglycosides, cephalosporins, amphotericin B, bacitracin and vancomycin)
- Diuretics
- Non-steroidal anti-inflammatory drugs (NSAIDs)
- Antihypertensives (e.g. angiotensin-converting enzyme [ACE] inhibitors and angiotensin receptor blockers)
- Chemotherapy (e.g. cisplatin, carboplatin, methotrexate)
- Contrast media, such as used in medical imaging
- Recreational drugs (e.g. heroin and amphetamines)
- HIV medication, such as protease inhibitors
- Ulcer medication (cimetidine)

common cause. Where a patient presents with AKI, the patient care records should be immediately reviewed for medication as a possible cause.

The term AKI is now more commonly used than acute kidney failure. It is also more accurate as it reflects injury that can precede failure, including its reversibility if the cause can be identified early. Given that several AKI presentations are due to pre-renal processes, conditions such as sepsis should be the focus of active treatments by healthcare professionals, with focus on the 'Sepsis 6' bundle of care to decrease the risk of AKI from this cause (McGregor, 2014). The degree of treatment will depend on the stage of the AKI, defined in Table 11.2.

Table 11.2   Stages of acute kidney injury.

Stage	Criteria
1	Creatinine rise of 26 µL or more within 48 hours OR Creatinine rise of 50–99% from baseline within 7 days[a] (1.50–1.99 × baseline) OR Urine output[b] < 0.5 mL/kg/h for more than 6 hours
2	100–199% creatinine rise from baseline within 7 days[a] (2.00–2.99 × baseline) OR Urine output[b] <0.5 mL/kg/h for more than 12 hours
3	200% or more creatinine rise from baseline within 7 days[a] (3.00 or more × baseline) OR Creatinine rise to 354 µL or more with acute rise of 26 µL or more within 48 hours or 50% or more rise within 7 days OR Urine output[b] <0.3 mL/kg/h for 24 hours or anuria for 12 hours

[a] The rise is known (based on previous blood tests) or presumed (based on history) to have occurred within 7 days.
[b] Measurement of urine output may not be practical in a primary care population but can be considered in a person with a catheter.

185

Management of AKI can be undertaken in conjunction with the renal team at the local admitting hospital and should be started as soon as possible and within 24 hours of detection of the AKI. Where there is uncertainty around the cause, admission of the patient for further investigation and identification of the cause is warranted. For Stage I AKI, urgent removal of the cause is a priority, including deprescribing or reducing the dose of that medication. Appropriate hydration is required to support the kidney and referral to the *British National Formulary* for guidance on prescribing in renal impairment may be warranted. Close monitoring of renal function is required to ensure that the AKI resolves adequately (NICE, 2013).

Chronic kidney disease

Chronic kidney disease is a progressive deterioration of kidney function over time, anaemia marked by reduction of estimated glomerular filtration (eGFR) and a corresponding rise in the creatinine levels in the blood. This deterioration is hastened by comorbid factors such as diabetes and hypertension. Diagnosis of CKD is made when eGFR is less than 60 mL/min/1.73m^2 , or there is proteinuria (identified through a urinary albumin:creatinine ratio [UrACR] of more than 3 mg/mL), or persistent haematuria (two out of three dispsticks show 1+ or more blood after local infection has been excluded). Figure 11.2 shows an example of a blood test result indicating CKD which has the renal failure pattern of reduced eGFR and a rise in serum creatinine. There is an absence of AKI staging and if compared against previous test results would be expected to show a chronic deterioration or a long-term (but possibly stable) CKD presentation.

Chronic kidney disease is often a silent disease that is picked up as part of testing for other diseases, such as essential hypertension or diabetes, or during a normal medical check. The blood panel urea and electrolytes (U&E) is a commonly requested and relatively low-cost investigation used in a wide variety of clinical presentations that warrant investigation. The possibility of an acute-on-chronic deterioration should be considered when there is a sudden deterioration, as per the guidance related to AKI presentations. Dependent on the urine ACR and eGFR, CKD can be given a grade of 1–5, as described in Table 11.3 (NICE, 2015). CKD warrants caution in prescribing and regular appraisal for signs of deterioration.

Management of CKD

The prescribing of iron is not routinely required for renal anaemias ('anaemia of chronic disease') but care should be taken to exclude other types of anaemia, such as iron deficiency. If renal anaemia is suspected, arrange referral to a nephrology specialist for further investigation and management.

As indicated in Figure 11.1, hypocalcaemia and increased parathyroid hormone secretion are seen in renal disease, so checking these levels is recommended in CKD 1–3b stages (NICE, 2015). Calcium abnormalities may present as an acute crisis and should be rapidly appraised and clinically correlated. Prescribing vitamin D3 and calcium, available in a combined formulation for ease of administration, should be considered in renal patients to try and correct these abnormalities.

Specimen: SERUM

Investigation	Normal	Result
Serum electrolytes		
Serum sodium	133.0–146.0 mmol/L	141 mmol/L
Serum potassium	3.5–5.3 mmol/	4.8 mmol/L
Serum creatinine	59.0–104.0 µmol/L	162 µmol/L
Serum chloride	95.0–108.0 mmol/L	104 mmol/L

Serum urea

Specimen: SERUM   Collected: 25 Sep 2017 09:00

Investigation	Normal	Result
Serum urea	2.5–7.8 mmol/L	11.9 mmol/L

eGFR using creatinine (CKD-EPI) per 1.73 m^2

Specimen: SERUM   Collected: 25 Sep 2017 09:00

Investigation	Normal	Result
eGFR using creatinine (CKD-EPI) per 1.73 m^2	>60.0 mL/min	34 mL/min If Afro-Caribbean, multiply result by 1.159

Figure 11.2   Blood tests that indicate chronic kidney disease.

Table 11.3   Categories of CKD.

eGFR (mL/min/1.73 m^2)	Urinary ACR (mg/mmol)		
	A1 (<3) Normal to mildly increased	A2 (3–30) Moderately increased	A3 (>30) Severely increased
G1 ≥90 Normal and high	≤1	1	≥1
G2 60–89 Mild reduction related to normal range for a young adult	≤1	1	≥1
G3a 45–59 Mild to moderate reduction	1	1	2
G3b 30–44 Moderate to severe reduction	≤2	2	≥2
G4 15–29 Severe reduction	2	2	3
G5 <15 End-stage kidney failure	4	≥4	≥4

The aim of treatment of CKD is to slow the rate of decline of renal function and this will involve managing comorbid conditions such as diabetes and hypertension. Medications such as angiotensin-converting enzyme (ACE) inhibitors and angiotensin receptor blockers (ARBs), perhaps paradoxically since they also have renotoxic potential, are known as renoprotective agents as, their therapeutic action is to reduce blood pressure, and slow the rate of progression of CKD. If using these medicines, a follow-up U&E blood test should be made 1–2 weeks after starting or changing dosing, in order to screen for acute renal toxicity produced by these drugs (see Box 11.1). The drugs may need to be stopped if there is significantly reduced eGFR. Failure to deprescribe can be a common pitfall of using these drugs.

Electrolyte abnormalities resulting from poor renal function

Hyponatraemia (low serum sodium)

As the most abundant extracellular cation in the body, sodium exerts a large influence on the plasma osmolality and therefore the extracellular fluid volume. The physiological control of serum sodium concentration is achieved by adjusting water intake (through thirst) and water excretion (through antidiuretic hormone). Hyponatraemia is defined as a serum sodium concentration of less than 135 mmol/L. Box 11.2 defines the various levels of severity of hyponatraemia. The rate of onset can also be classified as acute (<48 h) or chronic (≥48 h).

Box 11.2   Levels of hyponatraemia

Mild	130–135 mmol/L
Moderate	125–129 mmol/L
Severe	<125 mmol/L

Healthy kidneys are able to produce urine with a much higher osmolality than plasma, thereby excreting solutes while conserving water, and adjusting the excretion of electrolytes and water to control plasma osmolality.

Kidney disease may result in failure to maintain electrolyte balance, as the kidneys lose the ability to produce urine of a different osmolality to the plasma. In this situation, if fluid intake is greater than urine output, there will be water retention and a dilutional (volume overload) hyponatraemia.

Treatment of severe hyponatraemia will require hospital admission and infusion with hypertonic saline (Ball et al., 2016).

Hypokalaemia (low serum potassium) and hyperkalaemia (high serum potassium)

Potassium is the main intracellular cation and is integral to the maintenance of an electrochemical gradient across cell membranes, and the normal functioning of electrically excitable tissues such as nerve and muscle. Abnormalities in serum potassium levels can therefore cause serious, sometimes fatal, cardiac dysrhythmias and should be considered life-threatening.

Urinary retention and incontinence

Clinical consideration

Urinary retention is often really uncomfortable, and the clue may be that the patient struggles to sit still or is in a lot of pain. The intervention will be catheterisation, but you want to make sure the cause (maybe a medicine) has been determined before removal of the catheter!

Urinary incontinence can occur as a result of structural or other abnormalities or with no underlying pathology. Medications that can contribute to incontinence include diuretics, muscle relaxants, sedatives, narcotics and antihistamines. Assessment of prescribed medications and reduction in dosing or deprescribing may be an option to address incontinence and is an important consideration. Acute incontinence can also be caused by urinary tract infection and assessment for the infection and antimicrobial treatment may be an appropriate management option.

Initiation of urination is dependent upon the parasympathetic nervous system and relies upon co-ordination of simultaneous detrusor muscle (in the body of the bladder) contraction and sphincter muscle (at the neck of the bladder) relaxation.

In the male, enlargement of the prostate can cause urethral compression, since the prostate wraps around the urethra. Clinically this may present as changes in urinary habit, including struggling to start urinating, weak urinary stream, multidirectional spray and postvoiding dribble.

In females, a clear clinical history will help differentiate between stress incontinence, urgency urinary incontinence or a mixed presentation (Hsu and Pierre, 2019; NICE, 2019). Subtypes of incontinence are also detailed in national guidelines, including those associated with overactive bladder syndrome or OAB (Barkin et al., 2017).

Drugs which may exacerbate urinary incontinence include alpha-1 adrenoceptor antagonists, beta-adrenoceptor antagonists, antipsychotics, anticholinergics, antiparkinsonism drugs, antidepressants, benzodiazepines, diuretics and hormone replacement therapy. Contributing conditions may include spinal surgery, bladder prolapse, multiple sclerosis and Parkinson disease. Fluid volume may be increased in heart failure and bladder irritation may be seen in diabetes mellitus where glucosuria is present. Given the potential for bladder pathology to result in urine backflow to the kidneys, assessment for AKI is sensible in acute presentations.

There are several non-pharmacological steps which can be taken to support the management of urinary incontinence, including pelvic floor exercises, reduction of dietary caffeine and surgical options in some cases.

As a second line and pharmacological treatment, duloxetine may be a consideration in people over 18 years of age. Duloxetine inhibits the reuptake of serotonin and noradrenaline.

Urinary retention can cause an overflow incontinence as the bladder becomes distended and starts to empty by passive overflow. The bladder distension can be very painful and patients often present in great discomfort. Acute intervention will be with urinary catheterisation to relieve the retention and pharmacological therapy may be used to support a trial without catheter process, for example, modified-release alfuzosin (alpha-blocker) in men over 65 years of age.

Drug-induced renal damage

As previously highlighted, nephrotoxic drugs are a common but avoidable cause of acute kidney injury that also potentially contribute to or accelerate the development of chronic kidney disease. Figure 11.3 provides examples of medications which can cause or contribute to kidney damage. Healthcare professionals and workers should be aware that administration of drugs can cause a rapid deterioration in a patient's condition, as detailed in the section on acute kidney injury. If kidney function is compromised by a drug, it is also likely that the concentration of the causative agent and other drugs in the patient's circulation may rise to toxic levels, resulting in other adverse effects. Prescribing information which will allow for adaptive prescribing considerations is contained within electronic prescribing systems or within the *British National Formulary* (BNF).

Drugs that act on the renal system
Diuretics

Diuretics increase the excretion of fluid and are used to treat a number of different pathologies, most commonly hypertension and congestive heart failure (both acute and chronic). Diuretics act by reducing the reabsorption of filtered salts and water from the nephrons back into the bloodstream, consequently increasing the excretion of both in the urine. The result is increased quantity of urine and increased frequency of micturition. This removal of extracellular fluid will lower blood volume, and therefore pressure and reduce oedema.

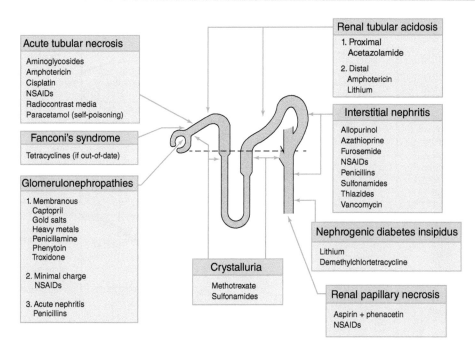

Figure 11.3 Adverse effects of drugs on the kidney.

Table 11.4 Subclasses of diuretics and their clinical uses.

Subclass	Common uses
Loop diuretics, e.g. furosemide, bumetanide	• Fluid retention/oedema due to chronic heart failure • Resistant hypertension (not as a first-line agent)
Thiazides and related diuretics, e.g. bendroflumethiazide, indapamide	• Hypertension, not first-line agent, commonly used in diabetes patients • Mild to moderate heart failure
Osmotic diuretics, e.g. mannitol	• Cerebral oedema and raised intraocular pressure
Potassium-sparing and aldosterone antagonists. e.g. amiloride, spironolactone	*Spironolactone* • Oedema (as monotherapy) • Potassium conservation when used as an adjunct to thiazide or loop diuretics for hypertension, congestive heart failure or hepatic ascites *Amiloride* • Oedema • Ascites in cirrhosis of the liver • Nephrotic syndrome • Moderate to severe heart failure (adjunct) • Resistant hypertension (adjunct) • Primary hyperaldosteronism in patients awaiting surgery • Given with thiazide or loop diuretics to preserve serum potassium levels
Carbonic anhydrase inhibitors, e.g. acetazolamide	• Reduction of intraocular pressure • Glaucoma • Epilepsy

There are several subclasses of diuretic, including loop diuretics, thiazide and related diuretics, osmotic diuretics, potassium-sparing and aldosterone-antagonists and carbonic anhydrase inhibitors (see Table 11.4).

Diuretics affect electrolyte and water balance within the nephrons by acting on cotransporter pumps, antagonising the effects of aldosterone or inhibiting transport of bicarbonate. When sodium

189

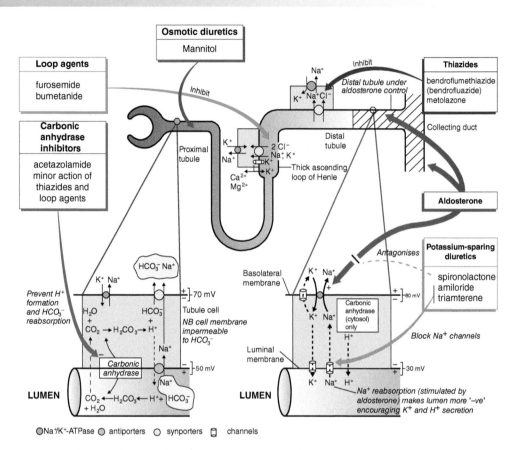

Figure 11.4 The site of action of various diuretics in the nephron.

excretion (natriuresis) is increased, water excretion (diuresis) will follow, leading to reduction of body fluid volume. Manipulation of this mechanism is the key action of diuretics and this can occur at various points in the nephron (the proximal tubule, the loop or the distal tubule) (Figure 11.4). The pharmacological choices may include use of one or more diuretics, dependent on the desired pharmacological effect, as they can act synergistically.

Clinical consideration

Diuretics will affect electrolyte levels, so careful consideration must be given to the use of these drugs and high doses avoided if at all possible.

Loop diuretics

Loop diuretics act on the thick ascending limb of the loop of Henle to inhibit the sodium–potassium–chloride (Na–K–Cl) cotransporter. This transporter normally returns a high sodium and chloride load from the nephron back to the blood, so inhibition of this pump has the potential to reduce sodium and chloride reabsorption very significantly. This causes loss of both fluid (diuresis) and sodium (natriuresis) in the urine. The additional sodium retained in the tubule travels to the distal convoluted tubule, and stimulates the aldosterone-sensitive sodium transporter which causes the reabsorption of sodium in exchange for potassium. The resulting increase in potassium excretion can cause hypokalaemia, which is a serious complication and a consideration in the use of loop diuretics.

In the UK, a loop diuretic such as furosemide is commonly prescribed for heart failure or hypertension. In acute heart failure, loop diuretics administered intravenously can be a life-saving intervention where congestive heart failure has resulted in pulmonary oedema, hypoxia and associated cerebral irritation.

Clinical consideration

Paramedics can use furosemide to treat acute heart failure presentations, although first-line treatment should be with nitrates. If using furosemide, be careful to check the mg/mL, as different manufacturers produce different concentrations. As furosemide is given IV, the nitrate spray or sublingual tablet will be a quicker administration and may buy you time to site a cannula.

The pharmacology of the loop diuretics is shown in Table 11.5.

Thiazide diuretics

Thiazide diuretics such as bendroflumethiazide and hydrochlorothiazide exert their effect on the proximal portion of the distal convoluted tubule (DCT), which normally reabsorbs around 5% of the filtered sodium (this limits the impact of thiazide diuretics on sodium excretion compared with the loop diuretics). The thiazides inhibit the sodium and chloride cotransporter situated on the DCT cells. This reduces the reabsorption of sodium and chloride ions, increasing their delivery to the sodium/potassium exchangers further along the distal tubule, causing increased secretion of potassium and hydrogen into the tubule, in exchange for sodium reabsorption. This results in an increased excretion and therefore lower serum levels of potassium and hydrogen, which can lead to hypokalaemia and a metabolic alkalosis. The thiazides also cause increased calcium reabsorption by nephrons, which can raise serum calcium levels.

Oral bendroflumethiazide is a thiazide commonly used in the treatment of hypertension. It is advised not to take this medication late in the day, as it increases urine volume and may cause nocturia. Occasionally serum electrolyte and lipid levels may be altered when starting medicines in this group and these should be monitored after starting treatment.

Table 11.6 details the pharmacology of bendroflumethiazide.

Osmotic diuretics

Osmotic diuretics, including mannitol and isosorbide, are reserved to treat life-threatening cerebral oedema that can occur, for example, after traumatic brain injury. When swelling occurs in the brain, reduction of blood flow and compression of brain tissue can occur without rapid treatment to free up some room inside the rigid skull. Osmotic diuretics are freely filtered by the glomerulus, are minimally reabsorbed by the renal tubules and have no other pharmacological effects. The presence of these osmotically active particles in the filtrate generates an osmotic pressure, promoting the movement of water into the renal tubule. Osmotic diuretics exert their effects in the proximal convoluted tubule, the thin descending loop of Henle and the collecting ducts, as these are the segments that are highly permeable to water. In the presence of an osmotic diuretic, water moves into the tubule, producing a diuresis.

The osmotic action of mannitol is also used in the management of raised intracranial or intraocular pressure, as it remains within the circulation, raising plasma osmolarity, resulting in movement of water from the target tissues (brain, eye) into the circulation. The diuretic effects are subsequently exerted in the kidney. Other uses include prevention of renal injury during major cardiac and vascular surgery as well as promotion of diuresis following renal transplantation, poisoning, rhabdomyolysis or haemolysis.

Table 11.5   Pharmacology of loop diuretics.

Drug name	Furosemide	Bumetanide
Mode of action	Inhibition of the sodium–potassium–chloride (Na–K–Cl) cotransporter	
Route of administration	Oral, intramuscular, intravenous	Oral
Indications	*Adult*	
	Oedema and resistant oedema Resistant hypertension	Oedema and resistant oedema
	Child	
	Oedema in heart failure, renal disease and hepatic disease Pulmonary oedema Oliguria	Oedema in heart failure, renal disease and hepatic disease Pulmonary oedema (severe cases)
Contraindications	*Anuria* Comatose and precomatose states associated with liver cirrhosis Renal failure due to nephrotoxic or hepatotoxic drugs Severe hypokalaemia Severe hyponatraemia Previous anaphylactic reaction	
Precautions	Can exacerbate diabetes (but hyperglycaemia less likely than with thiazides) Can exacerbate gout Hypotension should be corrected before initiation of treatment Hypovolaemia should be corrected before initiation of treatment Urinary retention can occur in prostatic hyperplasia Lower initial doses of diuretics should be used in the elderly because they are particularly susceptible to the side-effects. Dose should then be adjusted according to renal function Can cause acute urinary retention in children with obstruction of urinary outflow If there is an enlarged prostate, urinary retention can occur, although this is less likely if small doses and less potent diuretics are used initially; an adequate urinary output should be established before initiating treatment Hypokalaemia is dangerous in severe cardiovascular disease and in patients also being treated with cardiac glycosides In hepatic failure, hypokalaemia caused by diuretics can precipitate encephalopathy *Pregnancy and breast feeding* Furosemide crosses the placental barrier and should not be given during pregnancy unless there are compelling medical reasons. Furosemide is contraindicated in breast feeding as it passes into breast milk and may inhibit lactation Bumetanide should be avoided during the first trimester. Bumetanide has no data on breast feeding and therefore should not be used in lactating mothers unless essential	
Side-effects (common and very common ONLY)	Dizziness Electrolyte imbalance Fatigue Headache Metabolic alkalosis Muscle spasms (secondary to electrolyte disorders) Nausea	

(Continued)

Table 11.5 (Continued)

Drug name	Furosemide	Bumetanide
Interactions	The dosage of concurrently administered cardiac glycosides, diuretics, antihypertensive agents or other drugs with hypotensive potential may require adjustment as a more pronounced fall in blood pressure must be anticipated if given concomitantly with furosemide. The toxic effects of nephrotoxic drugs may be increased by concomitant administration of potent diuretics such as furosemide. Some electrolyte disturbances (e.g. hypokalaemia, hypomagnesaemia) may increase the toxicity of some other drugs (e.g. digoxin and drugs inducing QT interval prolongation syndrome)	As for furosemide. Should not be administered concurrently with lithium, as diuretics reduce the clearance rate of lithium, leading to increased risk of toxic effects. Should not be given concurrently with cephaloridine or amphotericin as increased risk of toxic effects
Absorption	Approximately 65% of the dose is absorbed after oral administration	Rapidly and almost completely absorbed from the gastrointestinal tract (bioavailability 80–95%)
Distribution	Furosemide is up to 99% bound to plasma proteins	95% bound to plasma proteins Plasma elimination half-life 0.75–2.6 h
Metabolism	Liver	Liver No active metabolites are known
Elimination	Mainly excreted in the urine, largely unchanged. Remainder via bile in faeces. This route significantly increases in renal failure	~50% excreted unchanged via the kidneys. Remainder via bile in faeces
Monitoring	Patients receiving loop diuretics should undergo regular monitoring of their serum sodium and potassium levels; this is particularly important in the following patient groups: <ul><li>the elderly population.</li><li>patients with impaired renal function and creatinine clearance below 60 mL/min per 1.73m² body surface area</li><li>patients with a coexisting disease which may cause electrolyte deficiencies (e.g. liver disease, anorexia nervosa)</li><li>patients receiving chronic corticosteroid or digoxin therapy. Digoxin has a very narrow therapeutic range and potassium deficiency can trigger or exacerbate digoxin toxicity</li></ul>	
Ototoxicity	Rapid intravenous administration of furosemide can cause tinnitus and permanent hearing loss (ototoxicity). Intravenous administration rates should not usually exceed 4 mg/min, but single doses of up to 80 mg may be administered more rapidly; a lower rate of infusion may be necessary in renal impairment	

Source: British National Formulary 2021.

Drugs used to treat urinary retention and urinary incontinence

The pharmacotherapy targets for these conditions are the receptors responsible for bladder control – adrenergic and muscarinic receptors. Adrenergic alpha-1 receptors in the smooth sphincter muscle in the neck of the bladder cause contraction of the sphincter when activated, preventing bladder emptying. Inhibition of this sphincter is necessary to allow bladder emptying. Parasympathetic control of the body of the bladder results in contraction of the bladder when acetylcholine acts on muscarinic receptors in the bladder muscle. Blockers (antagonists) of alpha-1 receptors such as tamsulosin and doxazosin are used in the treatment of acute and chronic urinary retention, as they prevent the contraction of the bladder sphincter, helping to relieve urinary retention (Figure 11.5). Since normal bladder voiding involves parasympathetic contraction of the bladder while simultaneously relaxing the sphincter muscle by inhibiting the sympathetic influence on

Table 11.6   Pharmacology of thiazide diuretics.

Drug name	Bendroflumethiazide
Mode of action	Inhibition of the sodium chloride cotransport protein with the proximal part of the distal convoluted tubule (DCT)
Route	PO
Indications	*Adult* Oedema Hypertension *Child* Hypertension Oedema in heart failure, renal disease and hepatic disease Pulmonary oedema
Contraindications	Addison disease Hypercalcaemia Hyponatraemia Refractory hypokalaemia Symptomatic hyperuricaemia
Cautions	Diabetes Gout Hyperaldosteronism Hypokalaemia – dangerous in severe cardiovascular disease and in patients also being treated with cardiac glycosides Lower initial doses of diuretics should be used in the elderly Malnourishment Nephrotic syndrome Systemic lupus erythematosus *Pregnancy and breast feeding* • Crosses the placenta and its use may be associated with hypokalaemia, increased blood viscosity and reduced placental perfusion, so should be avoided • Small amounts pass into breast milk – should be avoided in breast-feeding mothers • Suppresses lactation
Common side-effects	Alkalosis due to hypochloraemia Constipation Diarrhoea Dizziness Electrolyte imbalance Headache Hyperuricaemia Nausea Postural hypotension Urticaria
Interactions	Antiarrhythmics Antidepressants Antidiabetics Antiepileptics Antifungals Antihypertensives Antipsychotics Calcium salts Corticosteroids Cytotoxic agents Hormone antagonists Lithium Vitamins

194

(Continued)

Table 11.6   (Continued)

Drug name	Bendroflumethiazide
Absorption	Completely absorbed from the gastrointestinal tract Diuresis is initiated in about 2 h and lasts for 12–18 h or longer
Distribution	>90% bound to plasma proteins
Metabolism	Variable degree of hepatic metabolism
Elimination	~30% excreted unchanged in urine with the remainder excreted as metabolites

Source: British National Formulary 2021.

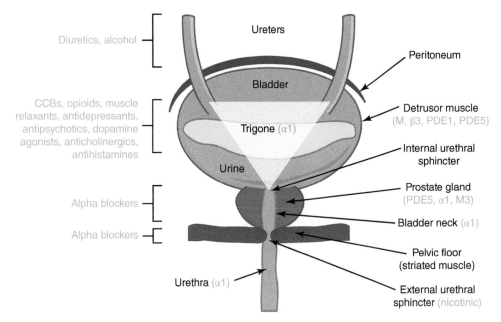

α: alpha-adrenergic; β: beta-adrenergic; CCB: calcium channel blocker; M: muscarinic; PDE: phosphodiesterase; UI: urinary incontinence.

Figure 11.5   Sites of drug action in the urinary tract.

it, combination treatment with both cholinergic agents and alpha-blockers can significantly improve bladder emptying when compared to treatment with alpha-blocker therapy alone (Filson et al., 2013). The pharmacology of these agents is shown in Table 11.7.

Conclusion

As an allied healthcare professional, you will undoubtedly be involved in the care of a number of patients with one or multiple types of renal disorder. These disorders can be very complex and can have detrimental effects on a patient's activities of daily living. The causes of renal disorders can be multifactorial and often are interlinked with other comorbidities, such as cardiovascular disease and diabetes. The incidence of AKI continues to rise despite multiple public health campaigns and NHS initiatives. As such, it is crucial that healthcare professionals involved in supporting this patient group to manage their disease have a sound understanding of the pathophysiological and pharmacological evidence base that underpins the promotion of safe and effective care.

Table 11.7   Pharmacology of two alpha-1 receptor antagonists used for urinary tract disorders.

Drug	Doxazosin	Tamsulosin
Mode of action	Alpha-1 receptor antagonist	Alpha-1 receptor antagonist
Route	Oral	PO
Indications	*Adult* Benign prostatic hyperplasia (BPH) Hypertension	*Adult* Benign prostatic hyperplasia *Child* Dysfunctional voiding (administered on expert advice)
Contraindications	Previous anaphylactic response to drug History of micturition syncope (in patients with BPH) History of postural hypotension	Previous anaphylactic response to drug History of micturition syncope (in patients with BPH) History of postural hypotension
Cautions	Care with initial dose (risk of postural hypotension) Cataract surgery (risk of intraoperative floppy iris syndrome) Elderly Heart failure Pulmonary oedema due to aortic or mitral stenosis *Pregnancy and breast feeding* No evidence of teratogenicity; use only when potential benefit outweighs risk Accumulates in milk in animal studies	Cataract surgery (risk of intraoperative floppy iris syndrome) Concomitant antihypertensives (reduced dosage and specialist supervision may be required) Elderly *Pregnancy and breast feeding* Tamsulosin is not indicated for use in women
Common side-effects	Arrhythmias Chest pain Cough Cystitis Dizziness Drowsiness Dry mouth Dyspnoea Gastrointestinal discomfort Headache Hypotension Muscle complaints Nausea Oedema Palpitations Vertigo	Dizziness Sexual dysfunction
Interactions	Phosphodiesterase inhibitors – additional vasodilation CYP 3A4 inhibitors such as clarithromycin, indinavir, itraconazole, ketoconazole, nefazodone, nelfinavir, ritonavir, saquinavir, telithromycin or voriconazole. Results in slower metabolism and higher plasma level of drug	Phosphodiesterase inhibitors (due to vasodilatory effects). CYP 3A4 inhibitors such as clarithromycin, indinavir, itraconazole, ketoconazole, nefazodone, nelfinavir, ritonavir, saquinavir, telithromycin or voriconazole. Results in slower metabolism and higher plasma level of drug
Absorption	Absorbed from the intestine. Bioavailability 66%	Absorbed from the intestine. Bioavailability almost 100%
Distribution	98% bound to plasma proteins, so limited distribution	99% bound to plasma proteins, so limited distribution
Metabolism	Extensively metabolised in the liver	Low hepatic first-pass effect, metabolised slowly
Elimination	In urine	In urine

Source: British National Formulary 2021.

Skills in practice: identifying the need for furosemide use

- Is this definitely acute heart failure (and not pneumonia?)
- Why are you using a diuretic instead of nitrates?
- Have you checked your JRCALC clinical guidelines for indications, cautions and contraindications?
- Have you checked the vial using the 5 Rs (right drug, right dose, right time, right route, right person)?
- If you haven't done so, check your JRCALC clinical guidelines for the required dose level.
- Site a cannula and flush it for patency.
- Draw up the medicine and administer as a slow push.

Episode of care

You are dispatched to a 65-year-old male feeling short of breath. You and your crewmate attend a local address in a ground floor flat. On entering the venue, you can hear a bubbly chest from down the hallway and the male patient appears diaphoretic and tachypnoeic.

His observations show a marked tachycardia but no arrhythmia and signs of an old myocardial infarction in the anterior leads. There are no other ischaemic or acute changes. His heart rate is 125 beats per minute, his blood pressure is 210/130 mmHg, his temperature is 37.0 °C and his oxygen saturations are 65% on room air. You suspect acute heart failure.

Your management includes sitting the patient up, applying oxygen therapy and then a salbutamol nebuliser to ease the respiratory distress. You now consider which treatments you are going to start first.

Do you start with sublingual glyceryl trinitrate or intravenous diuretics?

The red flags that may indicate the need for fluid offloading are:
- severe hypertension
- hypoxia
- audible pulmonary oedema.

The red flags which may indicate someone is in acute urinary retention include:
- not passing urine
- lower abdominal pain
- history of back pain (including cauda equina syndrome and pyelonephritis).

The following are a list of conditions associated with the renal tract. Take some time and write notes about each of the conditions. Think about the medications that may be used to treat these conditions and be specific about the pharmacokinetics and pharmacodynamics. Remember to include aspects of patient care. If you are making notes about people you have offered care and support to, you must ensure that you have adhered to the rules of confidentiality.

The condition	Your notes
Acute kidney injury	
Chronic kidney disease	
Electrolyte imbalance	
Oedema	
Urinary retention	

Glossary

Acute	A word meaning short-term and of rapid onset, usually requiring a rapid response.
Albumin	A type of protein that occurs in the blood.
Alphacalcidol	A vitamin D supplement.
Anaemia	A shortage of red blood cells in the body, causing tiredness, shortage of breath and pale skin. One of the functions of the kidneys is to make EPO (erythropoietin), which stimulates the bone marrow to make blood cells. In kidney failure, EPO is not made and anaemia results.
Bicarbonate	A substance that is normally present in the blood which is measured in the biochemistry blood test. A low blood level of bicarbonate shows there is too much acid in the blood.
Biochemistry blood test	A test that measures the blood levels of various different substances. Substances measured in people with kidney failure usually include sodium, potassium, glucose, urea, creatinine, bicarbonate, calcium, phosphate and albumin.
Bladder	The organ in which urine is stored before being passed from the body.
Blood level	A measurement of the amount of a particular substance in the blood, sometimes expressed in mmol/L (millimoles per litre) or μmol/L (micromoles per litre) of blood.
Blood pressure	The pressure that the blood exerts against the walls of the arteries as it flows through them. Blood pressure measurements consist of two numbers. The first is the systolic blood pressure, the second, the diastolic blood pressure.
Blood vessels	The tubes that carry blood around the body. The main blood vessels are the arteries and veins.
BP	Abbreviation for blood pressure.
CAPD	Abbreviation for continuous ambulatory peritoneal dialysis. A continuous form of peritoneal dialysis in which patients perform the exchanges of dialysis fluid by hand. The fluid is usually exchanged four times during the day, and is left inside the patient overnight.
Catheter	A flexible plastic tube used to enter the interior of the body. A catheter is one of the access options for patients on haemodialysis. For patients on peritoneal dialysis, a catheter allows dialysis fluid to be put into and removed from the peritoneal cavity. A catheter may also be used to drain urine from the bladder.
Chronic	A word meaning long-term and of slow onset, not usually requiring immediate action.
CKD	Abbreviation for chronic kidney disease. This is an abnormality in the kidneys that is present for more than 3 months, and is graded stages 1, 2, 3a, 3b, 4 and 5 for minor to severe kidney disease.
Clearance	The removal of substances from the body by the kidneys. In kidney failure, clearance is inadequate and toxins can build up in the blood.
Creatinine	A waste substance produced by muscle metabolism. The clearance of creatinine is also used as an indicator of kidney function.
Cystitis	A type of infection that causes inflammation of the bladder.
Cytomegalovirus (CMV)	A virus that normally causes only a mild 'flu-like' illness.
Dehydration	A condition in which there is a lower than normal body water content.
Diabetes mellitus	A condition (also known as sugar diabetes or simply as diabetes) in which the glucose level in the blood is poorly controlled, resulting in chronically high blood glucose. This can lead to kidney failure over the long term kidney failure.

Dialysis	An artificial process by which the toxic waste products of food and excess water are removed from the body. Dialysis therefore takes over some of the work normally performed by healthy kidneys. The name *dialysis* comes from a Greek word meaning 'to separate', i.e. to separate out the 'bad things' in the blood from the 'good things'.
Diuretic drugs	The medical name for water tablets. These drugs increase the amount of urine that is passed. Two commonly used diuretics are furosemide and bumetanide.
eGFR	Abbreviation of estimated glomerular filtration rate. Measurement of how much blood is filtered by the kidneys, calculated from the blood level of creatinine.
End-stage renal failure (ESRF)	A term for advanced chronic kidney failure. People who develop ESRF will die within a few weeks unless treated by dialysis or transplantation. These treatments control ESRF but cannot cure it.
End-stage renal disease (ESRD)	An alternative name for end-stage renal failure.
Established renal failure (ERF)	An alternative name for end-stage renal failure or end-stage renal disease.
Fluid overload	A condition in which the body contains too much water. It is caused by drinking too much fluid, or not losing enough. Fluid overload occurs in kidney failure because one of the main functions of the kidneys is to remove excess water. Fluid overload often occurs with high blood pressure. Excess fluid first gathers around the ankles (ankle oedema) and may later settle in the lungs (pulmonary oedema).
GFR	Abbreviation of glomerular filtration rate. Measurement of how much blood is filtered by the kidneys; if the GFR is low, there is kidney disease.
Glomerulus	One of the tiny filtering units inside the kidney.
Glomerulonephritis	Inflammation of the glomeruli, which is one of the causes of kidney failure.
Haemodialysis	A form of dialysis in which the blood is cleaned outside the body, in a machine called a dialysis machine or kidney machine. The machine contains a filter called the dialyser or artificial kidney. Each dialysis session lasts for 3–5 hours, and sessions are usually needed three times a week.
Kidneys	The two bean-shaped body organs where urine is made. They are located at the back of the body, below the ribs. The two main functions of the kidneys are to remove toxic wastes and to remove excess water from the body. The kidneys also help to control blood pressure, control the manufacture of red blood cells and keep the bones strong and healthy.
Kidney failure	A condition in which the kidneys are less able than normal to perform their functions of removing toxic wastes, removing excess water, helping to control blood pressure, control red blood cell manufacture and to keep the bones strong and healthy. Kidney failure can be acute or chronic. Advanced chronic kidney failure is called end-stage renal failure (ESRF).
Liver function tests (LFTs)	Blood tests that show how well the liver is working.
Marker	A substance that is used as an indicator of physiological function. Both creatinine and urea are markers for kidney function.
Nephr-	Prefix meaning relating to the kidneys.
Nephron	Small filtering unit in the kidney, made up of blood vessels (glomeruli) and tubules.

199

Nephritis	A general term for inflammation of the kidneys. Also used as an abbreviation for glomerulonephritis (GN). A kidney biopsy is needed to diagnose nephritis.
Nephrology	The study of the kidneys.
Oedema	An abnormal build-up of fluid, mainly water, in the tissues. People with kidney failure are prone to fluid overload leading to oedema. The two most common places for water to collect in the body are around the ankles (ankle oedema) and in the lungs (pulmonary oedema).
Potassium	A mineral that is normally present in the blood, and which is measured in the biochemistry blood test. Either too much or too little potassium can be dangerous, causing the heart to stop. People with kidney failure may need to restrict the amount of potassium in their diet.
Pulmonary oedema	A serious condition in which fluid builds up in the lungs, causing breathlessness. People with kidney failure develop pulmonary oedema if fluid overload is not treated promptly.
Pyelonephritis	Inflammation of the drainage system of the kidneys, one of the causes of kidney failure. It can be diagnosed by an ultrasound scan or by an intravenous pyelogram (IVP).
Renal	Adjective meaning relating to the kidneys.
Renal artery	The blood vessel which carries blood from the heart to the kidneys.
Sodium	A mineral that is normally present in the blood, and which is measured in the biochemistry blood test. Sodium levels are not usually a problem for people with kidney failure and are quite easily controlled by dialysis.
Uraemia	An abnormally high level of nitrogenous wastes in the blood. Symptoms may include nausea, weight loss, high blood pressure and/or trouble sleeping.
Ureters	The tubes that take urine from the kidneys to the bladder.
Urethra	The tube that takes urine from the bladder to the outside of the body.
Urinary catheter	A plastic tube inserted into the bladder for the removal of urine.
Urination	The passing of urine out of the body.
Urine	The liquid produced by the kidneys, consisting of nitrogenous waste products, electrolytes and water.
Water tablets	The common name for diuretic drugs.

References

Ball, S., Barth, J. and Levy, M. (2016).Emergency management of severe symptomatic hyponatraemia in adult patients. *Endocrine Connections* **5**(5): g4–g6.

Barkin, J., Habert, J. and Wong, A. (2017). The practical update for family physicians in the diagnosis and management of overactive bladder and lower urinary tract symptoms. *Canadian Journal of Urology* **24**(5S1): 1–11.

Filson, C.P., Hollingsworth, J.M., Clemens, J.Q. and Wei, J.T. (2013). The efficacy and safety of combined therapy with alpha-blockers and anticholinergics for men with benign prostatic hyperplasia: a meta-analysis. *Journal of Urology* **190**(3): 2153–2160.

Hu, J.S. and Pierre, E.F. (2019). Urinary incontinence in women: evaluation and management. *American Family Physician* **100**(6): 339–348.

McGregor, C. (2014). Improving time to antibiotics and implementing the 'Sepsis 6'. *BMJ Open Quality* **2**: u202548.

National Institute for Health and Care Excellence (NICE). (2013). *Clinical guideline 169: Acute kidney injury. Prevention, detection and management up to the point of renal replacement therapy.* London: National Institute for Health and Care Excellence.

National Institute for Health and Care Excellence (NICE). (2015). *Chronic kidney disease. Early identification and management of chronic kidney disease in adults in primary and secondary care.* London: National Institute for Health and Care Excellence.

National Institute for Health and Care Excellence (NICE). (2019). *Clinical guideline NG123. Urinary incontinence and pelvic organ prolapse in women: management.* London: National Institute for Health and Care Excellence.

Further reading

Renal and ureteric colic: https://cks.nice.org.uk/topics/renal-or-ureteric-colic-acute/
Incontinence in children: https://cks.nice.org.uk/topics/bedwetting-enuresis/
Chronic kidney disease: https://cks.nice.org.uk/topics/chronic-kidney-disease/
Hyponatraemia: https://cks.nice.org.uk/topics/hyponatraemia/
Lower urinary tract symptoms in men: https://cks.nice.org.uk/topics/luts-in-men/

Multiple-choice questions

1. What is the name of the loop within the kidney nephron?
   (a) The loop of Destiny
   (b) The loop of Henry
   (c) The loop of Henle
   (d) The loop of Bowman

2. Each of the tubes which connect the kidney to the urinary bladder is a:
   (a) Ureter
   (b) Urethra
   (c) Uterus
   (d) Uvula
3. Which of the following is an example of a pre-renal pathophysiology?
   (a) Fibromuscular dysplasia
   (b) Acute tubular necrosis
   (c) Acute interstitial nephritis
   (d) Benign prostatic hyperplasia
4. Which of the following is an example of an intrarenal pathophysiology?
   (a) Fibromuscular dysplasia
   (b) Low BP from a haemorrhage
   (c) Cardiogenic shock from a myocardial infarction
   (d) Acute glomerulonephritis
5. Which of the following is an example of a postrenal pathophysiology?
   (a) Heart failure
   (b) Anaphylaxis
   (c) Renal calculus
   (d) Acute tubular necrosis
6. Which of the following is an example of a pre-renal pathophysiology?
   (a) Bladder tumour
   (b) Extensive burns
   (c) Renal calculi
   (d) Benign prostatic hyperplasia
7. Which of the following is an example of a postrenal pathophysiology?
   (a) Heart failure
   (b) Anaphylaxis
   (c) Sepsis
   (d) Bladder tumour
8. Which of the following drugs have nephrotoxic potential?
   (a) Propranolol
   (b) Mannitol
   (c) Aspirin
   (d) Salbutamol

9. Acute kidney injury is characterised by which change in blood measurement?
   (a) A reduced estimated glomerular filtration rate (eGFR)
   (b) A raised estimated glomerular filtration rate (eGFR)
   (c) A raise in hepatic transaminases
   (d) A decrease in hepatic transaminases

10. Plasma level of which nitrogenous chemical tends to rise in acute kidney injury?
   (a) Uric acid
   (b) Acetic acid
   (c) Creatinine
   (d) Basophils

11. What is the medical term for reduced urine output?
   (a) Azotemia
   (b) Polydipsia
   (c) Polyuria
   (d) Oliguria

12. What is the name of an increase in plasma level of nitrogenous waste products?
   (a) Oliguria
   (b) Azotemia
   (c) Ketoacidosis
   (d) Metabolic alkalosis

13. What is the blood vessel that encircles the nephron?
   (a) Vasa recta
   (b) Vas deferens
   (c) Inferior vena cava
   (d) Renal artery

14. How much urine does an average adult produce per hour?
   (a) 0.5–1 mL/kg/h
   (b) 50–100 mL/kg/h
   (c) 500–1000 mL/kg/h
   (d) 5000–10000 mL/kg/h

15. Which system, when activated, may worsen ischaemia caused by renal artery stenosis?
   (a) Hepatorenal system
   (b) Renin-angiotensin-aldosterone system
   (c) Reno-diverse system
   (d) Glomerular-tubular-interstitial system

Chapter 12

Medications and diabetes mellitus

Hayley Croft and Olivia Thornton

Aim

This chapter aims to describe medicines used by patients with diabetes and their effects on blood glucose, including medicines used to treat complications that could present to paramedics when attending to a patient with diabetes.

Learning outcomes

After reading this chapter the reader will be able to:

1. Discuss the role of insulin and glucagon in maintaining blood glucose homeostasis
2. Recognise a range of antihyperglycaemic agents used in diabetes and describe their effect on blood glucose levels and potential adverse effects
3. Recognise the signs and symptoms of common diabetic emergencies and their causes
4. Describe the management of common diabetic emergencies, including hyperglycaemia and hypoglycaemia.

Test your knowledge

1. How are blood glucose levels regulated in the body?
2. What strategies could you use to determine if a patient was experiencing high or low blood glucose?
3. What groups of patients are vulnerable to experiencing fluctuations in blood glucose levels?
4. What drugs are you aware of that may be used to increase or decrease blood glucose levels?

Fundamentals of Pharmacology for Paramedics, First Edition. Edited by Ian Peate, Suzanne Evans, and Lisa Clegg.
© 2022 John Wiley & Sons Ltd. Published 2022 by John Wiley & Sons Ltd.

Introduction

Insulin is necessary for normal carbohydrate, protein and fat metabolism. Diabetes mellitus (DM) is defined as a group of chronic disorders characterised by high blood sugar (hyperglycaemia), arising from insulin deficiency or insulin resistance, or both. DM is known for its association with long-term damage and organ impairment. Although their names suggest two types of the same disease, the pathophysiology of type 1 and type 2 diabetes mellitus is different.

People with type 1 diabetes mellitus (T1DM) do not produce enough insulin and rely on exogenous insulin administration for survival. In type 2 diabetes mellitus (T2DM), the body's cells cannot respond to insulin as well as they should. In later stages of T2DM, the body may also not produce enough insulin. People with T2DM are not completely dependent on insulin administration for survival. However, many of these individuals will experience decreased insulin production and may therefore require supplemental insulin use, particularly during times of stress (Petersons, 2018).

Gestational diabetes mellitus (GDM) arises when the woman's insulin reserves are insufficient to meet the extra demands of pregnancy. Screening for hyperglycaemia during pregnancy is important in detecting gestational diabetes as women may be asymptomatic. If left untreated, complications of gestational diabetes such as fetal macrosomia (big baby syndrome) and neonatal hypoglycaemia may not be recognised and managed appropriately. Many women with GDM develop T2DM later in life (Sherwin and Svancarek, 2021).

People with diabetes can experience an acute decline in control of their condition if their blood glucose levels and insulin are out of balance. Although many patients will be educated on strategies to correct the problem, sometimes they will not be able to help themselves, and a rapid response to a diabetic emergency may be necessary, to assess and attend to patients with life-threatening metabolic disturbance.

Hormonal control of blood glucose

Glucose is the primary source of fuel for all cellular ATP energy. Glucose is obtained from dietary sources of carbohydrate, from liver stores of glycogen (the main storage form of glucose in the body) or synthesised from non-carbohydrate precursors (gluconeogenesis). Blood glucose concentration is maintained within a relatively narrow range despite wide fluctuations in dietary intake, under the control of the endocrine pancreas which produces two major hormones, insulin and glucagon, that regulate its mobilisation and storage (Figure 12.1).

Under normal circumstances, nutrient intake stimulates secretion of insulin from pancreatic beta cells in the islets of Langerhans. Insulin lowers blood glucose by facilitating movement of glucose across cell membranes for use as an energy source. Insulin also regulates glucose levels by suppression of hepatic glucose output, increased uptake of glucose in muscle and reduced fat breakdown. When there is no nutrient intake, blood glucose level is maintained by glucagon, a peptide hormone produced by

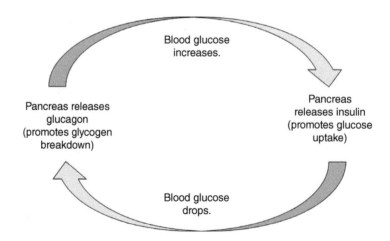

Figure 12.1   Interplay between insulin and glucagon in control of blood glucose.

Box 12.1 Major actions of insulin and glucagon in the body.

Insulin has the following anabolic effects.
- Drives glucose into cells
- Decreases production glucose by liver
- Inhibits fat breakdown (lipolysis)
- Increases conversion of glucose to triglycerides (fats)
- Drives potassium into cells

Glucagon has the following catabolic effects.
- Increases hepatic glucose output

MIMS Australia, 2020a, 2020b.

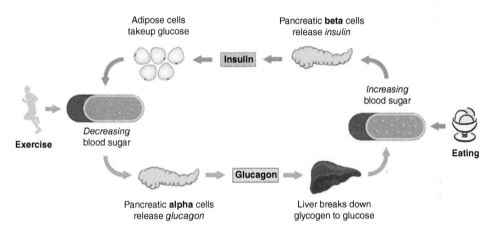

Figure 12.2 Major actions of insulin and glucagon in the body.

pancreatic alpha cells. Glucagon provides the major counter-regulatory mechanism for insulin in maintaining glucose homeostasis. It raises blood glucose concentration by stimulating hepatic glucose production. The major actions of insulin and glucagon in the body are outlined in Box 12.1.

While insulin and glucagon exert short-term glucose control, as shown in Figure 12.2, other hormones exert long-term effects on blood glucose, including glucocorticoid hormones (e.g. cortisol), growth hormone, thyroid hormones and catecholamines (adrenaline and noradrenaline).

Monitoring diabetes

Patients with diabetes will require ongoing monitoring of various aspects of disease. One of the main aims of diabetes treatment is to keep the blood glucose levels within target range. Blood glucose monitoring is used as an educational tool to aid understanding of glycaemic control by the patient, family, carers and health personnel, including paramedics. For many, it is an important aspect of the day-to-day care of a patient with diabetes which enables adjustment of medication, food and drink intake and physical activity, and response to hypo- or hyperglycaemia.

While home monitoring of blood glucose levels shows the short-term fluctuations, a glycated haemoglobin (HbA1c) check provides a longer-term measure of blood glucose over 10–12 weeks, as it indicates the percentage of haemoglobin molecules that have reacted with excess blood glucose to become glycated. For health professionals, information about blood glucose levels and HbA1c is used to optimise diabetic control to eliminate symptoms of hyperglycaemia, with the longer-term aim of preventing diabetic complications such as blindness, kidney damage, amputation, heart attack and stroke.

In the prehospital setting, however, blood glucose and blood ketone levels are the most useful indicators, and blood glucose measurement should be considered in all patients with an altered level of consciousness (Sherwin and Svancarek, 2021).

Measuring blood glucose

Blood glucose levels are measured in millimoles per litre of blood (mmol/L). Normal blood glucose levels are between 4.0 and 7.8 mmol/L (Diabetes Australia, 2021). The usual target blood glucose level range depends on the individual and factors such as the type of diabetes, their medications and medical conditions, diet, activity level and age.

The measurement is made by applying a small amount of blood to a disposable test strip. An electronic meter is then used to read the strip and display the blood glucose level. Some newer devices use a sensor applied to the upper arm which captures interstitial fluid glucose readings, and other monitoring systems are embedded into insulin pump devices.

Skills in practice: Tips for measuring blood glucose levels

- Always use gloves.
- Pretest topical alcohol swab is not routinely required but may be used when necessary to clean test site.
- Check expiry date on individual test strips and ensure they have not been damaged.
- Use a lancing device to obtain a blood sample from the side of the fingertip. It may be appropriate to massage the finger in the direction of the fingertip to make it easier to obtain a blood sample.
- Although alternative sites (e.g. palm, upper forearm, thigh, calf) may be used to obtain a blood sample, testing from these sites is less accurate when blood glucose levels are falling or rising rapidly, and fingertip testing is appropriate for non-routine blood glucose testing.
- Apply blood sample to test strip.
- Ensure the lancet is disposed of in a sharps container.

Paramedics may find that a patient's blood glucose reading is unexpectedly high or low, and it may be difficult to identify the reason(s) for this. Changes in activity level, food intake or medication can cause blood glucose readings to alter and illness, pain and stress are common causes of changes in blood glucose patterns. However, it is also important to consider circumstances in which a blood glucose reading may be inaccurate, such that the results shown do not reflect the true blood glucose level. This is particularly important when the patient's signs and symptoms do not match the blood glucose reading.

Clinical consideration: Factors that may interfere with the accuracy of blood glucose measurements

- Poor quality of test strips, e.g. test strips are expired/out of date, poor storage and handling, ageing
- Wrong strips or incorrect technique
- Not enough blood applied to test strip
- Residual substance on unwashed hands prior to testing
- Testing site still damp from pretest topical alcohol
- Altitude, temperature and humidity.
- Test site location: side of fingertip usually used; alternative sites may be used when blood glucose is stable but not when it is changing rapidly (e.g. after eating or exercise, when hypoglycaemic or ill).

Measuring ketones

Ketones are produced when the body metabolises fats, which can occur in patients with inadequate insulin, since glucose is not transported into cells and metabolised under those conditions. Ketones can be detected in blood or urine, and high ketones can indicate diabetic ketoacidosis (DKA), a severe complication of lack of insulin. Not all patients will need to be tested for ketones, and although DKA can occur in any patient with diabetes, it is rare in T2DM, so patients with T1DM and those with DKA symptoms are most likely to be tested. Blood ketone testing may be performed using at-home test kits or meter systems in a very similar way to blood glucose levels, by using specific test strips.

Drug use in diabetes

Treatment of diabetes involves lifestyle measures, including diet and physical activity, and self-blood glucose monitoring (SBGM), as well as antihyperglycaemic medications (oral and/or injectable). Paramedics should be familiar with therapeutic approaches to managing diabetes and the factors that can lead to an emergency.

Insulin replacement therapy

When diet and other therapies provide insufficient control of hyperglycaemia, insulin replacement therapy is required. In health, basal insulin secretion constitutes approximately 50% of total insulin secreted, with the remainder secreted as a rapid bolus response to food. Endogenous insulin is secreted into the hepatic portal vein and acts directly on the liver, which does not occur when insulin is injected into peripheral sites. The aim of insulin replacement therapy is to mimic, as far as possible, normal 'basal bolus' physiological insulin response by pancreatic beta cells.

Insulin is measured in international units, and while most formulations are 100 units per mL (U/mL), some newer formulations contain 200 U/mL, 300 U/mL or 500 U/mL. Insulin is considered a high-risk medicine and varying strength of formulations may be a source of medication error.

Insulin administration

As a protein, insulin is rapidly destroyed by proteases in the gastrointestinal (GI) tract, and therefore requires parenteral administration. Insulin is usually administered by injection into the subcutaneous tissue layer of the abdomen. This is generally the area that provides the fastest absorption. It may also be injected subcutaneously in the upper arm or anterolateral aspects of the thigh or buttocks. Although not recommended for routine use, insulin can be given intramuscularly under certain circumstances, such as diabetic ketoacidosis. The injection site is rotated with every injection to avoid injection site reactions such as lipodystrophy (abnormal distribution of fatty tissue under the skin). Rotations are usually within the one area (e.g. a systematic pattern within the abdomen), aiming to ensure each injection site is at least one finger-width away from the previous injection, and not used more than once every 4 weeks (American Diabetes Association, 2003).

Clinical consideration: insulin administration

Factors that may affect insulin absorption include the following.

Injection site: insulin may absorb at different rates depending on where it is injected. It is absorbed fastest from the abdomen, followed by the upper arms, outer thigh and buttocks. Fatty areas under the skin (lipohypertrophy) and/or scar tissue may cause slower or more erratic absorption.

Muscle: insulin injected into muscle rather than subcutaneous tissue will be absorbed faster.

Physical activity: exercise increases the rate of insulin absorption from the injection site.

Table 12.1   Properties of insulin preparations.

	Examples	Onset	Peak	Duration	Other
Ultra-short OR rapid-acting analogue insulin	Insulin aspart, insulin glulisine, insulin lispro	10–15 mins	1–2 hours	2–5 hours	Preparations are colourless/clear solutions
Short-acting human insulin	Neutral insulin	30 mins	2.5–5 hours	5–8 hours	Preparations are colourless/clear solutions
Intermediate-long-acting biphasic insulin	Isophane/NPH	1–2 hours	4–12 hours	12–18 hours	Suspension of soluble insulin complexed with protamine sulfate. Preparations are cloudy in appearance
Long-acting analogue insulin	Insulin detemir, insulin glargine	2 hours	'Peakless'	Up to 24 hours	Preparations are colourless/clear solutions
Ultra-long-acting	Insulin degludec	2 hours	'Peakless'	Up to 42 hours	Only used in fixed-dose combination with insulin aspart

Source: Adapted from AMH (2020a) and MIMS Australia (2020b).

Insulin preparations

There are several types of insulin preparations as shown in Table 12.1. Insulin dosages are titrated to the glycaemic response of the individual, their food intake and level of physical activity.

Mixed/premixed insulins are a combination of ultra-short-acting and intermediate/long-acting insulins, usually administered once or twice daily. Premixed insulins are useful for elderly people who may have difficulty mixing their own insulins, but the major disadvantage is inflexibility in dosing adjustment.

Some longer-acting insulins continue to exert blood glucose-lowering effects for up to 24 hours or longer. These insulin preparations may contribute to hypoglycaemic emergencies for several hours after their administration.

The appropriate insulin dosage is dependent on the glycaemic response of the individual and requires adjustment in certain situations.

Clinical consideration: Dosing insulin in certain situations

Intercurrent illness: there may be increased requirements for insulin during illness, increased temperature and/or inflammation.

Exercise: lower doses of insulin may be required.

Surgery: additional insulin may be required during surgery and recovery.

Fasting: even during fasting, basal insulin is usually required, at an adjusted dose.

Adverse effects of insulin

Hypoglycaemia (blood glucose level below 4 mmol/L) is the most important adverse effect of insulin. The onset of hypoglycaemia may be abrupt and dangerous, and if prolonged or repeated can lead to neurological damage. It may be caused by administering too much insulin, inadequate food intake or intense exercise. Excessive alcohol consumption may prolong or delay hypoglycaemia. Insulin, as an anabolic hormone, can also lead to weight gain, which may impact compliance with insulin replacement therapy, as well as increasing the risk of cardiometabolic disease.

Metformin

Metformin acts by inhibiting the production of glucose (gluconeogenesis) by the liver and inhibiting the breakdown of stored glycogen to glucose (glycogenolysis). The drug improves insulin sensitivity and glucose uptake by peripheral tissues such as skeletal muscle and delays intestinal glucose absorption. Metformin is a preferred first-line treatment option for patients with T2DM and may be particularly useful for patients who are overweight as it tends to produce gradual weight loss. Metformin may be used as monotherapy or in combination with other antihyperglycaemic agents (AMH, 2020b; American Diabetes Association, 2019).

Metformin is administered orally, and steady-state concentrations are reached in 24–48 hours at usual clinical doses. It is not bound to plasma proteins and does not undergo hepatic metabolism so its half-life is largely dependent on renal function. In patients with decreased renal function, the plasma half-life of metformin is prolonged. Metformin is available in immediate-release formulations usually given 2–3 times daily or extended-release preparations usually given once daily in the evening.

Metformin is associated with GI adverse effects (flatulence, diarrhoea, nausea, vomiting, metallic taste in the mouth, abdominal cramps). These effects are usually mild and transient and can be minimised by starting at a low dose, gradual dose titration and taking after food. Hypoglycaemia is less likely to occur when metformin is used as a single agent, but can occur when used in combination with other antihyperglycaemic agents that cause hypoglycaemia. Vitamin B12 malabsorption leading to vitamin B12 deficiency with long-term metformin use can occur (AMH, 2020b).

Rarely, metformin may be associated with metabolic (lactic) acidosis and should not be given to patients with other risk factors for this condition, including hypoxic conditions such as respiratory and heart failure, kidney disease, procedures that require iodine contrast media, excessive alcohol intake or poorly controlled diabetes (Misbin, 2004).

Lactic acidosis is a form of metabolic acidosis associated with a build-up of lactate in the body and low blood pH. It is a rare but serious side-effect of metformin therapy. Lactic acidosis occurs rarely after metformin at normal therapeutic doses but is more of a risk in patients with conditions that can themselves cause lactic acidosis, or where metformin accumulates, such as in patients with renal impairment.

Sulfonylureas

Sulfonylureas include glibenclamide, gliclazide, glimepiride and glipizide. They act by directly stimulating pancreatic islet beta cells to increase insulin release. Consequently, they are only effective in patients with functioning pancreatic beta cells. The rise in plasma insulin concentration results in decreased hepatic glucose production and increased peripheral utilisation of glucose. These drugs may be used as monotherapy or in combination with other antihyperglycaemic agents (Petersons, 2018).

Sulfonylureas are not alike and differ in their potency, duration of action, activity of metabolites and route of elimination (AMH, 2020c). They are well absorbed after oral administration. After absorption, sulfonylureas bind almost completely to plasma proteins, especially albumin. Glibenclamide is completely metabolised in the liver, and its metabolites, which continue to have some hypoglycaemic action, are excreted via a dual pathway in both bile and urine (MIMS Australia, 2020c). Other sulfonylureas are extensively metabolised in the liver and their metabolites are predominantly excreted in the urine (MIMS Australia, 2020c).

Sulfonylureas may cause weight gain (which may be particularly problematic in overweight patients with T2DM) and hypoglycaemia. Hypoglycaemia is associated more with long-acting agents, the highest risk being with glibenclamide, which can provoke long-lasting hypoglycaemic reactions.

The risk of hypoglycaemia is increased by taking sulfonylureas without food, alcohol consumption, renal impairment and coadministration of other antihyperglycaemic agents (AMH, 2020c).

Incretin mimetics

Incretins are peptide hormones produced by cells of the intestinal mucosa in response to food. After their release into the gastrointestinal tract (GIT), incretins, such as glucagon-like peptide-1 (GLP-1), are responsible for a cascade of events culminating in secretion of insulin. This effect, known as the incretin effect, depends on the nutrient composition of the food in the GIT and accounts for at least 50% of the total insulin secreted after oral glucose (Nauck et al., 1986).

Incretins have a short half-life due to rapid inactivation by dipeptidyl peptidase (DPP-4). The incretin effect is blunted in some people with T2DM (Hinnen, 2017). There are two approaches to increasing the activity of the incretin GLP-1 in the body. Oral DPP-4 inhibitors, known as gliptins, reduce the degradation of endogenous GLP-1, and injectable GLP-1 receptor agonists produce the effect that GLP-1 itself would produce at the receptors.

DPP-4 inhibitors

These include sitagliptin, vildagliptin and saxagliptin. DPP-4 is the enzyme responsible for the breakdown of physiologically released incretin hormones. Inhibition of the enzyme leads to elevated and prolonged GLP-1 levels. As a result, glucose-dependent insulin secretion is increased and there is a reduction in glucagon production. The main effect is a reduction in postprandial glucose levels.

DPP-4 inhibitors are available in stand-alone formulations or in fixed-dose combinations with metformin. They are not first line treatments.

These drugs have been linked with pancreatic agents but are used as add-on agents in dual or triple therapy. Adverse effects should be avoided in patients with acute pancreatitis or history of pancreatitis. They rarely cause hypoglycaemia except in combination with other antihyperglycaemic agents (AMH, 2020d).

GLP1 receptor agonists

GLP-1 receptor agonists include exenatide, liraglutide and dulaglutide. These agonists share sequence similarity with endogenous GLP-1 but exhibit increased resistance to degradation by DPP-4. The shorter-acting agonists such as exenatide and liraglutide offer improved control of postprandial hyperglycaemia, while longer-acting formulations such as exenatide extended-release, dulaglutide and albiglutide further improve fasting plasma glucose and HbA1c. In addition to their positive effects on glycaemic control, these drugs help with weight and blood pressure reduction. They are usually used as add-on therapy for patients with T2DM who do not achieve adequate blood glucose control with one first-line drug.

Administered GLP1-agonists achieve concentrations greater than endogenous GLP-1 levels and delay gastric emptying, making nausea and vomiting the most common side-effects, especially if the patient does not modify their usual food intake. This effect is usually transient and improves as treatment continues. These effects can also be minimised by slow introduction of the GLP-1 agonist (AMH, 2020e; Rasalam et al., 2019).

SGLT-2 inhibitors

Sodium-glucose cotransporter-2 (SGLT-2) inhibitors include empagliflozin, dapagliflozin and ertugliflozin. They act by inhibiting the transporter, located in the proximal convoluted tubule (PCT) of the nephron, resulting in increased glucose excretion. SGLT-2 inhibitors may be used in combination with other antihyperglycaemic agents in dual- or triple-therapy regimens for patients who do not achieve the desired HBA1c with first-line agents.

These drugs are not effective for patients with impaired renal function and may be associated with genitourinary infection due to the increased glucose in the urine. Patients should also be advised that their urine will test positive for glucose and because of the osmotic diuresis produced, they should consume more water to maintain hydration. SGLT-2 inhibitors do not cause hypoglycaemia except in combination with other antihyperglycaemic agents. SGLT-2 inhibitors should be stopped 3 days prior to surgery due to perioperative risks (dehydration, UTI, renal impairment). These agents may have additive effects with other diuretics, leading to dehydration (AMH, 2020f; Chesterman and Thynne, 2020).

SGLT-2 inhibitors may cause ketoacidosis even if blood glucose level is normal. Patients who present unwell should be monitored for signs of ketoacidosis, including severe vomiting and abdominal pain. Monitoring for ketones should be performed.

Thiazolidinediones

Thiazolidinediones, also known as 'glitizones', are less frequently used by patients with diabetes because of their adverse effects. Some drugs in this class have been withdrawn in some countries due to their association with increased risk of fractures, heart failure and bladder cancer. Pioglitazone is still included in management guidelines and acts to improve utilisation of glucose in peripheral tissues. Weight gain and swollen feet are common adverse effects of pioglitazone and it is important to assess the risk of fluid retention before increasing the dosage and stop treatment immediately if heart failure is diagnosed (AMH, 2020g).

Alpha-glucosidase inhibitors

Acarbose works by inhibiting an enzyme, alpha-glucosidase, that breaks down carbohydrates (AMH, 2020h). It therefore delays the digestion of carbohydrates and the absorption of glucose into the bloodstream. The tablets are taken just before a meal or chewed with the first few mouthfuls of food. Acarbose has a limited role in management of diabetes due to its lower efficacy, but it may be a useful addition in situations when control of blood glucose remains poor despite dietary modifications. The use of acarbose is limited by dose-dependent GI adverse effects such as diarrhoea, flatulence and abdominal pain.

When acarbose is used in combination with a sulfonylurea or insulin, hypoglycaemia may occur. If it does, the patient must take glucose (e.g. glucose gel, glucose tablets) to restore normal blood glucose concentration.

Acarbose does not affect the absorption of glucose or fructose. Therefore, if hypoglycaemia occurs, it should be treated with glucose. Sucrose (e.g. fruit juice, milk) is ineffective to treat hypoglycaemia as its absorption may be delayed.

Drug use in diabetic emergencies

Hypoglycaemic emergency

During hypoglycaemia, the brain is most vulnerable as it is unable to make or store glucose and therefore requires an uninterrupted supply in the bloodstream to maintain normal function. People with diabetes are at risk of a hypoglycaemic event because the medications used to manage diabetes reduce blood glucose and because the normal physiological responses that counter low blood glucose levels may be impaired (Box 12.2).

When blood glucose levels start to fall towards the lower end of the normal range, 4 mmol/L, there is a hormonal response which causes insulin secretion to cease and glucagon secretion to increase. Glucagon raises blood glucose levels by increasing hepatic glucose production. If blood glucose is not restored and levels drop beow the normal range, a sympathetic autonomic response is also triggered, which includes the release of adrenaline from the adrenal glands. Adrenaline produces many effects including suppression of insulin and stimulation of glucagon secretion and increased lipolysis in fatty tissue as shown in Figure 12.1. Other indications of a sympathetic response, such as raised heart rate and sweating, are often important signals to patients and healthcare professionals that they have become hypoglycaemic. If glucose levels drop still further, and particularly if the hypoglycaemia is prolonged, growth hormone and cortisol secretion is stimulated to further increase lipolysis in fatty tissue and promote ketogenesis and glucose production in the liver (Briscoe and Davis, 2006; Tesfaye and Seaquist, 2010).

Box 12.2   Medications most likely to cause iatrogenic hypoglycaemia.

These drugs elevate insulin levels independent of a patient's blood glucose level.

- Sulfonylureas
- Gliclazide
- Glibenclamide
- Glipizide
- Glimepiride
- Insulins

A person with diabetes is most likely to experience iatrogenic hypoglycaemia, that is, hypoglycaemia produced by the medications being used to control their hyperglycaemia. A hypoglycaemic episode can come about due to administration of more drug than is required under the circumstances that existed at the time. There are many reasons for a medication dose to exceed requirements on occasion, and only some medications are likely to produce this effect, as outlined in Box 12.2. While many medications will not cause iatrogenic hypoglycaemia when used alone, the risk of an episode of hypoglycaemia naturally increases when medications with glucose-lowering actions are used in combination.

Clinical consideration: Important medication interactions

- Alcohol decreases blood glucose levels and impairs the normal regulatory response, cognitive function and awareness of hypoglycaemia in the patient. The effect of alcohol on blood glucose levels may be present 6–12 hours after alcohol consumption, increasing the risk of severe hypoglycaemia.
- Many oral antihyperglycaemic medications do not cause hypoglycaemia when used alone, but may do so when used in combination with other diabetic medications.
- Beta-blockers, such as metoprolol and propranolol, may block important signs of acute hypoglycaemia (e.g. palpitations, tremor) as a result of blockade of the adrenergic receptors mediating these responses.

The risk of hypoglycaemia is highest where injected insulin is used to manage blood glucose levels and education surrounding its use is vital to avoid hypoglycaemia. People with T1DM may use injected insulin only, and those with T2DM may use insulin in conjunction with other injected or oral antihyperglycaemic medications. Where insulin is used, a person must know the amount of carbohydrate required for their specific insulin dose (carbohydrate counting), and time their meals depending on the type of insulin used (short-acting/regular/long-acting). Regular monitoring of blood glucose levels will enable a person to assess their insulin requirements based on their diet, exercise and lifestyle and will also allow early identification and self-treatment of hypoglycaemia at the first sign or symptom. The maintenance of euglycemia in a person with diabetes relies on education in all aspects of diabetes care, including hypoglycaemia risk factors, outlined in Box 12.3 (Briscoe & Davis, 2006).

The signs and symptoms of hypoglycaemia may be classified into two groups: neurogenic (autonomic nervous system activation) and neuroglycopenic (brain glucose insufficiency), outlined in Table 12.2. The neurogenic signs and symptoms, such as palpitations, trembling, dry mouth, sweating and nervousness, will often alert a person that blood glucose is low and are the consequence of an autonomic nervous system response.

Box 12.3   Hypoglycaemia risk factors

- Medication interactions, including alcohol
- Accidental or intentional overdose of antihyperglycaemic medication, especially insulin
- Unplanned reduction of food intake
- Missed or delayed meal
- Intensive exercise without increase in food intake
- Irregular or absent blood glucose monitoring
- Inability to identify or self-treat hypoglycaemia

Source: Modified from Briscoe and Davis (2006).

Table 12.2   Signs and symptoms of hypoglycaemia.

Brain glucose deficiency	Autonomic activation
Confusion	Hunger
Tiredness	Shakiness
Disorientation	Nervousness
Seizures	Tachycardia
Hypothermia	Hypertension
Coma	Diaphoresis/sweating

Neuroglycopenic symptoms come about as a result of inadequate glucose to the brain and include irritability, tiredness, difficulty thinking and confusion. Family members may recognise these signs of developing hypoglycaemia in the patient. When blood glucose levels are not corrected, the condition will progress to cerebral agitation, seizures, coma and death.

Treatment of hypoglycaemia requires the administration of glucose either directly or indirectly. The clinical context of a hypoglycaemia episode will determine the route of administration of glucose.

Mild to moderate hypoglycaemia may be effectively self-treated by the consumption of approximately 15 g of oral glucose. Oral glucose may be available in many forms including gels, tablets and jellybeans. Other foods that may be consumed are:

- ½ a can (150 mL) of regular soft drink (not diet) OR
- ½ a glass (125 mL) of fruit juice OR
- 3 teaspoons of sugar or honey.

It may take up to 15 minutes for blood glucose levels to rise to 4 mmol/L or above. If they are still below this after 15 minutes, then administration of another 15 g of glucose is recommended. The response to glucose is transient and if the next meal is not for more than 20 minutes, a small amount of carbohydrate should also be consumed, to maintain blood glucose. This could be:

- a slice of bread OR
- 1 glass of milk OR
- 1 piece of fruit OR
- 1 small tub of yoghurt.

Oral administration of glucose is not possible in cases of severe hypoglycaemia resulting in reduced consciousness, so these patients require an injectable form of glucagon or glucose (NDSS, 2021).

Management of severe hypoglycaemia

Glucagon

Glucagon is a hormone produced by the alpha cells of the islets of Langerhans of the pancreas. It stimulates the breakdown of liver glycogen to release glucose into the bloodstream. It can be given via intramuscular (IM), subcutaneous (SC) or intravenous (IV) routes. Glucagon is available in a kit that may be administered by a family member/carer or by ambulance personnel.

When the patient has recovered sufficiently to take oral foods, an immediate source of glucose and complex carbohydrates will be required. Be aware that an adverse effect of glucagon is nausea and vomiting which may make it difficult to ensure the patient consumes enough carbohydrate to prevent relapse.

Response to glucagon may be slow; most people will start to respond after 6 minutes. Where there are insufficient stores of liver glucose, e.g. in chronic malnourishment, glucagon may not be sufficient and intravenous glucose may also be required.

214

Skills in practice: preparation and administration of glucagon

- Only administer glucagon if the person has an altered level of consciousness and is unable to take glucose orally.
- Check expiry date.
- Do not mix the glucagon until you are ready to use it.
- Using universal precautions and aseptic technique, open the kit and mix the contents of the syringe (sterile water) with glucagon powder in the vial and shake gently to dissolve the powder. *Do not use if a gel has formed or if you see particles in the solution.* Using the same syringe, withdraw all the mixed solution and dispense any air bubbles back into the vial.
- Withdraw syringe from the vial and deliver 1 mL (1 mg) of glucagon subcutaneously or intramuscularly into one of the main injection sites (upper arms, thighs or buttocks).
- Ensure the used syringe is disposed of in a sharps container.

(MIMS Australia, 2020b).

Intravenous glucose

Administration of IV glucose requires a securely positioned cannula, ideally into a larger vein, as injection into the veins of the hand may cause superficial thrombophlebitis. Several different concentrations of glucose are available.

- Glucose 10% 150 mL or 20% 75 mL (15 g) by intravenous infusion over 15 minutes is the preferred intravenous treatment.
- Glucose 50% may also be administered by slow intravenous injection, but extreme caution must be used as extravasation can cause serious necrosis.

Response to IV glucose is rapid, but if blood glucose remains below 4 mmol/L 15 minutes after the first administration, a second dose may be administered. When the person has recovered sufficiently to take oral foods, a complex carbohydrate will be required (Diabetes, 2016).

Where a person uses a long-acting insulin, the action may last up to 24 hours (see Table 12.2). Due to the prolonged action of insulin and higher risk of relapse, it would be advisable to transport these people to hospital for close monitoring.

When a person experiences hypoglycaemia (especially severe hypoglycaemia) or has a history of hypoglycaemia, it is important to record details of the timing of the episode, medication dose and events leading up to the episode so adjustments to the treatment regimen can be made to prevent a recurrence. When this is not done, the risk of recurrent severe hypoglycaemia can be high.

Clinical consideration: hypoglycaemia unawareness

The blood glucose threshold at which a person will recognise hypoglycaemia is not static and may change depending on circumstances, a phenomenon known as 'relative hypoglycaemia'.

Hypoglycaemia usually produces recognisable signs and symptoms when blood glucose levels decrease below 4 mmol/L. However, people with persistently high blood glucose levels may experience hypoglycaemic signs and symptoms at higher blood glucose levels.

Of greater concern, though, is when people who have had a recent hypoglycaemic event may not experience symptoms until their blood glucose levels are significantly lower than 4 mmol/L. Often the characteristic autonomic symptoms that indicate low blood glucose are absent and the first sign of hypoglycaemia is confusion or loss of consciousness. This is termed 'hypoglycaemia unawareness' and can place people at risk of experiencing severe, life-threatening hypoglycaemia.

People over 60 years of age may have altered counter-regulatory responses as a result of ageing, long-standing diabetes, multiple comorbidities and medications. Because of this, older people may experience hypoglycaemia unawareness. Further, the initial signs and symptoms of brain glucose deficiency may be misinterpreted as indications of cerebral vascular events, dementia or urinary tract infection. Thus, hypoglycaemia unawareness, especially in older adults, may delay treatment and increase the risk of severe life-threatening hypoglycaemia (Martín-Timón and Javier del Cañizo-Gómez, 2015; Tesfaye and Seaquist, 2010).

Episode of care: hypoglycaemia

Peter, a 65-year old male, has a 20-year history of type 2 diabetes and until recently his blood glucose levels had been controlled by the oral diabetes medications metformin and empagliflozin. About 3 months ago, Peter commenced insulin therapy and his initial dose was 10 units of insulin glargine at night.

About 1 month ago, Peter began experiencing chest pain and was diagnosed with unstable angina which worried him as he hadn't experienced any problems with his heart before. His cardiologist commenced Peter on metoprolol 50 mg twice daily to reduce his angina symptoms. Peter's cardiologist also explained to Peter the link between diabetes and the risk of a heart attack. Concerned about this, Peter visited his general practitioner who agreed his long-term control of diabetes was not adequate. As a result, his doctor increased his dose of insulin glargine to 15 units at night.

Peter is now taking the following medications.

- Metformin XR 2 g at night
- Empagliflozin 10 mg at night
- Aspirin 100 mg in the morning
- Metoprolol 50 mg morning and night
- Telmisartan 40 mg in the morning
- Atorvastatin 40 mg in the morning
- Insulin glargine 15 units night

Motivated by his recent diagnosis, Peter determined to start exercising and lose a bit of weight. He began walking after work and stopped eating snacks before his evening meal. After about a week of his new lifestyle regimen, he had lost about 1 kg of weight which made him feel great.

At about 4 am one morning about a week later, Peter's wife Janet woke to the sounds of loud snoring. When she tried to wake Peter, he pushed her away and started speaking incoherently. Janet called the ambulance, and on arrival and paramedics measured his blood glucose level (BGL) as 2 mmol/L. They administered 1 mL (1 mg) of glucagon and Peter slowly responded until after 20 minutes his BGL had increased to 4 mmol/L. Peter then ate a jam sandwich and promptly booked an appointment with his doctor.

At the appointment, Peter described the events and admitted that he wasn't monitoring his BGL regularly and couldn't provide his nightly and morning BGL readings. He explained that he had been feeling tired and light-headed when he went to bed that night, but thought his new heart medication was responsible. The doctor reduced his insulin dose back to 10 units at night and his metformin and empagliflozin were moved to a morning dose. Peter was also referred to a diabetes educator for information about blood glucose monitoring, hypoglycaemia symptoms and self-treatment.

Hyperglycaemic emergency
Diabetic ketoacidosis

Diabetic ketoacidosis (DKA) is a medical emergency that is characterised by elevated blood glucose and ketones accompanied by metabolic acidosis. DKA can occur in both type 1 and type 2 diabetes (where insulin is used). The consequences of untreated DKA are renal failure, cerebral oedema, coma and death.

Diabetic ketoacidosis occurs due to an absolute or relative insulin deficiency. Because of this deficiency, glucose does not enter cells for use as a fuel and the body, effectively in a state of starvation, is forced to switch to alternative fuel sources. This lack of glucose supply to the cells initiates a counter-regulatory response and glucagon, adrenaline, noradrenaline, cortisol and growth hormone are secreted. These hormones increase glucose production and lipolysis. The resulting hyperglycaemia produces an osmotic diuresis as the kidney is unable to reabsorb the excess filtered glucose, and the additional water loss results in dehydration and loss of electrolytes such as sodium, potassium and chloride. Free fatty acids are utilised during lipolysis as alternative fuel sources, but the keto acids produced as by-products of this process accumulate rapidly, causing metabolic acidosis (Nyenwe and Kitabchi, 2016). Important differential diagnoses for DKA include hyperosmolar hyperglycaemia state (HHS) and euglycaemic ketoacidosis.

Clinical consideration: Hyperosmolar hyperglycaemia

Hyperosmolar hyperglycaemia state (HHS) is a potentially life-threatening situation that occurs in people with T2DM due to severe hyperglycaemia. It is rarer than DKA but has a higher mortality rate, partly because type 2 diabetes sufferers tend to be older, with more comorbidities, and partly because HHS produces venous blood clots.

Hyperosmolar hyperglycaemia state typically occurs in the presence of severe hyperglycaemia (>30 mmol/L), which causes increased urinary output leading to severe dehydration, hypovolaemia and plasma hyperosmolality (highly concentrated plasma) with high plasma sodium levels. The high sodium levels cause an altered level of consciousness and, in severe cases, coma. The key difference between HHS and DKA is that the former has little or no ketosis or metabolic acidosis. The absence of ketosis is explained by the fact that people with T2DM can still produce insulin which, while not enough to prevent hyperglycaemia, does suppress lipid metabolism and the production of ketones. Hyperglycaemia and dehydration will produce signs and symptoms similar to DKA without those associated with metabolic acidosis, such as abdominal pain, vomiting, fruity-smelling breath and Kussmaul respirations.

The causes and risk factors for developing HHS are the same as those that cause DKA: other medications, infection and other physiological stressors (Table 12.3). Non-adherence to diabetes therapy, including oral medicines, may precipitate HHS.

Treatment of HHS is also similar to DKA with the main aims of therapy being to correct dehydration and plasma osmolarity, electrolyte abnormalities and reduce BGL using insulin (Kitabchi et al., 2009).

Table 12.3   Factors precipitating DKA.

Factor	Causes
Insulin deficiency	Insulin pump failure Non-adherence to insulin therapy Unrecognised symptoms of new-onset diabetes
Medications and illicit drugs	Antipsychotics, e.g. olanzapine and quetiapine Corticosteroids, e.g. dexamethasone and prednisolone Sympathomimetic agents, e.g. pseudoephedrine and cocaine Alcohol abuse
Infection	Pneumonia, urinary tract infection,
Other physiological stressors	Pregnancy, myocardial infarction, trauma, surgery

The primary determinant of DKA is the absolute or relative lack of insulin, with undiagnosed diabetes, unawareness of symptoms in newly diagnosed diabetes or non-adherence to insulin therapy being the most common factors. Other factors include illicit drugs, alcohol abuse, infection and other physiological stressors (see Table 12.3).

Signs and symptoms

When body cells are deprived of glucose, polyphagia (increased appetite) occurs, often in the presence of weight loss. The BGL threshold for hyperglycaemia is generally accepted to be 14 mmol/L. Elevated serum ketones or the presence of ketones in the urine also may indicate DKA.

Hyperglycaemia causes polyuria (increased urination), resulting in polydipsia (increased thirst). Dehydration and hypovolaemia also cause tachycardia, hypotension, dry mouth and poor skin turgor.

Acidosis may cause Kussmaul breathing, which is a pattern of deep and forced breathing, an attempt to compensate by increasing the excretion of carbon dioxide via the lungs. The exhaled breath may smell fruity as it contains elevated levels of acetone, a type of ketone. Acidosis may also cause abdominal pain and vomiting. A reduced level of consciousness is a sign of severe DKA and is caused by both dehydration and acidosis. The signs and symptoms of DKA are outlined in Table 12.4 (Nyenwe and Kitabchi, 2016).

Table 12.4   Signs and symptoms of DKA.

Hyperglycaemia and dehydration
- Polyphagia
- Weight loss
- Polyuria
- Polydipsia
- Tachycardia
- Hypotension
- Dry mouth
- Poor skin turgor
- Altered level of consciousness

Metabolic acidosis
- Kussmaul breathing
- Abdominal pain
- Fruity breath
- Nausea and vomiting
- Altered level of consciousness

Source: Based on Nyenwe and Kitabchi (2016).

Clinical consideration: euglycaemic ketoacidosis

Euglycaemic ketoacidosis is a medical emergency in which elevated ketones and metabolic acidosis exist in the presence of either normal glucose levels or mild hyperglycaemia. This can occur in people with type 1 or type 2 diabetes. It is important to be aware of this condition as it may not present with the typical polyuria, polydipsia and marked dehydration. However, euglycaemic ketoacidosis may be life threatening because of metabolic acidosis, and medical evaluation and treatment are necessary.

Euglycaemic ketoacidosis occurs when the factors that trigger DKA are present and the person still continues with insulin treatment and/or glucose production is lowered and/or the excretion of glucose is higher. Lower glucose production occurs in the presence of glycogen depletion and higher glucose elimination may occur in the presence of SGLT-2 inhibitors.

218

Factors contributing to lower glucose production (glycogen depletion)	Factors contributing to higher excretion of glucose
Pregnancy (often third trimester)	Sodium-glucose cotransporter 2 inhibitors, e.g. empagliflozin and dapagliflozin
Fasting states, e.g. nausea and vomiting, post bariatric surgery	
Liver dysfunction	
(Barski et al., 2019)	

Management of hyperglycaemia

Treatment of hyperglycaemic emergencies involves the correction of dehydration, electrolyte abnormalities and hyperglycaemia. All persons suspected to be experiencing DKA, HHS or euglycaemic ketoacidosis should be transported to hospital. Careful treatment with close monitoring is necessary to avert a life-threatening crisis and specialist advice may be required.

Fluid replacement

Intravenous fluids should be started. Initially most people will receive 0.9% normal saline at 15–20 mL/kg/h, or 1–1.5 L in the first hour. The initial rehydration will improve blood volume and tissue perfusion. Administration of fluids 1 hour prior to administration of insulin is beneficial, as it prevents deterioration due to hypotension, improves insulin action and allows serum potassium to be measured prior to insulin administration. Maintenance treatment for hydration will depend on the level of hydration, electrolyte levels and urinary output. Half of the estimated fluid deficit should be replaced over 12–24 hours. When blood glucose levels fall to 11 mmol/L, saline solution should be replaced with 5% dextrose. Potassium, bicarbonate and phosphate levels should be monitored throughout treatment and replacement should be initiated where required.

Electrolyte replacement

Initial hydration can reduce BGL and potassium levels by a dilution effect. When adequate blood volume is achieved, further excretion of potassium occurs due to enhanced renal perfusion. When insulin therapy is initiated, the correction of acidosis causes potassium to move back into cells. It is therefore essential that electrolytes, particularly potassium, are monitored during treatment and replacement initiated where indicated.

Insulin therapy

Regular intravenous insulin infusion is recommended to reduce blood glucose levels. Administration usually starts 1–2 hours after fluids have been initiated and infusion rate should be titrated to response. When BGLs reach approximately 11 mmol/L, 5% dextrose is added to the intravenous fluids so a BGL of 8.3–11 mmol/L can be maintained (Diabetes, 2016).

Episode of care: Hyperglycaemia

Mrs Lavinia Howard has been a type 1 diabetic for approximately 6 months. Her diabetes was precipitated by a pancreatic cancer diagnosis and she has been managing it with a subcutaneous insulin pump.

Over the past week, Lavinia has been complaining of abdominal pain and constipation which has affected her appetite and caused her carbohydrate consumption to reduce significantly. Lavinia has been very diligent about monitoring her blood glucose levels and has returned BGLs of 3.5 mmol/L and 3.8 mmol/L. Due to the episodes of hypoglycaemia, Lavinia decided to turn off the insulin pump as, living alone, she was very worried about experiencing a serious hypoglycaemic episode. Lavinia visited her general practitioner complaining of constipation Her doctor prescribed laxatives and enemas for her constipation and measured her BGL, which returned a normal result.

Lavinia's constipation resolved and her appetite improved, as did her carbohydrate consumption. Lavinia, however, forgot to re-establish her insulin pump. The following day, she began to feel very nauseous and experienced two episodes of vomiting. She also noticed that she was urinating a lot but thought it was due to her increased appetite and fluid consumption. When Lavinia measured her BGL, she was alarmed to see the reading was 24 mmol/L and she called the ambulance for advice.

The paramedics measured her BGL and confirmed a reading of 22 mmol/L. Her blood pressure was 95/50 mmHg, heart rate 120 beats/min and her blood plasma was positive for ketones. The possibility of DKA was discussed and she was advised to go to hospital for treatment rather than simply re-establishing her insulin pump.

Conclusion

For prehospital care providers, abnormal blood glucose level is a common cause of patients presenting with altered mental status, with or without diabetes. One of the unintended complications of some medicines used for diabetes is iatrogenic hypoglycaemia, which must be managed promptly. This may occur after usual therapeutic doses, or may be related to inadvertent administration of the wrong dose or type of insulin. Conversely, use of medicines may also be implicated in poorly controlled or high blood sugar levels, for example when there are missed doses, or concurrent illness which causes blood glucose levels to fluctuate more widely. This chapter has described the medicines that could contribute to diabetic emergencies and medicines used to manage complications that could present to paramedics when attending to a patient with diabetes.

Find out more about these conditions.

Type 1 diabetes

Type 2 diabetes

Metabolic syndrome

Diabetes insipidus

Gestational diabetes mellitus (GDM)

Glossary

Analogue insulin	Insulin proteins created in a laboratory using recombinant DNA technology.
Adenosine triphosphate (ATP)	Source of energy used by cells.
Blood glucose level (BGL)	The concentration of glucose in the blood, measured in millimoles per litre (mmol/L).
Carbohydrate	A group of compounds (including starches and sugars) that are a major food source.
Catecholamines	A collective term for adrenaline, noradrenaline and dopamine.

Diabetes mellitus	An endocrine disorder affecting the regulation of blood glucose levels.
Dipeptidyl peptidase-4 (DPP-4)	A glycoprotein that breaks down a variety of substrates, including incretin hormones.
Enzyme	Protein that speeds up (catalyses) chemical reactions in the body.
Euglycaemia	Normal level of glucose in the blood.
Exogenous	Originating from outside the body.
Fatty acids	Dietary fats that have broken down into elements that can be absorbed into the blood.
Gastrointestinal (GI) tract	Organs of the digestive system that make up the continuous passage from mouth to anus.
Glucose-like peptide 1 (GLP-1)	An incretin hormone produced in the gut in response to food.
Gestational diabetes mellitus (GDM)	Diabetes mellitus first recognised during pregnancy.
Gluconeogenesis	Creation of glucose from non-carbohydrate substrates.
Glycogen	A carbohydrate (complex sugar) made from glucose.
Glycogenesis	Conversion of glucose to glycogen.
Glycogenolysis	Breakdown of glycogen in liver and muscle to glucose.
Hypoglycaemia	Lower than normal blood levels of glucose.
Hyperglycaemia	Higher than normal blood levels of glucose.
Iatrogenic	Caused by medical treatment.
Insulin resistance	When tissues (e.g. fat, liver, muscle) do not respond well to insulin and therefore do not effectively take up glucose from the blood.
Interstitial fluid	Body fluid found in the tissue spaces that surrounds the cells.
Ketones	Organic compounds that are by-products of fat metabolism, a process known as ketogenesis.
Lipolysis	Breakdown of stored lipids to release fatty acids into the bloodstream.
Parenteral	Medicines administered by a route that does not involve the gastrointestinal tract.
Plasma proteins	Protein molecules present in blood plasma which serve a variety of functions.
Postprandial	After a meal.
Steady-state drug concentration	Concentration at which the amount of drug being absorbed is the same as the amount cleared from the body when given continuously.
Thrombophlebitis	Inflammatory condition of a vein due to a blood clot.
Triglyceride	A form of fatty acid having three fatty acid components.

References

American Diabetes Association. (2003). Insulin administration. *Diabetes Care* **26**(Suppl. 1): s121–s124.

American Diabetes Association. (2019). Pharmacologic approaches to glycemic treatment: standards of medical care in diabetes – 2019. *Diabetes Care* **42**(Suppl. 1): s90–s102.

Australian Medicines Handbook (AMH). (2020a). *Insulins.* https://amhonline-amh-net-au.ezproxy.newcastle.edu.au/chapters/endocrine-drugs/drugs-diabetes/other-drugs-diabetes/insulins

Australian Medicines Handbook (AMH). (2020b). *Metformin.* https://amhonline-amh-net-au.ezproxy.newcastle.edu.au/chapters/endocrine-drugs/drugs-diabetes/other-drugs-diabetes/metformin

Australian Medicines Handbook (AMH). (2020c). *Sulfonylureas.* https://amhonline-amh-net-au.ezproxy.newcastle.edu.au/chapters/endocrine-drugs/drugs-diabetes/sulfonylureas?menu=vertical

Australian Medicines Handbook (AMH). (2020d). *Dipeptidyl peptidase-4 inhibitors.* https://amhonline-amh-net-au.ezproxy.newcastle.edu.au/chapters/endocrine-drugs/drugs-diabetes/dipeptidyl-peptidase-4-inhibitors?menu=vertical

Australian Medicines Handbook (AMH). (2020e). *Glucagon-like peptide-1 analogues.* https://amhonline-amh-net-au.ezproxy.newcastle.edu.au/chapters/endocrine-drugs/drugs-diabetes/glucagon-like-peptide-1-analogues?menu=vertical

Australian Medicines Handbook (AMH). (2020f). *Sodium-glucose co-transporter 2 inhibitors*. https://amhonline-amh-net-au.ezproxy.newcastle.edu.au/chapters/endocrine-drugs/drugs-diabetes/glucagon-like-peptide-1-analogues?menu=vertical

Australian Medicines Handbook (AMH). (2020g). *Pioglitazone*. https://amhonline-amh-net-au.ezproxy.newcastle.edu.au/chapters/endocrine-drugs/drugs-diabetes/other-drugs-diabetes/pioglitazone?menu=vertical

Australian Medicines Handbook (AMH). (2020h). *Acarbose*. https://amhonline-amh-net-au.ezproxy.newcastle.edu.au/chapters/endocrine-drugs/drugs-diabetes/other-drugs-diabetes/acarbose?menu=vertical

Barski, L., Eshkoli, T., Brandstatter, E. and Jotkowitz, A. (2019). Euglycemic diabetic ketoacidosis. *European Journal of Internal Medicine* **63**: 9–14.

Briscoe, V.J. and Davis, S.N. (2006). Hypoglycemia in type 1 and type 2 diabetes: physiology, pathophysiology and management. *Clinical Diabetes* **24**(3): 115–121.

Chesterman, T. and Thynne, T. (2020). Harms and benefits of sodium-glucose co-transporter 2 inhibitors. *Australian Prescriber* **43**: 168–171.

Diabetes (2016) Melbourne: Therapeutic Guidelines Limited. www-tg-org-au.ezproxy.newcastle.edu.au

Diabetes Australia. (2021). *Blood Glucose Monitoring*. www.diabetesaustralia.com.au/living-with-diabetes/managing-your-diabetes/blood-glucose-monitoring/

Hinnen, D. (2017). Glucagon-like peptide 1 receptor agonists for type 2 diabetes. *Diabetes Spectrum* **30**(3): 202–210.

Kitabchi, A.E., Umpierrez, G.E., Miles, J.M. and Fisher, J.N. (2009). Hyperglycemic crises in adult patients with diabetes. *Diabetes Care* **32**(7): 1335–1343.

Martín-Timón, I. and Javier del Cañizo-Gómez, F. (2015). Mechanisms of hypoglycemia unawareness and implications in diabetic patients. *World Journal of Diabetes* **6**(7): 912–926.

MIMS Australia. (2020a). *Glucagon*. www.mimsonline.com.au

MIMS Australia. (2020b). *Insulin*. www.mimsonline.com.au

MIMS Australia. (2020c). *Glibenclamide*. www.mimsonline.com.au

Misbin, R.I. (2004). The phantom of lactic acidosis due to metformin in patients with diabetes. *Diabetes Care* **27**(7): 1791–1793.

National Diabetes Services Scheme (NDSS). (2021). *Hypoglycaemia*. www.ndss.com.au/living-with-diabetes/managing-diabetes/hypoglycaemia/

Nauck, M.A., Homberger, E., Siegel, E. et al. (1986). Incretin effects of increasing glucose loads in man calculated from venous insulin and C-peptide responses. *Journal of Clinical Endocrinology and Metabolism* 63(2):492–498.

Nyenwe, E.A. and Kitabchi, A.E. (2016). The evolution of diabetic ketoacidosis: an update of its etiology, pathogenesis and management. *Metabolism* **65**(4): 507–521.

Petersons, C. (2018). Second steps in managing type 2 diabetes. *Australian Prescriber* **41**(5): 141–144.

Rasalam, R., Barlow, J., Kennedy, M., Phillips, P. and Wright, A. (2019). GLP-1 receptor agonists for type 2 diabetes and their role in primary care: an Australian perspective. *Diabetes Therapy* **10**: 1205–1217.

Sherwin, D.L. and Svancarek, B. (2021). *EMS Diabetic Protocols for Treat and Release*. Treasure Island: StatPearls Publishing.

Tesfaye, N. and Seaquist, E. (2010). Neuroendocrine responses to hypoglycemia. *Annals of the New York Academy of Sciences* **1212**: 12–28.

Multiple-choice questions

1. Which of the following adverse reactions is *not* a concern when taking metformin alone?
   (a) Hypoglycaemia
   (b) Metabolic acidosis
   (c) Vitamin B12 malabsorption
   (d) Gastrointestinal adverse effects including metallic taste in the mouth

2. Which of the following statements is *incorrect* with regard to insulin administration?
   (a) Administered via injection into subcutaneous tissue
   (b) Usual site of administration is the abdomen
   (c) Physical activity may increase the rate of insulin absorption from the site of administration
   (d) Insulin injected into muscle, rather than subcutaneous tissue, will absorb significantly slower

3. SGLT-2 inhibitors may be associated with which of the following adverse effects?
   (a) Ketoacidosis, even when BGLs appear within the normal range
   (b) Lactic acidosis, especially in patients with kidney damage
   (c) Hyperglycaemia
   (d) Weight gain

4. Which of the following statements is *incorrect* in relation to a paramedic attending to a patient with suspected hypoglycaemia?
   (a) DPP-4 inhibitors rarely cause hypoglycaemia except in combination with other antihyperglycaemic agents that cause hypoglycaemia
   (b) Sugars such as sucrose (e.g. fruit juice, milk) may be used to treat hypoglycaemia in patients using acarbose
   (c) Insulin glargine may contribute to hypoglycaemic emergencies for several hours after it has been administered
   (d) Sulfonylureas such as gliclazide commonly contribute to hypoglycaemia and weight gain

5. Which of the following would *not* be likely to interfere with the accuracy of blood glucose measurements?
   (a) Temperature and humidity
   (b) Residual substance on hands prior to testing
   (c) Use of metformin on the same day as testing
   (d) Incorrect use of test strips

6. Identify from the following medications which would *most* likely contribute to hypoglycaemia.
   (a) Oral metformin
   (b) Oral gliclazide
   (c) Oral sitagliptin
   (d) Subcutaneous exenatide

7. Identify which sign or symptoms of hypoglycaemia would most probbly be masked by the administration of beta-blockers.
   (a) Confusion
   (b) Tiredness
   (c) Tachycardia
   (d) Hunger

8. Which one of the following is not classified as a neuroglycopenic sign/symptom?
   (a) Sweating
   (b) Disorientation
   (c) Fatigue
   (d) Seizure

9. As a paramedic in the prehospital environment, identify which of the following scenarios is *most* correct.
   (a) BGL of 2.3 mmol/L, unconscious and unrousable treated with a slow infusion of intravenous glucose 10% 150 mL
   (b) BGL of 3.2 mmol/L, confused but able to swallow treated with 1 mL (1 mg) subcutaneous injection of glucagon
   (c) BGL of 3 mmol/L, irritable and confused, refusing to eat, treated with glucose gel inserted onto mucosa for absorption
   (d) BGL of 2.8 mmol/L, unconscious, history of fasting treated with 1 mL (1 mg) subcutaneous injection of glucagon

10. Which of the following are not contributing factors to hyperglycaemia and diabetic ketoacidosis (DKA)?
    (a) Pneumonia, prednisolone therapy, pseudoephedrine therapy
    (b) Metoprolol therapy, heart disease, non-adherence to metformin
    (c) Surgery, insulin pump failure, quetiapine therapy
    (d) Pregnancy, non-awareness of diabetes symptoms, refusal to use insulin
11. Which of the following are symptoms of hyperglycaemia and metabolic acidosis?
    (a) Dry skin, cool extremities, abdominal pain, vomiting and lethargy
    (b) Headache, breathing difficulties, chest wheezes and high body temperature
    (c) Sweating, tachycardia, hunger, confusion and tremors
    (d) Slurred speech, facial droop, incontinence and altered level of consciousness

Chapter 13

Medications used in the respiratory system

Jason McKenna

Aim

The aim of this chapter is to familiarise the reader with key pathophysiological processes in respiratory emergencies and the pharmacological management often utilised in prehospital care.

Learning outcomes

After reading this chapter the reader will:

1. Have gained an understanding of the key pathophysiological and clinical characteristics of common respiratory emergencies
2. Be able to describe the principal characteristics and mechanisms of action of the key pharmacological agents used in each of these problems
3. Be able to effectively manage various respiratory emergencies utilising the pharmacological agents described in this chapter
4. Be able to describe the various side-effects associated with the medication classes and how to safely consider these when applying pharmacology management to any respiratory conditions.

Test your knowledge

1. Describe the main components of the respiratory system and their functions.
2. Describe how the autonomic nervous system innervates the respiratory system and its two opposing branches of control.
3. List the similarities and differences between asthma and COPD.
4. List the medication classes utilised to manage respiratory emergencies.
5. Describe the mechanism of action of the pharmacological agents used to manage respiratory emergencies.

Fundamentals of Pharmacology for Paramedics, First Edition. Edited by Ian Peate, Suzanne Evans, and Lisa Clegg.
© 2022 John Wiley & Sons Ltd. Published 2022 by John Wiley & Sons Ltd.

Introduction

Respiratory disease is the third most common cause of death (after cardiovascular disease and cancer) and affects around one in five people. Hospital admissions for lung disease are three times higher than other admissions, with chronic obstructive pulmonary disease (COPD), pneumonia and lung cancer the leading causes of death. The incidence and mortality due to respiratory diseases are higher within socially deprived areas and among disadvantaged groups where there are higher rates of occupational hazards, smoking, increased air pollution and poor housing conditions (NHS England, 2020).

Dyspnoea can be the initial life-threatening symptom of respiratory failure and its importance is highlighted by the Airway, Breathing, Circulation (ABC) approach in emergency medicine (Lindskou et al., 2019). Patients in respiratory distress are at increased risk of morbidity and mortality, often seek emergency care from prehospital services, and are subsequently transported to emergency departments via ambulance. Prehospital personnel play a prominent role in the triage, treatment and transport of patients with respiratory distress, and evidence shows that prehospital interventions decrease mortality among these patients (Prekker et al., 2014).

Anatomy and physiology

The respiratory system's primary roles are to deliver oxygen (O_2), essential for glycolysis (energy production), and removal of carbon dioxide (CO_2), the waste product of respiration (Figure 13.1). There are two processes involved in this: (1) air is moved into and out of the lungs through a process called

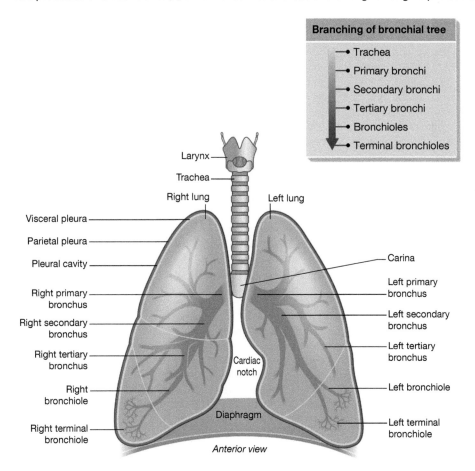

Figure 13.1   The respiratory system. Source: Nair, M. and Peate, I. (2015). *Pathophysiology for Nurses at a Glance*. Chichester: John Wiley & Sons, Ltd.

mechanical ventilation, and (2) gas exchange across the alveolar–capillary membrane in a process called diffusion. The respiratory system has an important role in protection against pathogens, acid–base balance and phonation.

The respiratory system can be divided into the upper respiratory tract and the lower respiratory tract. The upper respiratory tract encompasses the nose, nasal cavity, mouth, pharynx, epiglottis and larynx. Inhaled air is warmed and moistened as it swirls within the nasal cavity due to scroll-shaped bones known as the nasal conchae. Mucous membranes lining the respiratory tract clean the inhaled air by trapping foreign particles and pollutants. During swallowing, the epiglottis closes like a trap door, routing food down the oesophagus away from the trachea. Failure of this process will lead to aspiration of food contents into the lungs.

Below the glottis are the structures of the lower airway and lungs. These include the trachea, bronchial tree (primary bronchi, secondary bronchi and bronchioles), alveoli and lungs. The right lung has three lobes and the left lung has two lobes and the heart lies within the cardiac notch adjacent to the left lung. The conducting airways include the trachea which bifurcates at the carina into the two main bronchi which divide into smaller secondary bronchi, ultimately leading to the terminal bronchioles. The bronchi are made up of complete rings of cartilage combined with smooth muscle and lined with pseudostratified ciliated epithelium. Further down the bronchial tree, lesscartilage exists and additional smooth muscle is found. Terminal bronchioles lead to respiratory bronchioles, which represent the transition zone between the conducting airways and the gas exchange part of the respiratory system. The respiratory bronchioles lead to alveolar ducts and finally to the alveolar sacs which are entirely composed of alveoli.

There are around 300 million alveoli in the two lungs; they are the functional components of the respiratory system and are the chief component of lung tissue. The wall of an alveolus comprises a single layer of epithelial cells and elastic fibres. These fibres allow the alveolus to stretch and contract during breathing. The exchange of oxygen and carbon dioxide in the lungs takes place in the alveoli in a process known as diffusion (Paramothayan, 2019).

Each alveolus is encircled by a fine network of capillaries which are arranged so that air in the alveolus is separated by a thin respiratory membrane from the blood in the alveolar capillaries. Oxygen crosses from the alveoli and enters the blood via diffusion because the PO_2 (partial pressure of oxygen) of alveolar air is greater than the PO_2 within the blood. This is known as a pressure gradient and oxygen molecules diffuse across the membrane to equalise the gradient. Simultaneously, carbon dioxide molecules leave the blood by diffusing across the membrane into the alveoli in the same manner due to the partial pressure of carbon dioxide (PCO_2) in venous blood being higher than the PCO_2 within the alveoli (Peate, 2015).

The diffusion of gases at the capillary-alveolar level can be affected in a number of ways. Some respiratory diseases destroy and collapse the alveolar walls, resulting in the formation of fewer but larger alveoli. The degenerative process reduces the total area available for diffusion. In some diseases the alveolar-capillary membrane becomes thick or less permeable which forces gas molecules to travel farther, reducing the rate of diffusion. An example of such a disease is pulmonary oedema. In this condition, fluid collects in the alveoli and pulmonary interstitial space. This forces gases to diffuse through a thicker than normal layer of fluid and tissue (Paramothayan, 2019).

Nervous system control

The autonomic nervous system can be subdivided into the sympathetic nervous system (SNS) and parasympathetic nervous systems (PNS). One division carries impulses which inhibit certain functions whereas the other division usually carries impulses which enhance a function. As a rule, the SNS prepares the body for 'action' and is commonly referred to as the 'flight or fight' response. In contrast, the PNS reduces muscular activity, conserves energy and produces selective localised responses such as increased gastrointestinal activity and is commonly referred to as the 'rest and digest' response. The two systems operate at the same time, but at any given time one is normally more dominant (Sanders et al., 2019).

Figure 13.2 shows the two branches of the autonomic nervous system and their systemic effects. Within the respiratory system, the postganglionic SNS nerves secrete the neurotransmitter norepinephrine which acts on beta-2 receptors within airway smooth muscle, causing relaxation and bronchodilation of the airways. In contrast, the PNS secretes the neurotransmitter

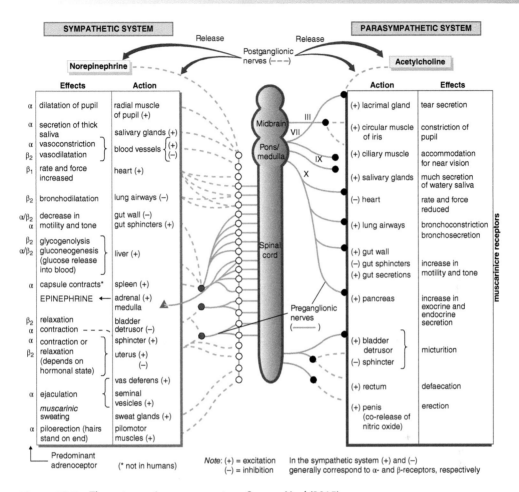

Figure 13.2   The autonomic nervous system. Source: Neal (2015).

acetylcholine which acts on muscarinic receptors in lung tissue, causing bronchoconstriction and increased bronchosecretions (Neal, 2015).

Reflection

Medications used to treat respiratory conditions will often take advantage of the body's natural physiology. Consider how some of the medications in this chapter inhibit or enhance autonomic nervous system control to elicit a response.

Common respiratory emergencies
Asthma

Asthma is a disease that affects the airways which carry air in and out of the lungs. In asthma, the airways become oversensitive and they react to things that would not typically cause an issue, such as dust particles or cold air. These are also known as triggers.

When the airways react to triggers, the smooth muscles of the airway walls constrict, making the airway narrow and leaving little room for air to flow in and out of the lungs. The lining of the airway passages then becomes swollen and a sticky mucus is produced which clogs up the breathing passages.

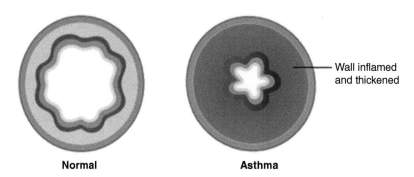

Normal   Asthma

Figure 13.3   Normal airway vs asthmatic airway. Source: Nair, M. and Peate, I. (2015). *Pathophysiology for Nurses at a Glance*. Chichester: John Wiley & Sons, Ltd.

With narrowing of the airways, it becomes hard for air to move in and out of the lungs and the chest muscles have to work much harder to breathe. Constriction of the muscles around the airways can occur rapidly (Figure 13.3) and this is the most common cause of asthma symptoms.

Asthma cannot be cured, but with appropriate treatment it can be well managed so there is no reason why individuals with asthma should be unable to live a full and active life, free from symptoms. Anybody can develop asthma but it often commences in childhood. In 2016 the World Health Organization (WHO) estimated that globally, over 339 million people had asthma, with over 400 000 deaths in the same year attributed to the disease (WHO, 2020). It is especially common in Ireland, where more than 380 000 adults and children have asthma, which equates to approximately 7.75% of the population (Asthma.ie, 2020).

In the initial acute phase, smooth muscle spasm is accompanied by excessive secretion of mucus that may clog the bronchi and bronchioles and exacerbate the attack. The late chronic phase is characterized by inflammation, oedema, fibrosis and necrosis of bronchial epithelial cells. A host of mediator chemicals, including histamine, prostaglandins, leukotrienes, platelet-activating factor and thromboxane, take part (Figure 13.4) (Tortora and Derrickson, 2014).

Status asthmaticus is a severe, protracted asthmatic attack which cannot be stopped with conventional management and is a life-threatening emergency. Just as an individual with COPD (see Table 13.2) usually does not call for an ambulance unless their condition has changed noticeably, a

A person with asthma does not ring for an ambulance unless the event is considerably worse than their typical attack. Assume status asthmaticus until proven otherwise.

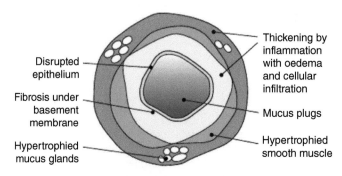

Figure 13.4   Inflammatory changes in the airway. Source: Rees, J., Kanabar, D. and Pattani, S. (2010). *ABC of Asthma*, 6th edn. Chichester: Wiley-Blackwell.

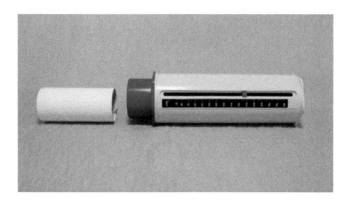

Figure 13.5   Peak flow meter. Source: Paramothayan (2019).

person with asthma does not ring for an emergency ambulance unless the event is considerably worse than their typical attack. It is practical to assume that an asthmatic who feels sick enough to call for an emergency ambulance is in status asthmaticus until proven otherwise (Pollak et al., 2018).

Signs and symptoms include anxiety, dyspnoea, wheezing, chest tightness, coughing, fatigue, tachycardia, diaphoresis and, in a severe life-threatening presentation, hypotension and a silent chest. Initial assessment should include a peak expiratory flow reading to help guide treatment (Figure 13.5). A mild/moderate acute asthma attack is managed by initiating oxygen therapy followed by administering an inhaled B2-agonist to help relax smooth muscle in the bronchioles and open the airways. This can be supplemented with a short-acting muscarinic antagonist, such as ipratropium bromide, if there is no improvement following initial therapy or if the patient has acute severe asthma (Table 13.1). One of the main contributors to severe asthma is inflammation, so early administration of intravenous hydrocortisone is indicated to reverse this process. For those who progress to life-threatening asthma, continue nebulised B2-agonist therapy in conjunction with intramuscular epinephrine (adrenaline) and/or a magnesium sulfate infusion (BTS/SIGN, 2019; JRCALC, 2019; PHECC, 2018).

Table 13.1   Signs and symptoms of acute asthma exacerbations.

Moderate acute asthma	Life-threatening asthma
• Increasing symptoms	In a patient with severe asthma any one of:
• PEF >50–75% best or predicted	• PEF <33% best or predicted
• No features of acute severe asthma	• SpO_2 <92%
	• Poor respiratory effort
Acute severe asthma	• Silent chest
	• Altered conscious level
Any one of:	• Exhaustion
	• Arrhythmia
• PEF 33–50% best or predicted	• Hypotension
• Respiratory rate ≥25/min	• Cyanosis
• Heart rate ≥110/min	
• Biphasic wheeze	
• Inability to complete sentences in one breath	
Near fatal asthma	
• Raised $PaCO_2$ and/or requiring mechanical ventilation with raised inflation pressures	

Source: BTS/SIGN (2019).
PEF, peak expiratory flow.

Skills in practice: obtaining a peak flow reading (DeVrieze et al., 2020)

Ensure patient is sitting or standing upright

1. Ensure peak flow marker is at the start point marked zero on the scale.
2. Attach the disposable mouthpiece to the peak flow meter.
3. Instruct the patient to take in a full, deep breath.
4. Place the mouthpiece between the patient's lips and hold level.
5. Instruct the patient to exhale in a single, fast, forceful expiration.
6. The marker should slide down the numbered scale.
7. Note the peak expiratory flow rate number obtained.
8. Obtain a total of three readings.
9. Record the best reading from the three attempts.

Chronic obstructive pulmonary disease

Chronic obstructive pulmonary disease includes at least two different clinical pathologies: chronic bronchitis and emphysema. Chronic bronchitis is defined as a sputum-producing cough for at least 3 months a year over a period of two consecutive years (Fayyaz, 2020).

The characteristic of the disease is excessive mucus production in the bronchial tree, which is almost constantly accompanied by a chronic or recurrent productive cough. A typical patient with chronic bronchitis is virtually always a heavy cigarette smoker, is typically overweight, and congested (Figure 13.6).

Blood gas levels have a tendency to be abnormal, with elevated $PaCO^2$ which is indicative of hypercapnia and decreased PaO_2 levels which indicates hypoxemia. Inhaled irritants cause chronic inflammation and growth in the size and number of goblet cells and mucous glands within the airway epithelium. The excessive, thick mucus that is produced narrows the airways and weakens ciliary function, causing inhaled pathogens to become embedded in airway secretions and reproduce quickly. In addition to a productive cough, signs and symptoms of chronic bronchitis are dyspnoea, wheezing, cyanosis and pulmonary hypertension.

Management of chronic bronchitis is similar to that for emphysema and frequently the patient will have related heart disease, including right-sided heart failure, known a Cor pulmonale.

Emphysema is a condition characterized by destruction of the walls of the alveoli, producing uncharacteristically large air sacs that remain full of air throughout exhalation. Emphysema damages or destroys the delicate structures of the terminal bronchioles. Clusters of alveoli combine into large blebs, or bullae, which are not as efficient as regular lung tissue due to having less surface area for gas exchange. This part of the tracheobronchial tree becomes so weak that its branches collapse during exhalation, trapping air in the alveoli. With less surface area for gas exchange, O_2 diffusion across the damaged respiratory membrane is impaired. Blood oxygen levels are slightly lowered and any minor exertion that increases the

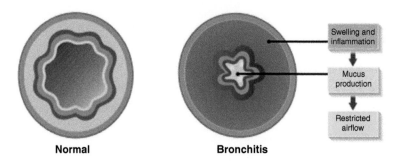

Figure 13.6 Inflammation and mucus production associated with bronchitis. Source: Nair, M. and Peate, I. (2015). *Pathophysiology for Nurses at a Glance*. Chichester: John Wiley & Sons, Ltd.

oxygen requirements of the cells leaves the patient dyspnoeic. As growing numbers of alveolar walls are damaged, lung elastic recoil declines due to the loss of elastic fibres, and an increasing amount of air becomes trapped in the lungs at the end ofe xhalation. Over several years, further effort during inhalation is required and it increases the size of the chest cage, resulting in a 'barrel chest'.

Emphysema is usually caused by a long-term irritation such as cigarette smoke, occupational exposure to dust and gases and air pollution. Some destruction of alveolar sacs may be caused by an enzyme imbalance. In most cases, COPD is avoidable because its greatest common cause is cigarette smoking or breathing second-hand smoke. Other causes include genetic factors and pulmonary infection (Pollak et al., 2018; Tortora and Derrickson, 2014).

Some COPD exacerbations are mild and self-limiting whereas others are severe, potentially life-threatening and require intervention. Prehospital management of a COPD exacerbation involves the use of oxygen therapy, nebulised bronchodilators (short-acting B2-agonists [SABA], short-acting muscarinic antagonists [SAMA] and intravenous corticosteroids) (JRCALC, 2019; PHECC, 2018). Caution should be exercised when administering oxygen therapy in patients with COPD as it may cause respiratory depression (NICE, 2018).

COPD patients are at risk of respiratory depression if overoxygenated. Maintain SpO$_2$ ≤92%.

Croup

Croup (laryngotracheobronchitis) is usually caused by a respiratory virus that is spread by person-to-person interaction, contact with contaminated nasopharyngeal secretions or by expelled large droplets. It mainly affects children between 6 months and 6 years old and it is the most frequent cause of upper airway distress in children. Croup affects the upper respiratory tract, leading to swelling and inflammation of the mucosal and submucosal tissues at the level of the cricoid ring, which is the narrowest part of the paediatric airway.

The diagnosis of croup is typically based on the physical examination and pertinent history. The child classically has a history of a runny nose, sore throat and a cough for a few days prior to the onset of croup symptoms which are frequently worse at night and when the child is agitated. These symptoms may be accompanied by a low-grade fever. Narrowing of the upper airway due to laryngeal swelling and inflammation leads to accompanying stridor, hoarseness and a 'seal-like' barking cough that may last up to10 days. The initial emergency management of croup is determined by the severity of the child's presenting symptoms.

- Mild croup is distinguished by an occasional cough, minimal respiratory distress and the absence of stridor when at rest.
- With moderate croup, the child's mental status and behaviour are normal, but inspiratory stridor and retractions are evident when the child is at rest and the level of respiratory distress has elevated.

Table 13.2   Clinical features differentiating COPD and asthma.

	COPD	Asthma
Smoker or ex-smoker	Nearly all	Possibly
Symptoms under age 35	Rare	Often
Chronic productive cough	Common	Uncommon
Breathlessness	Persistent and progressive	Variable
Night-time waking with breathlessness and/or wheeze	Uncommon	Common
Significant diurnal or day-to-day variability of symptoms	Uncommon	Common

Source: Adapted from Overview | Chronic obstructive pulmonary disease in over 16s: diagnosis and management | Guidance (2018).

- In severe croup there are mental status changes in conjunction with substantial respiratory distress and declining air entry, signifying looming respiratory failure. Intercostal and suprasternal accessory muscle retractions along with inspiratory and expiratory stridor are frequently present (Aehlert, 2017).

The treatment of croup depends on its severity. Maintain the child in a position of comfort sat upright and on a parent's lap if appropriate. A calm approach is recommended as any distress can lead to deterioration and complete airway occlusion. Patients with reduced oxygen saturations should receive supplemental oxygen therapy via flow-by method or humidified oxygen with a nebuliser mask (Sizar and Carr, 2020). Steroids are the mainstay of croup treatment and children may benefit from early steroid administration (JRCALC, 2019). In moderate and severe presentations where hypoxia and/or signs of severe obstruction are present, the administration of nebulised epinephrine is appropriate (PHECC, 2018) to decrease upper airway oedema with its faster onset of action over steroids. Children with the most severe croup symptoms benefit from medications with a rapid onset which may reduce the need for invasive interventions such as intubation (Bjornson et al., 2011).

Pneumonia

Pneumonia is not a single disease but a group of specific infections that cause acute inflammation of the respiratory bronchioles and alveoli. Pneumonia can be a result of bacterial, fungal or viral infection and related risk factors include cigarette smoking, extremes of age, exposure to cold and alcoholism. These diseases can be spread through interaction with infected individuals by respiratory droplets. Pneumonia can be classed as aspiration, bacterial, mycoplasmal or viral and usually manifests with classic signs and symptoms (Sanders et al., 2012). Pathophysiology, swelling of respiratory tissues, the production of pus and increased mucus secretion occur. The swelling can be dramatic and lead to airflow resistance due to narrowing of the airways. In conjunction, the alveoli lose the ability to function when they fill with fluid or pus (consolidation) which occurs in pneumonia. People with chronic illnesses, the elderly and those who smoke are at increased risk of developing pneumonia. Individuals who produce excessive mucus or do not ventilate effectively, such as asthmatics, COPD patients, the immunocompromised and those who are bedridden or sedentary, are at an increased risk of developing pneumonia (Pollak et al., 2018).

The classic signs and symptoms of pneumonia include pleuritic chest pain, a productive cough and fever that produces rigor which is typically related to a bacterial infection. It also may cause non-specific complaints, particularly in older and weakened patients. These non-specific complaints can include headache, sore throat, fatigue and a non-productivecough (Sanders et al., 2012). Auscultation may reveal crackles typically at the lung base unilaterally, but in advanced cases breath sounds may be diminished or absent. Due to dehydration, sputum may be thick and discoloured (Pollak et al., 2018).

Management of pneumonia in the prehospital field is primarily supportive, ensuring adequate oxygenation and assessing for sepsis. Patients who present with sepsis may also require intravenous fluids, antibiotics and antipyretics (JRCALC, 2019; PHECC, 2018).

Pneumothorax

A pneumothorax is defined as a collection of air trapped inside the pleural cavity outside the lung and happens when air gathers between the visceral and parietal pleurae within the thorax. As the air gathers within the pleural space, it applies pressure to the lung, causing it to collapse, and the grade of collapse will determine the patient's clinical presentation. Air can enter the pleural space by two possible mechanisms: due to trauma which causes air to enter the thorax via an open wound in the chest wall, or via a rupture of the visceral pleura causing air to escape from the lung.

A traumatic pneumothorax is a result of penetrating or blunt trauma and can be further classified as a simple, tension or open pneumothorax. A simple pneumothorax occurs when the air trapped with the pleural space does not apply pressure to the mediastinal structures such as the heart, great blood vessels, trachea and oesophagus. A tension pneumothorax is present when the volume of air trapped within the pleural space increases to the point where the contents of the mediastinum are compressed. This is a time-sensitive emergency which should be corrected immediately when identified. In an open pneumothorax, air enters the thorax via an open wound in the chest wall (McKnight and Burns, 2020).

Non-traumatic pneumothorax can be characterised as primary or secondary. A primary spontaneous pneumothorax (PSP) happens suddenly without any known precipitating event, whereas a secondary spontaneous pneumothorax (SSP) occurs due to pre-existing lung disease such as COPD or a congenital disease. Individuals with severe asthma along with tall, thin smokers are prone to blebs which are weak spots that can rupture when under stress. These blebs can rupture simply by coughing or by aggressive bag-valve-mask ventilation.

The majority of patients with a pneumothorax will not require an immediate intervention, such as a needle chest decompression. Patients with an open pneumothorax should have the wound covered with a three-sided occlusive dressing. Oxygen therapy may be required and the patient should be reassessed regularly for signs of a tension pneumothorax developing which should be decompressed when identified (Pollak et al., 2018).

Pulmonary oedema

Pulmonary oedema is characterised as an abnormal build-up of extravascular fluid within the lungs. This leads to reduced gas exchange within the alveoli, causing dyspnoea and hypoxia which can potentially progress to respiratory failure. Pulmonary oedema can be classified as cardiogenic or non-cardiogenic based on the underlying process leading to fluid accumulation in the lungs. In cardiogenic pulmonary oedema, the heart is not sufficiently moving blood through the pulmonary circulation due to injury or disease (see Chapter 10). This leads to increased pulmonary venous pressure and increased hydrostatic pressure resulting in a fluid shift (Malek and Soufi, 2020). In non-cardiogenic pulmonary oedema, there is an increase in pulmonary vascular permeability leading to fluid moving from the intravascular space to the interstitial and alveolar spaces. The main causes of non-cardiogenic pulmonary oedema are acute respiratory distress syndrome (ARDS), allergic reaction, acute kidney injury (AKI), aspiration, drowning, inhalation injury, fluid overload and intracranial haemorrhage (neurogenic pulmonary oedema) (Sureka et al., 2015).

Acute pulmonary oedema is an emergency in which immediate intervention is required. It is characterised by dyspnoea, hypoxia and crackles on auscultation as a result of increasing fluid accumulation within the lungs, which is impairing lung compliance and gas exchange.

Management of patients with pulmonary oedema focuses on improving symptoms and treatment of the underlying condition (Malek and Soufi, 2020), but the management differs depending on the underlying pathology (Manne et al., 2012). Pharmacological therapy for acute cardiogenic pulmonary oedema includes oxygenation, nitrates and the administration of diuretics. To supplement the pharmacological treatment, the use of continuous positive airway pressure (CPAP) in the management of acute pulmonary oedema has been shown to decrease mortality and the need for intubation (Williams et al., 2013). Oxygen therapy should be administered to any patient with acute pulmonary oedema and guided by a target oxygen saturation level of 94–98%. Sublingual glyceryl trinitrate (GTN) can be administered to reduce preload and afterload, therefore improving cardiac output and reducing pulmonary congestion (Kim et al., 2020).

Diuretics remain the backbone of acute pulmonary oedema management (Malek and Soufi, 2020); however, with the introduction of prehospital CPAP, the administration of intravenous diuretics has been moved further down the treatment algorithms. Diuretics are recommended in acute cardiogenic pulmonary oedema patients who are in severe respiratory distress with signs of systemic fluid retention (JRCALC, 2019; PHECC, 2018). Loop diuretics, such as furosemide, are normally the diuretics of choice and have been used in prehospital care for many years (Purvey and Allen, 2017). For patients in respiratory distress, initiate non-invasive ventilation in conjunction with medical management by nitrates and diuretics based on systolic blood pressure and the degree of pulmonary congestion (Mebazaa et al., 2015). Management of non-cardiogenic pulmonary oedema focuses on addressing the underlying cause, providing supportive care including oxygen therapy and CPAP if required (Clark and Soos, 2020).

Reflection

Treatment of cardiogenic and non-cardiogenic pulmonary oedema differs. Why would the pharmacological agents used to manage cardiogenic pulmonary oedema not have the same effect on patients with non-cardiogenic pulmonary oedema?

Classes of medications

In this section the various classes of medications used to manage respiratory emergencies in the prehospital field are discussed.

Bronchodilators

Bronchoconstriction is common in individuals with respiratory diseases such as asthma, COPD and cystic fibrosis, which may require bronchodilators. Bronchodilators are fundamental in the management of obstructive airway diseases, and their mechanism of action either enhances (agonist) or inhibits (antagonist) the actions of the autonomic nervous system to elicit a response which reverses asthma symptoms or improves lung function in COPD patients (Almadhoun and Sharma, 2020).

Airway smooth muscle tone is largely controlled by the parasympathetic nervous system via cholinergic and non-cholinergic innervation. Parasympathetic fibres release acetylcholine, causing constriction of the smooth muscle layer surrounding the airways. Increased vagus nerve activity has a significant role in provoking airway obstruction in asthma and COPD patients and is a reversible element of airway obstruction (Cotes, 2006; Matera et al., 2020). Bronchodilator therapy often reduces the symptoms of airflow obstruction by relaxing smooth muscle in the bronchi and bronchioles, decreasing dyspnoea and improving quality of life (Williams and Rubin, 2018).

The types of bronchodilators utilised in prehospital care are:

- beta-2 adrenergic receptor agonists (B2-agonists)
- muscarinic receptor antagonists (anticholinergics)
- sympathomimetics
- electrolytes and minerals.

Beta-2 adrenergic receptor agonists (B2-agonists)

Beta-2 agonists are the fundamental therapy for respiratory diseases such as asthma and COPD. Beta-agonists bind to beta-receptors on cardiac and smooth muscle tissues, especially bronchial smooth muscle where they cause relaxation of the muscle. Drugs defined as agonists work by binding to a receptor and stimulating it to produce the anticipated therapeutic effect. The patient subsequently experiences improved airflow for a time.

Beta-adrenoceptors usually bind to circulating epinephrine and to norepinephrine released by sympathetic adrenergic nerves. Therefore, beta-agonists mimic the actions of sympathetic adrenergic stimulation (sympathomimetic) acting through beta-adrenoceptors (Klabunde, 2012). B2-agonists work by binding to B2-receptors in airway smooth muscle where they set in progress a chain of events similar to that produced by the action of the natural neurotransmitters. In other words, they mimic norepinephrine and normal sympathetic nervous system response.

The onset of action and duration of B2-agonists determine their classification. The classifications are shortacting beta-agonists (SABA) and long-acting beta-agonists (LABA). SABAs have a short half-life and are primarily used for rapid relief of symptoms. LABAs, in contrast, have a longer half-life and deliver continuous symptomatic relief, however, they are not routinely used in prehospital care.

The most familiar SABAs are:

- salbutamol (Ventolin®);
- terbutaline (Bricanyl®).

234

Short-acting beta-agonists start to work within a few minutes of being inhaled and last from 4–6 hours. They are used for rapid symptom relief and are given in high doses in cases of acute exacerbations of airway obstructive disease. The use of high-dose inhaled B2-agonists as first-line agents in patients with acute asthma is recommended and should be administered as early as possible via an oxygen-driven nebuliser (BTS/SIGN, 2019). Patients with COPD also benefit from symptom relief with SABA therapy during an exacerbation; however, caution should be applied when using an oxygen-driven nebuliser to maintain an oxygen saturation level of 92% (GOLD, 2020). Side effects of SABA's are associated with their sympathomimetic action. These include tachycardia, tachyarrythmias, and tremors.

Muscarinic receptor antagonists (anticholinergics)

Muscarinic receptor antagonists produce bronchodilation by inhibiting muscarinic acetylcholine receptors in bronchial smooth muscle. Acetylcholine is a neurotransmitter secreted from terminal parasympathetic fibres which bonds with M3 muscarinic receptors within bronchial smooth muscle, producing bronchoconstriction. Muscarinic receptor antagonist drugs block the bronchoconstriction effects of acetylcholine (anticholinergic) on M3 muscarinic receptors within bronchial smooth muscle (GOLD, 2020) and are often combined with a B2-agonist for the management of serious bronchial airway narrowing (Long et al., 2020). M3 receptors are also located within bronchial glands which secrete mucus when stimulated. Antimuscarinics compete with acetylcholine and antagonise the normal parasympathetic effect reducing bronchial mucus secretion.

235

There are two types of muscarinic receptor antagonists: short-acting muscarinic antagonists (SAMA) and long-acting muscarinic antagonists (LAMA). LAMAs are not routinely used in prehospital care.

Short-acting muscarinic antagonists

Short-acting muscarinic antagonists, similar to SABAs, are utilised in both acute and chronic management of asthma and COPD. Ipratropium bromide is the most commonly used and blocks all muscarinic receptors. Its onset of action is within minutes, with peak activity taking place at 1–2 hours and a duration of action of approximately 4 hours in the majority of patients (Ejiofor and Turner, 2013). Common side-effects of SAMAs include gastrointestinal motility disorder, headache, dizziness, nausea, cardiac arrhythmias and throat complaints such as dry mouth and coughing (Joint Formulary Committee, 2019a).

Skills in practice: preparing and administering nebulised medications

1. Select appropriately sized nebuliser device for the patient.
2. Using aseptic technique, mix medication into nebuliser chamber.
3. Attach nebuliser chamber to mask and ensure tight seal.
4. Connect oxygen tubing to port on the oxygen flowmeter.
5. Adjust oxygen flowmeter to 4–8 L/min and ensure visible mist is obtained.
6. Place mask over patient's mouth and nose, ensuring tight seal.
7. Instruct patient to take deep steady breaths to disperse medications throughout the bronchial tree.

Clinical consideration: inhalation therapy

There are a number of devices available for administering medications via inhalation. These include the nebuliser mask, hand-held nebuliser, metred dose inhaler and spacer devices. Some prehospital services carry multiple devices which can be utilised to deliver medications to the patient. Consider the devices available to you and which patients are better suited to each one.

Sympathomimetics: epinephrine (adrenaline)

Epinephrine is a synthetic preparation of the naturally occurring catecholamine produced by the adrenal glands which has bronchodilation and vasoconstricting properties. It is a potent alpha- and beta-adrenergic stimulant although its effect on beta-receptors is more profound. Stimulation of alpha-receptors within blood vessels causes vasoconstriction, increasing vascular resistance and blood pressure. Through its beta-receptor stimulation, epinephrine increases the rate (chronotropic) and force (inotropic) of myocardial contraction and causes bronchodilation by relaxing bronchial smooth muscle. In children with severe croup, nebulised epinephrine causes localised vasoconstriction which reduces the upper airway oedema and stridor. In addition to the above conditions, epinephrine is the main drug administered during cardiac arrest management due to its chronotropic and inotropic effects (Paramothayan, 2019; PubChem, 2021).

Side-effects of epinephrine are related to its sympathomimetic action and include tachycardia, tachyarrhythmias, anxiety, hypertension, palpitations, tremors and angina-like symptoms (Joint Formulary Committee, 2019b).

236

Epinephrine comes in multiple presentations and concentrations. <u>Double check</u> the dose and route prior to administration.

Electrolytes and minerals: magnesium sulfate

Magnesium sulfate ($MgSO_4$) is an electrolyte important for many biochemical reactions which occur in the body. It is also an adjunct medication for the management of severe life-threatening asthma exacerbations and has a role as a cardiovascular drug, an antiarrhythmic and an anticonvulsant. $MgSO_4$ causes bronchodilation by inhibiting acetylcholine release from cholinergic nerve endings, histamine release from mast cells and calcium influx to the cytosol. Through this inhibitory action, $MgSO_4$ induces bronchial smooth muscle relaxation (Song and Chang, 2012). In a systematic review of randomised control trials, asthmatic patients treated with $MgSO_4$ had a reduction in hospital admission and improved lung function (Paramothayan, 2019). When administered intravenously, it has an immediate onset of action with a duration of action of around 30 minutes. If the intramuscular route is used, the onset of action is around 60 minutes with a duration of action of 3–4 hours (HPRA, 2019).

Side-effects of $MgSO_4$ are hypotension, confusion, drowsiness, decreased deep tendon reflexes, muscle weakness, slurred speech, nausea, vomiting, thirst, flushing, respiratory depression, arrythmias, coma and cardiac arrest. Bradycardia can happen during administration which can be reduced by slowing the rate of infusion (Joint Formulary Committee, 2019c).

Diuretics

Loop diuretics, such as furosemide, are the most powerful diuretics and are widely utilised for the management of pulmonary and systemic oedema. They bind to chloride receptors in the ascending loop of Henle within the kidneys, inhibiting reabsorption of chloride and sodium. This leads to a hypertonic state where water is retained within the loop of Henle and eliminated by the bladder (Sniecinski et al., 2007). Loop diuretics are administered in cases of cardiogenic pulmonary oedema with intravenous administration relieving dyspnoea and reducing preload in acute presentations.

Side-effects of loop diuretics are electrolyte imbalances, dizziness, headache, hypotension, fatigue, muscle spasms, nausea, vomiting and metabolic alkalosis (Joint Formulary Committee, 2019d).

Nitrates

Nitrates, such as glycerol trinitrate, cause smooth muscle relaxation by releasing nitric oxide, resulting in dilation of systemic veins and reduction of preload. These actions reduce intravascular pressure within the lungs, allowing fluid within interstitial lung tissue to cross into pulmonary capillaries, thus reducing pulmonary oedema. Higher doses of nitrates lead to arterial dilation, resulting in reduced afterload and blood pressure. Dilation of the coronary arteries results in increased coronary blood flow. These actions collectively improve oxygenation and reduce cardiac workload.

Nitrates can cause hypotension due to the methods of action mentioned above, so blood pressure monitoring is essential prior to administration: nitrates should be withheld if systolic blood pressure is <90 mmHg.

There are a number of formulations of nitrates but in prehospital care the most commonly used is the sublingual route via dissolvable tablet or aerosol pump spray. Nitrates are usually well tolerated with the most common side-effects being headache, flushing, dizziness and transient hypotension (Purvey and Allen, 2017).

Steroids

Corticosteroids are synthetic equivalents of the natural steroid hormones produced in the adrenal gland, which include glucocorticoids (cortisol) and mineralocorticoids (aldosterone). Glucocorticoids have anti-inflammatory, immunosuppressive and vasoconstrictive properties, whereas mineralocorticoids regulate electrolytes and water balance via an effect on ion transport within the renal tubules.

Corticosteroids are utilised in the management of conditions in almost all areas of medicine and have both endocrine and non-endocrine indications. Their non-endocrine role takes advantage of the potent anti-inflammatory and immunosuppressive properties of the medication to manage patients with a wide range of inflammatory and immunological conditions (Hodgens and Sharman, 2020). Two examples of corticosteroids used in prehospital care are dexamethasone and hydrocortisone. In respiratory conditions, steroids are indicated for the management of acute inflammation in asthma exacerbations, COPD exacerbations, anaphylaxis and croup (JRCALC, 2019; PHECC, 2018). Side-effects of corticosteroids are hypertension, vertigo, abdominal distension, headache, hiccups, nausea and hyperglycaemia (HPRA, 2020).

Clinical consideration: corticosteroids

Prolonged therapy with corticosteroids can cause serious life-threatening side-effects. Adrenal atrophy can develop due to supplemental steroid use and can persist for years after ceasing the medication. Patients who stop taking their corticosteroids abruptly can present with an adrenal crisis resulting in hypoglycaemia, hypotension and death (Joint Formulary Committee, 2019e).

Episode of care: COPD exacerbation

You are dispatched to a 67-year-old female patient with shortness of breath. On arrival, you enter the living room of the house and observe the patient sitting in an armchair at the other side of the room. She is sitting upright with both hands on her knees and she has a home nebuliser mask on. You notice that she has a very slight build and a flushed complexion, and from your position you can easily see that she is breathing fast while utilising accessory muscles. As you glance around the room, you notice signs of recent smoking and several empty nebuliser pods sitting on the table along with other medication boxes. When you introduce yourself, the patient replies with one word and a head nod to acknowledge your greeting.

On examination, the patient is tachypnoeic with bibasal absent breath sounds, a nearly inaudible expiratory wheeze in all other fields and significant accessory muscle use. Her pulse oximetry is reading 86%, her pulse is fast and regular, she has dry skin and hypertension, her temperature is 36.8°C, and her blood glucose is 8.6 mmol/L. You obtain a 12-lead ECG which shows sinus tachycardia with right ventricular hypertrophy.

The patient's daughter tells you that her mum's breathing has been getting worse for the last 4 days and that she went to the GP 3 days ago. The GP started prophylactic antibiotics and a course of oral prednisolone. Along with this, the patient is prescribed salbutamol, Atrovent®, Spiriva® and ramipril for daily management of COPD and hypertension.

What do you think is the cause of the COPD exacerbation?

What is the significance of the respiratory examination findings?

Why did the GP prescribe prophylactic antibiotics and oral prednisolone?

Smoking is a major cause of COPD and a common trigger of exacerbations. COPD patients are also prone to chest infections due to excessive mucus accumulation within the airways which can trigger severe symptoms. When assessing any respiratory patient, the absence of breath sounds should raise a red flag. In asthmatic and COPD patients, this can be due to significant bronchospasm and mucus plugging resulting in minimal air movement. These patients should be handled with caution as they can deteriorate very quickly.

- Patients with COPD exacerbations should be managed with a step-wise approach beginning with a B2-agonist such as salbutamol. B2-agonists start to work quickly, causing bronchial smooth muscle relaxation and aiding airflow through the lungs.
- In moderate exacerbations B2-agonists can be supplemented with a short-acting muscarinic antagonist such as ipratropium bromide. These medications also aid bronchial smooth muscle relaxation and reduce bronchial secretions which clog the airways.
- Inflammation plays a major role in exacerbations and COPD patients will often be prescribed corticosteroids to alleviate this. Parenteral corticosteroids have a slow onset of action, so in severe exacerbations early administration is recommended.

238

Medical gases

Oxygen (O_2) is an odourless, colourless, tasteless gas which is necessary for life and is an important part of patient care. It is essential in the management of hypoxic patients as it raises their O_2 levels by increasing the inspired percentage of O_2, the concentration within the alveoli, the arterial O_2 levels, and increases the volume of O_2 delivered to systemic tissues and cells. O_2 should be administered to hypoxic patients only, as per Table 13.3, and to maintain their O_2 saturation level within the normal range (Weekley and Bland, 2020). The normal target O_2 saturation for adults is 94–98%, for patients with COPD the normal target O_2 saturation is 88–92%, and for paediatric patients aim for an O_2 saturation greater than 96% (JRCALC, 2019; PHECC, 2018). O_2 administration is commonly based upon pulse oximetry readings, but pulse oximetry can provide false readings in cases of carbon monoxide poisoning, anaemia and shock (Weekley and Bland, 2020). Hyperoxia should be avoided.

Oxygen devices

There are numerous oxygen delivery devices available which can be divided into 'low-flow' devices and 'high-flow devices'. Table 13.4 lists some of the various types and the O_2 flow rates associated with them.

Table 13.3   Indications for oxygen administration.

Chronic	Acute
Chronic obstructive pulmonary disease	Shock
Cystic fibrosis	Sepsis
Pulmonary fibrosis	Major trauma
Sarcoidosis	Cardiac arrest
Asthma exacerbation	Anaphylaxis
Lung cancer	Carbon monoxide poisoning
Sickle cell disease	Myocardial ischaemia[a]
	Acute pulmonary oedema

SpO_2 < 94% for all acutely unwell or injured patients.

SpO_2 < 92% for patients with an acute exacerbation of COPD.

SpO_2 < 96% for all paediatric patients.

[a]Studies have shown that routine oxygen therapy in myocardial infarction patients with a normal range SpO_2 is not associated with any clinical benefit (Sepehrvand et al., 2018).

Table 13.4   Oxygen delivery devices.

| Low-flow devices | | High-flow devices | |
Devices	O$_2$ rate		O$_2$ rate
Nasal cannula	2–6 L/min	Non-rebreather mask	10–15 L/min
Venturi mask	2–15 L/min	Bag-valve-mask ventilator	15 L/min
Simple face mask	5–8 L/min	High-flow nasal cannula	Up to 60 L/min
		Continuous positive airway pressure (CPAP)	Up to 25 L/min

Source: Weekley and Bland (2020).

Devices frequently used to administer O$_2$ in prehospital care are the nasal cannula, non-rebreather mask, bag-valve-mask ventilator and, less frequently, the Venturi mask and CPAP device. The O$_2$ delivery device used should be appropriate to the patient's needs and tolerances. Those with mild hypoxia may be managed with a low-flow O$_2$ device, such as the nasal cannula which can deliver O$_2$ concentrations of 24–4%. The simple face mask is appropriate for patients who are suffering from moderate hypoxia as it can deliver O$_2$ concentrations of 40–60%. The disadvantage of the face mask is that it requires a tight seal which can be confining for the patient and muffle their speech. The non-rebreather mask can deliver 80–100% concentration of O$_2$. When the patient inhales, the O$_2$ within the reservoir bag is drawn into the mask and subsequently the patient's lungs. As the patient exhales, the rubber flaps at the side of the mask open to allow air to escape. This means the non-rebreather mask is a closed system and if the O$_2$ flow rate cannot inflate the reservoir bag, the patient could potentially suffocate (Bledsoe and Claden, 2012).

239

Conclusion

Respiratory distress is a common reason for people to request emergency ambulance assistance. With ever improving methods of care, people with respiratory diseases are living longer than ever before. This has a knock-on effect for prehospital services when these patients have an exacerbation of their illness. Evidence supports that prehospital management of respiratory diseases improves outcomes and reduces mortality. Therefore, prehospital practitioners should have a good understanding of the pathophysiological and pharmacological processes that underpin respiratory emergencies and their management.

Find out more

The following is a list of respiratory conditions or conditions that affect the respiratory system which are also encountered in the prehospital field. Take some time to review these conditions, paying close attention not only to the pharmacological management but also the medications (if any) which the patient may be prescribed by their doctor to manage their symptoms.

Condition	Notes
Cystic fibrosis	
Lung cancer	
Motor neuron disease	
Acute respiratory distress syndrome	
Bronchiectasis	

References

Aehlert, B. (2017). *Pediatric Advanced Life Support Study Guide*, 4th edn. Sudbury: Jones and Bartlett Learning, LLC.
Almadhoun, K. and Sharma, S. (2020). *Bronchodilators*. www.ncbi.nlm.nih.gov/books/NBK519028/
Asthma.ie. (2020). *Asthma Basics*. www.asthma.ie/get-help/learn-about-asthma/asthma-basics/asthma-basics
Bjornson, C., Russell, K.F., Vandermeer, B., Durec, T., Klassen, T.P. and Johnson, D.W. (2011). Nebulized epinephrine for croup in children. *Cochrane Database of Systematic Reviews* **10**: CD06619.

Bledsoe, B. and Clayden, D. (2012). *Prehospital Emergency Pharmacology*, 7th edn. Harlow: Pearson, 226–228.

BTS/SIGN. (2019). *British Guideline on the Management of Asthma*. www.sign.ac.uk/sign-158-british-guideline-on-the-management-of-asthma

Clark, S. and Soos, M. (2020). *Noncardiogenic Pulmonary Edema*. www.ncbi.nlm.nih.gov/books/NBK542230/

Cotes, J. (2006). *Lung Function, 6th edn. Malden: Oxford: Blackwell Publishing*.

DeVrieze, B., Modi, P. and Giwa, A. (2020). *Peak Flow Rate Measurement*. www.ncbi.nlm.nih.gov/books/NBK459325/

Ejiofor, S. and Turner, A.M. (2013). Pharmacotherapies for COPD. *Clinical Medicine Insights: Circulatory, Respiratory and Pulmonary Medicine* **7**: 17–34.

Fayyaz, J. (2020). *How is Chronic Bronchitis Defined?* www.medscape.com/answers/297108-6913/how-is-chronic-bronchitis-defined

GOLD. (2020). *Pocket Guide to COPD Diagnosis, Management, and Prevention*. https://goldcopd.org/wp-content/uploads/2020/03/GOLD-2020-POCKET-GUIDE-ver1.0_FINAL-WMV.pdf

Hodgens, A. and Sharman, T. (2020). *Corticosteroids*. www.ncbi.nlm.nih.gov/books/NBK554612/

HPRA. (2019). *Summary of Product Characteristics: Magnesium Sulphate*. www.hpra.ie/img/uploaded/swedocuments/Licence_PA0549-020-001_20062019112032.pdf

HPRA. (2020). *Summary of Product Characteristics: Solu-Cortef Powder*. www.hpra.ie/img/uploaded/swedocuments/Licence_PA0822-137-001_13112020120319.pdf

Joint Formulary Committee. (2019a). *BNF 78: September 2019-March 2020*. London: Pharmaceutical Press, 245–247.

Joint Formulary Committee. (2019b). *BNF 78: September 2019-March 2020*. London: Pharmaceutical Press, 224.

Joint Formulary Committee. (2019c). *BNF 78: September 2019-March 2020*. London: Pharmaceutical Press, 1051.

Joint Formulary Committee. (2019d). *BNF 78: September 2019-March 2020*. London: Pharmaceutical Press, 225-226.

Joint Formulary Committee. (2019e). *BNF 78: September 2019-March 2020*. London: Pharmaceutical Press, 672–673.

Joint Royal Colleges Ambulance Liaison Committee (JRCALC). (2019). *Clinical Guidelines 2019*. Bridgwater: Class Professional Publishing.

Kim, K., Kerndt, C. and Schaller, D. (2020). *Nitroglycerin*. www.ncbi.nlm.nih.gov/books/NBK482382/

Klabunde, R. (2012). *Beta-Adrenoceptor Agonists (B-Agonists)*. www.cvpharmacology.com/cardiostimulatory/beta-agonist

Lindskou, T.A., Pilgaard, L., Søvsø, M.B. et al. (2019). Symptom, diagnosis and mortality among respiratory emergency medical service patients. *PLoS One* **14**(2): e0213145.

Long, B., Lentz, S., Koyfman, A. and Gottlieb, M. (2020). Evaluation and management of the critically ill adult asthmatic in the emergency department setting. *American Journal of Emergency Medicine* **44**: 441–451.

Malek, R. and Soufi, S. (2020). *Pulmonary Edema*. www.ncbi.nlm.nih.gov/books/NBK557611/

Manne, J.R., Kasirye, Y., Epperla, N. and Garcia-Montilla, R.J. (2012). Non-cardiogenic pulmonary edema complicating electroconvulsive therapy: short review of the pathophysiology and diagnostic approach. *Clinical Medicine and Research* **10**(3): 131–136.

Matera, M.G., Page, C.P., Calzetta, L., Rogliani, P. and Cazzola, M. (2020). Pharmacology and therapeutics of bronchodilators revisited. *Pharmacological Reviews* **72**(1): 218–252.

McKnight, C. and Burns, B. (2020). *Pneumothorax*. www.ncbi.nlm.nih.gov/books/NBK441885/

Mebazaa, A., Yilmaz, M.B., Levy, P. et al (2015). Recommendations on pre-hospital and early hospital management of acute heart failure: a consensus paper from the Heart Failure Association of the European Society of Cardiology, the European Society of Emergency Medicine and the Society of Academic Emergency Medicine. *European Journal of Heart Failure* **17**(6): 544–558.

Neal, M. (2015). *Medical Pharmacology at a Glance*, 8th edn. Chichester: John Wiley & Sons.

NHS England. (2020). *Respiratory Disease*. www.england.nhs.uk/ourwork/clinical-policy/respiratory-disease/

NICE. (2018). *Chronic obstructive pulmonary disease in over 16s: diagnosis and management*. www.nice.org.uk/guidance/ng115>

Paramothayan, S. (2019). *Essential Respiratory Medicine*. Hoboken: John Wiley & Sons Ltd.

Peate, I. (2015). *Anatomy and Physiology for Nurses at a Glance*. Chichester: Wiley Blackwell.

PHECC. (2018). *Clinical Practice Guidelines – Advanced Paramedic*, 7th edn. Naas: Pre-Hospital Emergency Care Council (PHECC).

Pollak, A., Elling, B. and Aehlert, B. 2018. *Nancy Caroline's Emergency Care in the Streets*. 8th ed. Burlington: Jones & Bartlett Learning.

Prekker, M.E., Feemster, L.C., Hough, C.L. et al. (2014). The epidemiology and outcome of prehospital respiratory distress. *Academic Emergency Medicine* **21**(5): 543–550.

PubChem. (2021). *Epinephrine*. https://pubchem.ncbi.nlm.nih.gov/compound/Epinephrine

Purvey, M. and Allen, G. (2017). Managing acute pulmonary oedema. *Australian Prescriber* **40**(2): 59.

Sanders, M., Lewis, L., Quick, G. and McKenna, K. (2012). *Mosby's Paramedic Textbook*, 4th edn. St Louis: Elsevier Mosby JEMS.

Sanders, M., McKenna, K., Tan, D., Pollak, A. and Mejia, A. (2019). *Sanders' Paramedic Textbook*, 5th edn. Burlington: Jones and Bartlett Learning.

240

Sepehrvand, N., James, S.K., Stub, D., Khoshnood, A., Ezekowitz, J.A. and Hofmann, R. (2018). Effects of supplemental oxygen therapy in patients with suspected acute myocardial infarction: a meta-analysis of randomised clinical trials. *Heart* **104**(20): 1691–1698.

Sizar, O. and Carr, B. (2020). *Croup*. www.ncbi.nlm.nih.gov/books/NBK431070/

Sniecinski, R.M., Wright, S. and Levy, J.H. (2007). *Cardiovascular Pharmacology*. St Louis: Elsevier Inc.

Song, W.J. and Chang, Y.S. (2012). Magnesium sulfate for acute asthma in adults: a systematic literature review. *Asia Pacific Allergy* **2**(1): 76.

Sureka, B., Bansal, K. and Arora, A. (2015). Pulmonary edema – cardiogenic or noncardiogenic? *Journal of Family Medicine and Primary Care* **4**(2): 290.

Tortora, G. and Derrickson, B. (2014). *Principles of Anatomy and Physiology*, 14th edn. Hoboken: Wiley.

Weekley, M. and Bland, L. (2020). *Oxygen Administration*. www.ncbi.nlm.nih.gov/books/NBK551617/

Williams, B., Boyle, M., Robertson, N. and Giddings, C. (2013). When pressure is positive: a literature review of the prehospital use of continuous positive airway pressure. *Prehospital and Disaster Medicine* **28**(1): 52.

Williams, D.M. and Rubin, B.K. (2018). Clinical pharmacology of bronchodilator medications. *Respiratory Care* **63**(6): 641–654.

World Health Organization. (2020). *Asthma*. www.who.int/news-room/fact-sheets/detail/asthma

Further reading

Cukic, V., Lovre, V., Dragisic, D. and Ustamujic, A. (2012). Asthma and chronic obstructive pulmonary disease (COPD) – differences and similarities. *Materia Socio-Medica* **24**(2): 100.

Multiple-choice questions

1. Ventilation is:
   (a) The movement of gases between cells
   (b) Movement of air into and out of the lungs
   (c) The total volume of air in forced expiration
   (d) The process of administering inhaled medication.

2. Diffusion of gases across a membrane occurs due to:
   (a) Differences in gas pressure gradients
   (b) Total lung volume capacity
   (c) Pulmonary blood flow rate
   (d) Respiratory rate and heart rate.

3. COPD patients with dyspnoea should have oxygen therapy administered to achieve an O_2 saturation of:
   (a) 94–98%
   (b) ≤92%
   (c) >96%
   (d) 94%.

4. Wheezes most commonly suggest:
   (a) Secretions in large airways
   (b) Abnormal lung tissue
   (c) Airless lung areas
   (d) Narrowed airways.

5. Which of the following would *not* be found in a patient with chronic bronchitis?
   (a) Weight loss
   (b) Pulmonary hypertension
   (c) Cyanosis
   (d) Right-sided heart failure

6. Which of these drugs are M3-receptor antagonists?
   (a) Bronchodilators
   (b) Antimuscarinics

(c) Antihistamines

(d) Sympathomimetics

7. Which of these drugs dilate constricted airways by relaxing smooth muscle?
   (a) Beta-2 adrenergic receptor agonists
   (b) Glyceryl trinitrate
   (c) H1-receptor antagonists
   (d) Hydrocortisone

8. In the emergency management of COPD, which of the following is the initial medication of choice?
   (a) Ipratropium bromide
   (b) Salbutamol
   (c) Hydrocortisone
   (d) Chlorphenamine

9. Muscarinic receptors antagonists cause:
   (a) Bronchodilation and increased mucus secretion
   (b) Bronchoconstriction and increased mucus secretion
   (c) Bronchodilation and reduced mucus secretion
   (d) Bronchoconstriction and reduced mucus secretion.

10. Which of the following is a synthetic form of an endocrine hormone?
    (a) Magnesium sulfate
    (b) Oxygen
    (c) Chlorphenamine
    (d) Hydrocortisone

11. Which of the following should be administered to an asthmatic patient who shows no improvement following a B2-agonist nebuliser?
    (a) A H1-receptor antagonist
    (b) An anticholinergic
    (c) A nitrate
    (d) An electrolyte

12. Which of the following is a sign of life-threatening asthma?
    (a) Peak expiratory flow = 50%
    (b) Respiratory rate of 25 bpm
    (c) Heart rate of 120 bpm
    (d) Hypotension

13. Which of the following is indicated for severe upper airway stridor?
    (a) Salbutamol
    (b) Epinephrine
    (c) Chlorphenamine
    (d) Ipratropium bromide

14. Which of the following oxygen delivery devices are 'high-flow' devices?
    (a) Nasal cannula
    (b) Simple face mask
    (c) Non-rebreather mask
    (d) Venturi mask

15. Which of the following patients requires oxygen therapy?
    (a) A 72-year-old with mild COPD exacerbation with an SpO_2 of 90%
    (b) A 24-year-old allergic reaction patient with isolated urticaria
    (c) A 56-year-old with carbon monoxide poisoning and an SpO_2 of 99%
    (d) A 2-year-old with upper airway stridor, mild distress and SpO_2 of 96%

Chapter 14

Medications used in the gastrointestinal system

George Bell-Starr and Ashley Ingram

Aim

The aim of this chapter is to provide the reader with an introduction to common pharmacological interventions and the gastrointestinal conditions that they may encounter.

Learning outcomes

After reading this chapter the reader will be able to:

1. Understand the pharmacological interventions commonly available to paramedics, their indications and contraindications
2. understand the pharmacological interventions available in a wider healthcare setting for various common gastrointestinal disorders
3. Develop a fundamental understanding of common gastrointestinal presentations, and their causes
4. Relate the signs and symptoms of common gastrointestinal conditions to their underlying pathophysiology.

Test your knowledge

1. Describe the components and main functions of the gastrointestinal tract.
2. Write down the common gastrointestinal disorders that you have encountered in clinical practice.
3. What are the common routes for the administration of gastrointestinal medications?
4. Identify common causes for constipation and potential interventions for this condition.
5. Consider some of the most common gastrointestinal medications you see prescribed to the patients you encounter.

Fundamentals of Pharmacology for Paramedics, First Edition. Edited by Ian Peate, Suzanne Evans, and Lisa Clegg.
© 2022 John Wiley & Sons Ltd. Published 2022 by John Wiley & Sons Ltd.

Introduction

Homeostasis is dependent on the consumption, absorption and metabolism of food and water. Paramedics will often come across disorders found within the gastrointestinal system, such as nausea and vomiting, peptic ulcers, constipation, diarrhoea, inflammatory bowel disease and gastro-oesophageal reflux disorder. Frequently those patients presenting to paramedics or the ambulance service may exhibit more severe conditions than those presenting to primary care. It is important to consider that patients may also present to this service as a result of not having resolved their condition with primary care providers or a failure to access primary care services. Approximately 40% of the UK population have at least one gastrointestinal symptom at any one time (NHS, 2019). This is comparable to other high-income countries. Medications such as omeprazole and lansoprazole (proton pump inhibitors) are often used in the treatment of gastrointestinal (GI) disorders and are the most commonly prescribed medication in the UK.

The chapter will be broken down into sections covering the disorders separately; these will feature an overview of the gastrointestinal disorder and the most likely medications utilised in its treatment and management. Furthermore, administrative considerations associated with pharmacological interventions commonly available to paramedics will be discussed. Additionally, specific cases pertinent to paramedic practice will be covered.

Anatomy and physiology of the gastrointestinal system

The GI tract begins at the mouth and ends at the anus. Its purpose is to mechanically and enzymatically digest food, absorb nutrients and water, protect the body from microbial invasion and expel faeces. Food enters the mouth where mechanical and enzymatic digestion begins and then is propelled down the oesophagus and into the stomach where digestion continues. As the food bolus passes through the small intestine, further digestion and absorption take place with the help of enzymes secreted by the stomach, small intestine, liver and pancreas. Most of the water absorption and formation of faeces occur in the large intestine, until it is temporarily stored in the rectum and defecated through the anus (Bruneau, 2017). See Figure 14.1 for an overview of the gastrointestinal tract.

Nausea and vomiting

Nausea and vomiting (emesis) are very common and have broad aetiology. Common causes include migraines, motion (car sickness), pregnancy and medications (such as opioids and cytotoxic agents). Due to this broad aetiology, it is very common for paramedics to assess and manage patients with nausea and/or vomiting secondary to their presenting condition.

A wide range of medications are used to treat nausea and vomiting, but not all are commonly available to paramedics. A cautionary approach should be taken in administering antiemetics prior to diagnosis as identification of the underlying cause might be delayed, particularly with children (NICE, 2020a). If an antiemetic is indicated, then the drug should be chosen according to the aetiology.

Clinical consideration: management of vomiting in the patient receiving palliative care

Nausea and vomiting are common symptoms in patients receiving palliative care. The paramedic should carefully consider the underlying pathology and whether this is reversible. Careful consideration should also be given to the side-effects of the chosen antiemetic. One of the most common reversible causes of vomiting is constipation (Albert, 2017). Paramedics may carry Ondansetron to use in the treatment of opiate-induced vomiting. This should be avoided for a constipated patient as the medication itself is constipating and may worsen a patient's condition. To serve as further examples, cyclizine would not be used in patients with heart failure as this could exacerbate the condition. Levomepromazine would be the choice if the cause of the vomiting and nausea was not obvious. Ondansetron may be useful if symptoms are likely to be caused by renal failure, chemotherapy or gastric cancers. The paramedic should seek GP support from either the patient's registered GP or out of hours so the most appropriate drug can be offered. Or the use of 'just in case' medication may be appropriate as this would have likely been considered (Blackmore, 2020).

The two key sites in the central nervous system involved with the vomiting reflex are the vomiting centre and the chemoreceptor trigger zone. The five neurotransmitters that provide feedback to these areas are:

- H1 receptors
- dopamine (D2)
- serotonin (5-HT3)
- acetylcholine (muscarinic)
- neurokinin (substance P).

Antiemetics are antagonists for these receptors, thus they block or dampen the biological response by binding to or blocking a receptor. Often they are simply called blockers, e.g. beta-blockers.

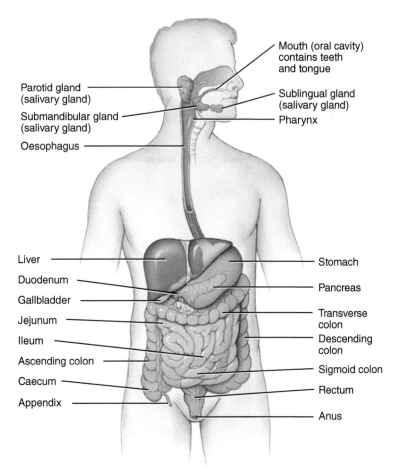

Figure 14.1   The gastrointestinal tract.

H1 receptor antagonists (antihistamines)

The most common type of antiemetic, these agents are primarily used to combat motion sickness and vertigo. However, they can also be used to treat opioid-induced sickness and morning sickness secondary to pregnancy (hyperemesis gravidarum).

Examples of H1 receptor antagonists include:

- promethazine
- doxylamine
- meclizine
- cyclizine.

All antihistamines cause anticholinergic effects which can include vasodilation, hallucinations and urinary retention. Cardiac toxicity effects induce tachycardia and prolonged QT may be seen on an electrocardiogram (ECG) (Brady et al., 2020).

Dopamine (D2) receptor antagonists

Dopamine receptors are located in the chemoreceptor trigger zone (CTZ) and respond to dopamine released from nerve endings. The most common cause of CTZ stimulation is from the GI tract, with the neurotransmitters dopamine and serotonin being released by GI irritation.

Dopamine receptor antagonists are most commonly used to treat the nausea and vomiting associated with chemotherapy or opioid administration. They are unlikely to be effective in reducing the nausea and vomiting caused by motion sickness.

Examples of D2 receptor antagonists include:

- prochlorperazine, commonly used to treat hyperemesis gravidarum
- metoclopramide
- domperidone.

Side-effects of these drugs can include diarrhoea, drowsiness and lower seizure thresholds. Metoclopramide should not be given to patients under the age of 18 years due to an increased risk of neurological events. Full monitoring including a 12-lead ECG should be considered post administration due to a risk of arrhythmia, QT prolongation, AV blocks and cardiac arrest (Brady et al., 2020).

Metoclopramide

JRCALC contraindicates the use of metoclopramide in patients younger than 18 years of age. The reasons behind this are as follows.

The European Medicines Agency's Committee on Medicinal Products for Human Use has reviewed the benefits and risks of metoclopramide. The review was done at the request of the French medicines regulatory agency, following concerns over side-effects and efficacy. The review confirmed the well-known risks of neurological effects such as short-term extrapyramidal disorders and tardive dyskinesia. The conclusion of the review was that these risks outweigh the benefits in long-term or high-dose treatment.

The EU review has recommended changes that include a restriction to the dose and duration of use to help minimise the risk of potentially serious neurological adverse effects. The risk of acute neurological effects is higher in children than in adults (Medicines and Healthcare products Regulatory Agency, 2014).

Serotonin (5-HT3) receptor antagonists

Serotonin receptor antagonists act upon receptors found within the vagus nerve, certain areas of the brain and the GI tract. These antagonists are the gold standard in controlling nausea and vomiting produced by chemotherapy; they can stop symptoms in up to 70% of people and reduce symptoms in the remaining 30% (NICE, 2016). Like D2 receptor antagonists, 5-HT3 receptor antagonists are ineffective in controlling motion sickness (Muth and Elkins, 2007).

Peptic ulcers

The phrase 'peptic ulcer' is used to describe any ulcer that develops in the stomach, duodenum or oseophagus (NHS, 2018). Ulcers form when there is an imbalance between the mucus layer (which protects the mucosa) and acid secretion (aids with digestion of proteins); where excessive acid is produced in combination with a reduction in mucus, erosion of the mucosa can occur and peptic ulcers can form (Neal, 2015). See Figure 14.2 for the common sites of peptic ulcer.

Factors that can cause this imbalance include:

- *Helicobacter pylori* infections
- long-term use of non-steroidal anti-inflammatory drugs
- in rare circumstances, tumours (both cancerous and non-cancerous) of the stomach or duodenum (National Institute of Diabetes and Digestive and Kidney Diseases, 2014).

Helicobacter pylori infections

Helicobacter pylori is a gram-negative rod found deep within the mucosal layer where a pH level of 7.0 is optimal for its growth. The bacteria can invade the cells of the mucosa, causing damage and reducing the production of the protective mucus layer. *H. pylori* can persist for years without treatment, and is associated with an increase in gastrin and thus stomach acid which further causes an imbalance between the damaging processes and the protective factors. Over half of the world's population is colonised with *H. pylori* and unless treated, it is likely to persist for life (Kusters et al., 2006).

If a patient tests positive for *H. pylori* then a trio of medications will be prescribed to eliminate the ulcer and the bacteria. These include a proton pump inhibitor (PPI) (e.g. lansoprazole or omeprazole) that will be used to try to reduce the amount of acid produced. Additionally, the antibiotic amoxicillin, alongside a further antibiotic such as metronidazole or clarithromycin, will be administered to further assist with healing of the damaged mucosa (BNF, 2020). Studies have suggested that due to antibiotic resistance, the efficacy of triple therapy is decreasing and new therapies are required (Fiorini et al., 2012).

The third medication that will probably be prescribed is an H2-receptor antagonist such as ranitidine. Similarly to the PPI, this is used to reduce the amount of acid the stomach produces. As well as this trio of medications, a further antacid such as aluminium hydroxide gel, calcium carbonate

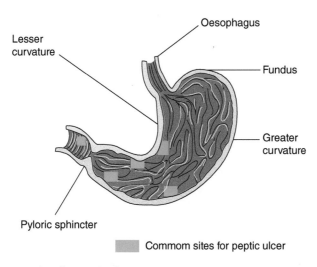

Figure 14.2   Common sites for peptic ulcer.

or magnesium hydroxide may be useful in the management of symptoms such as pain that may present with diarrhoea, stomach cramping and/or flatulence (NHS, 2018).

Non-steroidal anti-inflammatory drugs

There are several ways in which NSAIDs can damage the gastroduodenal mucosa. They can reduce the positive barrier properties of the mucus, suppress gastric prostaglandin synthesis (gastric prostaglandins help protect the mucosa) and interfere with the natural repair of mucosal injury.

Treatment for peptic ulcers not linked to *H. pylori* does not need an antibiotic. A H2-receptor antagonist such as ranitidine/cimetidine/famotidine is usually sufficient in promoting ulcer healing. Therefore, H2-receptor antagonists are often given prophylactically to prevent gastrointestinal complications.

Antacids are not commonly prescribed or encouraged as they only manage symptoms and do not eradicate the ulcer, although they can be given for symptom management.

Symptoms of peptic ulcer

Patients are most likely to present to a paramedic with a dull ache or burning sensation in their stomach, but this pain can be located anywhere between the umbilicus and sternum. This fact alone may mean that many patients are presented as having cardiac chest pain.

Common factors associated with the presentation of peptic ulcers include:

- the pain presenting frequently when the stomach is empty
- worsening over weeks or months
- discomfort fades temporarily after ingesting antacids.

In more serious cases a patient might present to the paramedic with a GI bleed. Approximately 50% of all GI bleeds are caused by gastric ulcers (Pirastehfar et al., 2010); it is likely that they will present with either coffee-ground vomiting or haematemesis.

Clinical consideration: Presentation of haematemesis

Ultan is a 26-year-old male. He is normally fit and well and takes no regular medication. He has felt nauseated for the last few days and has today vomited a small amount of what looked like coffee-ground vomit. His partner phoned 111 and an ambulance was dispatched to him.

Upon arrival you find a well-looking man. His observations are all within normal range. His abdominal exam is otherwise normal. He has some tenderness over his epigastria. He reports his bowels have been normal and daily. He has no other symptoms. He reports that he is prescribed no medication.

What further history or exam would be appropriate?

When questioned further, Ultan states that he has been training far harder than he normally does at the gym in anticipation for a triathlon he is due to compete in. He has found it increasingly hard to concentrate at work due to aches and pains post workout. He has been taking ibuprofen to combat this which has worked very well. He has been taking his full daily dose for around 3 weeks now.

What do you think is the likely cause of his haematemesis and abdominal pain? He is probably suffering with a peptic ulcer as a side-effect of his use of NSAIDs.

What would your next steps be for this patient?

Explain to the patient the risks with taking NSAIDs long term and advise that he stops.

If he is well, he can be followed up by his GP.

Constipation

Constipation is defined as bowel movements that are less frequent (less than every other day) or those that are hard, dry or lumpy to pass. Symptoms may include pain, bloating or the feeling of incomplete evacuation, nausea and abdominal discomfort (National Institute of Diabetes and Digestive and Kidney Diseases, 2018).

Constipation is ubiquitous; one study found up to 90% prevalence in patients on regular opioid medication (Canadian Agency for Drugs and Technologies in Health, 2014) whilst in the UK around 20% of adults complain of constipation. In the US, constipation accounts for 5.3 million prescriptions annually (National Institute of Diabetes and Digestive and Kidney Disease, 2014). Bowel habits can vary considerably in frequency without doing harm. Some people erroneously consider themselves constipated if they do not have a bowel movement each day, but this is not the case (NICE, 2020b).

Whilst most episodes of constipation will generally resolve with self-help, medication or a combination of both, constipation can be indicative of or the result of other health conditions.

Laxatives

Laxatives come as four predominantly different types of drugs. *Bulk-forming* laxatives work by increasing the 'bulk' or weight of faeces, which in turn stimulates the bowel; these include Fybogel (ispaghula husk) and methylcellulose. *Osmotic* laxatives draw water from the rest of the body into the bowel to soften faeces, making them easier to pass; the most common is lactulose. *Stimulant* laxatives stimulate the muscles that line the gut, helping them to move faeces along to the rectum; these include drugs such as bisacodyl and senna. Finally, *softener* laxatives work by letting water into faeces to soften it, making it easier to pass (NHS, 2019).

It is important for paramedics to consider abuse of these medications. A high index of suspicion should be considered with patients suffering from bulimia nervosa or anorexia. Medical complications of laxative abuse are often a result of chronic diarrhoea and the associated severe electrolyte disturbances. Potassium is the primary electrolyte in stool water. Patients may develop hypokalaemia, they may present with generalized muscle weakness, lassitude, skeletal muscle paralysis or rhabdomyolysis with renal impairment, and nerve palsies. More severe hypokalaemia can result in cardiac arrhythmias with an increased risk of sudden death (Roerig et al., 2010).

Bulk-forming laxatives

These work by increasing the 'bulk' or weight of faeces, which in turn stimulates the bowel. They are of particular value in adults with small hard stools if fibre cannot be increased in the diet. Symptoms of flatulence, bloating and cramping may be exacerbated. Adequate fluid intake must be maintained to avoid intestinal obstruction. Examples of these are Fybogel (ispaghula husk) and methylcellulose (BNF, 2020).

Osmotic laxatives

These agents increase the amount of water in the large bowel, either by drawing fluid from the body into the bowel or by retaining the fluid they were administered with. Lactulose is a semisynthetic disaccharide which is not absorbed from the GI tract. It produces an osmotic diarrhoea of low faecal pH and discourages the proliferation of ammonia-producing organisms. It is therefore useful in the treatment of hepatic encephalopathy. Macrogols (such as macrogol 3350 with potassium chloride, sodium bicarbonate and sodium chloride) are inert polymers of ethylene glycol which sequester fluid in the bowel; giving fluid with macrogols may reduce the dehydrating effect sometimes seen with osmotic laxatives (BNF, 2020).

Stimulant laxatives

These increase intestinal motility and often cause abdominal cramp; manufacturer advice is that they should be avoided in intestinal obstruction. The use of co-danthramer and co-danthrusate is limited to constipation in terminally ill patients because of potential carcinogenicity (based on animal studies) and evidence of genotoxicity.

Docusate sodium is believed to act as both a stimulant laxative and a faecal softener. Glycerol suppositories act as a lubricant and a rectal stimulant by virtue of the mildly

irritant action of glycerol, stimulating the muscles that line the gut, helping to move faeces forward to the rectum.

Stimulant laxatives include bisacodyl, sodium picosulfate and members of the anthraquinone group (senna, co-danthramer and co-danthrusate) (NICE, 2017).

Softener laxatives

These act by decreasing surface tension and increasing penetration of intestinal fluid into the faecal mass. Docusate sodium and glycerol suppositories have softening properties. Enemas containing arachis oil (groundnut oil, peanut oil) lubricate and soften impacted faeces and promote a bowel movement. Liquid paraffin has also been used as a lubricant for the passage of stools but manufacturer advice is that it should be used with caution because of its adverse effects, which include anal seepage and the risks of granulomatous disease of the GI tract or of lipoid pneumonia on aspiration (NICE, 2020a).

Again, it is important for paramedics to consider the abuse of these medications. A high index of suspicion should be considered with patients with bulimia nervosa or anorexia. Medical complications of laxative abuse are often a result of chronic diarrhoea and the associated severe electrolyte disturbances. Potassium is the primary electrolyte in stool water. Patients may develop hypokalaemia; they may present with generalised muscle weakness, lassitude, skeletal muscle paralysis, or rhabdomyolysis with renal impairment, and nerve palsies. More severe hypokalaemia can result in cardiac arrhythmias with an increased risk of sudden death (Roerig et al., 2010).

Episode of care: constipation

Derek, a 72-year-old male, lives alone since his wife died a year ago. She was the cook in the house and while he states he gets by, he feels now there is little point in cooking meals for just one person. His daughter who lives close by prepares him a home-cooked meal once a week. In between these times, Derek finds himself eating fast and convenience food. Derek fell 2 months ago and while he was not injured, he admits this has affected his confidence. He now finds he sits and watches television more than tending to the garden like he used to. He has developed gradually increasing, generalised abdominal pain and feels bloated more frequently. Due to being increasingly worried about this and unable to acquire a GP appointment, he called 111 which has dispatched an ambulance with the provisional diagnosis of dissecting aorta.

On arrival of the crew, Derek answers the door and looks well. The crew discuss his presentation and find out the information above. The paramedic discovers that his weekly bowel movements have reduced from 5–7 to three episodes and he often finds it difficult to pass motions.

During physical examination, the paramedic finds nothing of concern. The indicated observations are within normal ranges. Derek's current pain score is 3/10.

The paramedic notes this is probably chronic constipation as it has been ongoing for a few months now and that it may be exacerbated by poor diet and a more sedentary lifestyle. Derek has little medical history, he takes an antihypertensive and he had a dose of antibiotics for a urinary tract infection (UTI) around the time he was bereaved. He is fully independent at home but is showing signs of slowing since his fall.

There is no familial history of bowel cancer. Nevertheless, it is noted by the paramedic that this is a change in bowel habit for a patient over the age of 60 years and therefore he is indicated for NHS bowel screening. This is discussed with the patient who can self-refer to this service; however, Derek is not the best on computers so it is suggested that his daughter assist him with this.

It is discussed with Derek that there are many things he can do to help with his constipation.

Initially, secondary causes should be considered, particularly organic issues in a patient of this age, including but not limited to diabetes mellitus, strictures, haemorrhoids and hypothyroidism. These would need to be considered by the GP so referral to them is important. Derek has not started any new medication since this presentation so that can be excluded.

Lifestyle measures are then discussed with Derek as this may be the biggest cause of his consti-pation. He is advised to gradually increase his fibre intake and eat fruits high in sorbitol and to aim to drink 1500 mL of water daily which will have the added benefit of preventing UTIs. Upon discuss-ing this, it is again highlighted that Derek used to enjoy his garden and that he would grow many of his own vegetables. The paramedic feels it would be a good idea to arrange for a falls prevention team to visit the property to see if they can offer some aids to facilitate safer movement and allow Derek to enjoy his garden again. The paramedic also discussed this with Derek's daughter who states she may start to cook more frequently for him or assist him with his shopping to enable a better diet.

The paramedic discusses worsening advice with Derek and states that if his conditions get worse or do not resolve within a certain time frame after making these changes, he should report back to his GP. His GP is also notified regarding the bowel habit change.

Episode of care: suspected bowel perforation

Tamwar is a 55-year-old man. He saw his GP 10 days ago due to difficulty passing bowel motions. He was started on laxatives. Since then, he has still not passed a significant bowel motion. This afternoon he developed a sudden onset of abdominal pain. His wife called 999.

Upon arrival, the paramedic notes Tamwar is shouting out in pain. He is very pale, tachycardic, tachypnoeic, hypotensive and has a temperature of 39.0 °C. He is GCS 15 but the pain inhibits him from discussing his situation in detail to allow full assessment.

Abdominal assessment is difficult as the patient will not allow the paramedic to touch his abdomen. His abdomen is hard, the pain is predominantly in the left lower quadrant and there are no bowel sounds.

Typically bowel perforation results from insult or injury to the mucosa of the bowel wall resulting from rupture of the closed system. This then exposes the peritoneal cavity to gastrointestinal contents. Bowel perforation can be most commonly attributed to obstruction, trauma, invasive surgery or infec-tion as well as many other less frequent causes.

Red flags are difficult to determine as presentations can differ. Nevertheless, patients who pre-sent with abdominal pain and distension, especially with a pertinent history, should be assessed thoroughly as delayed diagnosis carries a high mortality rate. Even when appropriately managed, mortality is up to 70% when secondary complications such as peritonitis are present (Jones et al., 2020).

Gastro-oesophageal reflux disease

Gastro-oesophageal reflux disease (GORD) is a common condition, where acid from the stomach leaks up into the oesophagus. It usually occurs as a result of the ring of muscle at the bottom of the oesophagus becoming weakened. GORD causes symptoms such as heartburn and an unpleasant taste in the back of the mouth. It may just be an occasional nuisance for some people, but for others it can be a severe, lifelong problem. GORD can often be controlled with self-help measures but on occasion, medication may need to be prescribed. In very rare cases patients may require surgery (NHS Inform, 2020).

Current NICE guidance is to first request patients to change behaviours that may exacerbate the condition. For example, changing eating patterns/times, smoking cessation and raising the head of the bed when sleeping may help reduce or cure symptoms.

There are a number of drugs that can be a cause or a contributing factor to GORD, namely alpha-blockers, anticholinergics, benzodiazepines, beta-blockers, bisphosphonates, calcium channel blockers, corticosteroids, non-steroidal anti-inflammatory drugs (NSAIDs), nitrates, theophyllines and tricyclic antidepressants (NICE, 2019).

Drug interventions (patients with confirmed endoscope diagnosis)

Proton pump inhibitor

Proton pump inhibitors work by irreversibly inhibiting gastric H+K+ ATPase (the proton pump) in the stomach. They inhibit both basal and stimulated acid secretion (Therapeutics Initiative, 2016). In recent years there has been significant media coverage regarding the side-effects of PPIs and they have been linked to stomach cancer and an increased risk of hip fracture. It may be important for paramedics to consider if patients are indeed compliant with their prescribed PPI medication (NHS, 2017).

Examples of PPIs include omeprazole, lansoprazole, pantoprazole, rabeprazole, esomeprazole and dexlansoprazole.

Prokinetic/promotility/gastrointestinal stimulants (GIS)

These are drugs that increase motility of the gastrointestinal smooth muscle, without acting as a purgative. These drugs have different mechanisms of action but they all work to move the contents of the GI tract faster. They also decrease the reflux of stomach acid by strengthening the muscle of the lower oesophageal sphincter (International Foundation of Gastrointenstinal Disorders, 2018).

Examples of GIS medications include metoclopramide and domperidone (both are also commonly prescribed as antiemetics).

Sometimes an H2 antagonist (H2Ras) may be prescribed to GORD patients who are not responding to an initial dose of PPI. However, this is rare and this medication is discussed later under peptic ulcers.

Paramedic practice

While paramedics will encounter patients presenting with GORD, they are generally attending because the patient is experiencing chest pain. While differentiating between GORD and cardiac chest pain is beyond the scope of this chapter, it is best to be cautious. Chest pain should not be assumed to be gastric related.

Clinical consideration: chest pain mimics

There are many conditions which can cause chest pain. A presentation of GORD may be suggestive if it starts after eating, bringing up food or bitter-tasting fluids, feeling full and bloated.

A sprain or strain may be indicative if the pain starts after chest injury or chest exercise, and feels better when resting.

An anxiety- or hyperventilation-related pain may be indicated if the pain is triggered by worries or a stressful situation, heartbeat gets faster and sweating and dizziness occur.

The pain may be of respiratory origin if it gets worse when the patient breathes in and out, is coughing up yellow or green mucus, and has a high temperature.

The cause of the pain may be shingles if there is a tingling feeling on the skin, or a skin rash appears that turns into blisters.

Despite this, other risk factors should also be considered such as smoking status, obesity, hypertension, hypercholesterolaemia, age over 60 years and/or a history of myocardial infarction or failure, as well as familial history (NHS, 2020).

See Table 14.1 for a comparison of cardiac-related chest pain and gastric-related chest discomfort.

Table 14.1 Comparison of cardiac-related chest pain and gastric-related chest discomfort. Source: Adapted from Harvard Health Publishing (2018).

Common symptoms of cardiac-related chest pain	Common symptoms of gastric-related chest discomfort
Tightness, pressure, squeezing, stabbing or dull pain, most often in the centre of the chest	Burning chest pain that begins at the sternum
Pain that spreads to the shoulders, neck or arms	Pain that moves up toward the throat but doesn't typically radiate to shoulders, neck or arms
Irregular or rapid heartbeat	Sensation that food is coming back into the mouth
Cold, sweaty or clammy skin	Bitter or acidic taste at the back of the throat
Light-headedness, weakness or dizziness	Pain that worsens when the person lies down or bends over
Shortness of breath	The appearance of symptoms after a large or spicy meal
Nausea, indigestion and sometimes vomiting	
The appearance of symptoms with physical exertion or extreme stress	

Reflection

Over 16% of all ambulance conveyances to the emergency department (ED) are directly related to chest pain (Pedersen et al., 2019). Take some time and write some notes about a patient you have transported to the ED who might have been experiencing chest pain mimic. Are there any other questions you would have asked that patient?

Could you have changed your treatment plan?

Remember to adhere to all the rules of confidentiality when writing anything that includes patient information.

Clinical consideration: assessing diarrhoea

Diarrhoea is the passage of three or more loose or liquid stools per day (or more frequently than is normal for the individual).

- Acute diarrhoea is defined as lasting less than 14 days.
- Persistent diarrhoea is defined as lasting more than 14 days.
- Chronic diarrhoea is defined as lasting for more than 4 weeks.

Acute diarrhoea is usually caused by a bacterial or viral infection. Other causes include drugs, anxiety, food allergy and acute appendicitis.

Dehydration increases the risk of life-threatening illness and death, particularly in young infants and children, and older people. For this reason, care should be taken when assessing these patients, particularly in the presence of abdominal pain. Thorough assessment including hydration status should be considered. Red flags for dehydration include weakness, confusion, tachycardia, profound hypotension and oliguria/anuria.

Arrange *emergency admission to hospital* if:

- the person is vomiting and unable to retain oral fluids, or
- they have features of severe dehydration or shock (for more information, see clinical features of dehydration).

Other factors that influence the threshold for admission include (use clinical judgement):

- older age (people 60 years of age or older are more at risk of complications)
- home circumstances and level of support
- fever
- bloody diarrhoea
- abdominal pain and tenderness
- increased risk of poor outcome, for example:
  - coexisting medical conditions – immunodeficiency, lack of stomach acid, inflammatory bowel disease, valvular heart disease, diabetes mellitus, renal impairment, rheumatoid disease, systemic lupus erythematosus
  - drugs – immunosuppressants or systemic steroids, proton pump inhibitors, angiotensin-converting enzyme inhibitors, diuretics.

Adapted from NICE (2018).

Antidiarrhoeals

Antimotility agents are the class of drugs used for the management of diarrhoea. These agents act by modulating intestinal contractions and reducing frequency of bowel movements. The most effective antimotility agents are synthetic opiates, diphenoxylate with atropine (Lomotil®) and loperamide (Imodium®). Historically, opiates such as paregoric, tincture of opium and codeine were noted to be effective in the short-term treatment of diarrhoea, but their effects on the central nervous system and potential for drug dependency limited their use (Keystone, 2008).

Loperamide is the most commonly prescribed antimotility agent worldwide. In 2013, loperamide was added to the list of essential medications by the World Health Organization (WHO, 2014). Loperamide may be prescribed to patients who have a colostomy, Crohn's disease, ulcerative colitis and other common conditions such as irritable bowel syndrome (NHS, 2008).

Paramedics should consider that loperamide is an opioid medication and patients can develop dependency (Zarghami and Rezapour, 2017). It also has serious adverse effects and patients abusing the drug or those having overdosed can present with severe cardiotoxicity. Profound electrocardiogram (ECG) abnormalities (sinus bradycardia, wide QRS, prolonged PR interval, markedly prolonged QTc, Brugada-like ECG pattern), malignant ventricular arrhythmias and ventricular dysfunction have all been reported (Kohli et al., 2019).

Skills in practice: assessing bowel sounds

Auscultation of the bowel sounds is performed to detect altered bowel sound, vascular bruits or rubs. Peristalsis (the involuntary constriction and relaxation of the intestinal muscles) creates bowel sounds that might be altered or completely absent in the presence of disease or obstruction. This should be done before palpation as this may compromise assessment due to the palpation causing bowel sounds.

The patient should be positioned in a comfortable supine position lying at around 45°. Using a warmed stethoscope, the examiner should listen to multiple areas across the abdominal wall for several minutes. The stethoscope should be applied with a firm pressure, ensuring minimal discomfort is caused.

When bowel sounds are not clearly heard, the examiner should listen for a full 3 minutes to ensure that they are in fact, absent. Remember that the thickness of the abdominal wall may affect auscultation, and so the bowel sounds of an obese patient or a patient with ascites may be more difficult to hear.

Common causes of absent bowel sounds include:

- partial or complete blockage of the bowels
- strangulation of the bowel
- peritonitis.

Inflammatory bowel disease (IBD)

The cause of inflammatory bowel disease (IBD) remains unknown, but increasing evidence suggests that these conditions, like many chronic inflammatory disorders, involve immune-mediated tissue damage due to a variable interaction amongst genetic factors and environmental triggers. IBD is the collective term for the conditions that include Crohn's disease and ulcerative colitis (Rampton, 2008).

Crohn's disease

Crohn's disease is a chronic disease of the gastrointestinal tract with symptoms evolving in a relapsing and remitting manner. It is also a progressive disease that leads to bowel damage and disability. All segments of the GI tract can be affected, the most common being the terminal ileum and colon. Inflammation is typically segmental, asymmetrical and transmural. Most patients present with an inflammatory phenotype at diagnosis, but over time complications (strictures, fistulas, abscesses) will develop in half of patients, often resulting in surgery (Torres et al., 2017).

Ulcerative colitis

Patients with ulcerative colitis have mucosal inflammation starting in the rectum that can extend continuously to proximal segments of the colon. It usually presents with bloody diarrhoea and is diagnosed by colonoscopy and histological findings. The management is to induce and then maintain remission, defined as resolution of symptoms and endoscopic healing. Some patients can require colectomy for medically refractory disease or to treat colonic neoplasia (Ungaro et al., 2017).

255

Drug treatment for inflammatory bowel disease

There is currently no cure for IBD. Around 1 in 5 patients with ulcerative colitis will require surgery and as many as 3 in 4 patients with Crohn's disease may require surgery. Nevertheless, there are drugs that can help manage symptoms. These come under four main categories (NHS, 2020).

Aminosalicylates (5-ASAS)

These include sulfasalazine, mesalazine, Pentasa®, Mezavant® and olsalazine. These drugs contain 5-aminosalicylic acid, which is called 5-ASA for short. 5-ASA can help to reduce inflammation in the digestive tract by working directly on the lining of the bowel. 5-ASA drugs are chemically related to aspirin and work by reducing inflammation, allowing damaged tissue to heal. These are mainly used in the treatment of ulcerative colitis (Crohn's and Colitis UK, 2018).

Immunosuppressants

Immunosuppressants include adalimumab, azathioprine, golimumab, infliximab, methotrexate, steroids, tofacitinib and Entocort®.

Immunosuppressive drugs suppress actions of the immune system and its inflammatory response. These drugs are useful for very active IBD that does not respond to standard therapy and help maintain remission. An immunosuppressant is often combined with a steroid to speed up response during active disease (Gionchetti et al., 2017).

Corticosteroids

Corticosteroids such as prednisolone can be used with or instead of 5-ASAs to treat a flare-up if 5-ASAs alone are not effective. Like 5-ASAs, steroids can be administered orally or via a suppository or enema. Corticosteroids are not used as a long-term treatment to maintain remission because they can cause potentially serious side-effects such as osteoporosis and cataracts (NHS, 2020).

Biologic medicines (infliximab, adalimumab, golimumab and vedolizumab)

These drugs reduce inflammation of the intestine by targeting proteins the immune system uses to stimulate inflammation. These medicines block these receptors and reduce inflammation. They may be used to treat adults with moderate to severe ulcerative colitis if other options are not suitable or not working (NHS, 2020). It is useful for paramedics to have a generalised understanding of the above conditions. At times, patients with IBD may need hospitalisation and it would be sensible to discuss such patients with a general practitioner or other healthcare professional who may be more versed in these specific conditions. As a general rule, patients with IBD who have not responded to oral corticosteroid-based therapy as outpatients usually have to be admitted to hospital for inpatient supervised care (Baidoo, 2017).

Skills in practice: how to assess dehydration

Dehydration is common, specifically in the older person. There is a strong correlation between dehydration and increased mortality. The make-up of babies is 70% water. By the time patients are over the age of 65, years this has reduced to 50%. With age comes a decreasing sense of thirst and a reduced ability for the body to concentrate urine; this, coupled with a reduction in mobility, can mean that dehydration is a very real problem and one that paramedics should be investigating in the prehospital setting.

In hospital, a blood sample and measuring serum osmolality can show dehydration. However, this is not possible prehospital so a non-invasive alternative must be used.

First, it is important to consider risk factors for dehydration.

- Increasing age (Stookey, 2005; Warren et al., 1994)
- Gender – women are more at risk than men (Stookey, 2005; Stookey et al, 2005; Warren et al., 1994)
- Ethnicity – Afro-Caribbean Americans are at greater risk than white Americans (Stookey, 2005; Lancaster et al., 2003; Warren et al., 1994).

Second, it is important to consider that specific long-term conditions may cause certain patients to be at increased risk of dehydration

- Diabetes (Stookey et al., 2005)
- Hypertension (Stookey et al., 2005)
- Obesity (Stookey et al., 2005)
- Oral problems (Dyck, 2004)
- Functional limitations (Stookey et al., 2005)
- Dementia (Albert et al., 1989).

Non-invasive tests that may be done prehospital have little evidence to prove them as effective, therefore it would appear sensible for this advice to be seen as a guide only.

Simple observations such as orthostatic hypotension, increased heart rate and increased temperature may all be signs of patients at risk of dehydration.

paramedics should ask questions such as: do you have a headache; do your muscles feel weak; do you feel dizzy and or sick; does your mouth feel dry; do you feel thirsty?

Further to this, physical signs can also indicate dehydration, including increased skin turgor tested at various sites (often the back of the hand), although this may be non-specific due to the ageing process of skin, increased capillary refill time, a fissured and/or dry tongue and oral mucosa as well as a dry underarm. Also, dark urine colour and reduced urine output may also be signs of dehydration.

Whilst no single sign may completely rule out dehydration, a holistic approach should be considered to determine the likelihood of dehydration.

The following is a list of common conditions associated with patients who have GI disorders. Patients suffering with these disorders might present frequently to the ambulance service and having a deeper understanding of the condition and treatment pathways will allow you to offer optimal care to your patient.

Take some time to research and reflect on these conditions, possibly by thinking of patients you have treated who might have been suffering from them. Be detailed, look at the pharmacokinetics and pharmacodynamics and remember to look at all aspects of patient care.

Remember, though, if reflecting on specific patients, you must adhere to the rules of confidentiality.

Condition	Your notes
Barrett oesophagus	
Crohn's disease	
Gastro-oesophageal reflux disease	
Diverticulitis	

Conclusion

This chapter has provided an overview of common disorders within the gastrointestinal system and the medications used to treat them. Evidence has been provided for the use of each drug along with an understanding of the pharmacokinetics and pharmacodynamics, as well as considerations for administration and common adverse effects. Wider issues have been covered including patient management, non-pharmacological interventions relevant to paramedic practice and self-care.

References

Albert, S.G., Nakra, B.R., Grossberg, G.T. and Caminal, E.R. (1989). Vasopressin response to dehydration in Alzheimer's disease. *Journal of the American Geriatric Society* **37**(9):843–847.

Baidoo, L. (2017). Management of hospitalized patients with ulcerative colitis. *Gastroenterology and Hepatology* **13**(3): 180–183.

Blackmore, T. (2020). *Palliative and End of Life Care for Paramedics*. Bridgwater: Class Professional Publishing.

Brady, W.J., Lipinski, M.J., Darby, A. et al. (2020). *Electrocardiogram in Clinical Medicine*. Chichester: Wiley Blackwell.

British National Formulary (BNF). (2020). https://bnf.nice.org.uk/medicinal-forms/ispaghula-husk.html

Bruneau, E. (2017), Basic anatomy and physiology of the gastrointestinal tract. In: *Passing the Certified Bariatric Nurses Exam* (eds A. Loveitt, M. Martin and M. Neff). Chan: Springer.

Canadian Agency for Drugs and Technologies in Health. (2014). *Dioctyl sulfosuccinate or docusate (calcium or sodium) for the prevention or management of constipation: a review of the clinical effectiveness*. www.ncbi.nlm.nih.gov/books/NBK259243/

Crohn's and Colitis UK. (2018). *Aminosalicylates (5-ASAS)*. http://s3-eu-west-1.amazonaws.com/files.crohnsandcolitis.org.uk/Publications/5-ASAs.pdf

Dyck, M.J. (2004). Nursing staffing and resident outcomes in nursing homes. PhD thesis. Graduate College, University of Iowa.

Fiorini, G., Zullo, A., Gatta, L. et al. (2012). Newer agents for Helicobacter pylori eradication. *Clinical and Experimental Gastroenterology* **5**: 109–112.

Gionchetti, P., Rizzello, F., Annese, V. and Ardizzone, S. (2017). Use of corticosteroids and immunosuppressive drugs in inflammatory bowel disease: clinical practice guidelines of the Italian Group for the Study of Inflammatory Bowel Disease. *Digestive and Liver Disease* **49**(6): 604–617.

Harvard Health Publishing. (2018). *Heartburn vs. heart attack*. www.health.harvard.edu/heart-health/heartburn-vs-heart-attack

International Foundation of Gastrointestinal Disorders. (2018). *Medications*. https://aboutgastroparesis.org/medications.html

Jones, M.W., Kashyap, S. and Zabbo, C.P. (2020). *Bowel Perforation*. Treasure Island: StatPearls Publishing. www.ncbi.nlm.nih.gov/books/NBK537224/

Keystone, J.S. (2018). *Travel Medicine*, 4th edn. St Louis: Mosby Elsevier.

Kohli, U., Altujjar, M., Sharma, R. and Hassan, S. (2019). Wide interindividual variability in cardiovascular toxicity of loperamide: a case report and review of literature. *Heart Rhythm Case Reports* **5**(4): 221–224.

Kusters, J.G., Vliet, A.H.M.V. and Kuipers, E.J. (2006). Pathogenesis of Helicobacter pylori infection. *Clinical Microbiology Reviews* **19**(3), 449–490.

Lancaster, K.J., Smiciklas-Wright, H., Heller, D.A. et al. (2003). Dehydration in black and white older adults using diuretics. *Annals of Epidemiology* **13**(7): 525–529.

Medicines and Healthcare products Regulatory Agency. (2014). *Metoclopramide: risk of neurological adverse effects*. www.gov.uk/drug-safety-update/metoclopramide-risk-of-neurological-adverse-effects

Muth, E.R. and Elkins, A.N. (2007). High dose ondansetron for reducing motion sickness in highly susceptible subjects. *Aviation, Space and Environmental Medicine* **78**(7): 686–692.

National Health Service (NHS). (2008). *Loperamide*. www.nhs.uk/medicines/loperamide/

National Health Service (NHS). (2017). *Acid reflux drugs linked to increased stomach cancer risk*. www.nhs.uk/news/cancer/acid-reflux-drugs-linked-increased-stomach-cancer-risk

National Health Service (NHS). (2018). *Stomach ulcer*. www.nhs.uk/conditions/stomach-ulcer

National Health Service (NHS). (2019). *Laxatives*. www.nhs.uk/conditions/laxatives/

National Health Service (NHS). (2020). *Inflammatory bowel disease*. www.nhs.uk/conditions/inflammatory-bowel-disease/

National Health Service (NHS) Inform (2020). *Gastro-oesophageal reflux disease (GORD)*. www.nhsinform.scot/illnesses-and-conditions/stomach-liver-and-gastrointestinal-tract/gastro-oesophageal-reflux-disease-gord

National Institute of Diabetes and Digestive and Kidney Diseases. (2014). *Peptic ulcers: facts and figures*. www.niddk.nih.gov/health-information/digestive-diseases/peptic-ulcers-stomach-ulcers/definition-facts.

National Institute of Diabetes and Digestive and Kidney Diseases. (2018). *Constipation*. www.niddk.nih.gov/health-information/digestive-diseases/constipation/all-content#section1

National Institute for Health and Care Excellence (NICE). (2016). *Prevention of chemotherapy induced nausea and vomiting in adults: netupitant/palonosetron*. www.nice.org.uk/advice/esnm69/resources/prevention-of-chemotherapy-induced-nausea-and-vomiting-in-adults-netupitantpalonosetron-pdf-1502681113620421

National Institute for Health and Care Excellence (NICE). (2017) *Constipation in children and young people: diagnosis and management: guidance*. www.nice.org.uk/guidance/cg99/chapter/1-guidance.

National Insitute for Health and Care Excellence (NICE). (2018). *Diarrhoea – adult assessment*. https://cks.nice.org.uk/topics/diarrhoea-adults-assessment

National Institute for Health and Care Excellence (NICE). (2019). *Gastro-oesophageal reflux disease*. https://bnf.nice.org.uk/treatment-summary/gastro-oesophageal-reflux-disease.html

National Institute for Health and Care Excellence (NICE). (2020a). *Nausea and labyrinth disorders*. https://bnf.nice.org.uk/treatment-summary/nausea-and-labyrinth-disorders.html

National Institute for Health and Care Excellence (NICE). (2020b). *Constipation*. https://bnf.nice.org.uk/treatment-summary/constipation.html

Neal, M.J. (2015). *Medical Pharmacology at a Glance*, 8th edn. Oxford: Wiley-Blackwell.

Pedersen, C., Stengaard, C., Friesgaard, K. et al. (2019). Chest pain in the ambulance; prevalence, causes and outcome – a retrospective cohort study. *Scandinavian Journal of Trauma, Resuscitation and Emergency Medicine* **27**(1): 84.

Pirastehfar, M., Kaviani, M., Azari, A. and Saberifiroozi, M. (2010). Etiology and outcome of patients with upper gastrointestinal bleeding: a study from South of Iran. *Saudi Journal of Gastroenterology* **16**(4): 253.

Rampton, D. (2008). *Fast Facts: Inflammatory Bowel Disease*, 3rd edn. Abingdon: Health Press.

Roerig, J., Steffen, K. and Zunker, J. (2010). Laxative abuse: epidemiology, diagnosis and management. *Drugs* **70**(12): 1487–1503.

Stookey, J.D. (2005). High prevalence of plasma hypertonicity among community-dwelling older adults: results from NHANES III. *Journal of the American Dietetic Association* **105**: 1231–1239.

Stookey, J.D., Pieper, C.F. and Cohen, H.J. (2005). Is the prevalence of dehydration among community-dwelling older adults really low? Informing current debate over the fluid recommendation for 70+ adults. *Public Health Nutrition* **8**: 1275–1285.

Therapeutics Initiative. (2016). *Comparative effectiveness of proton pump inhibitors*. www.ti.ubc.ca/2016/06/28/99-comparative-effectiveness-proton-pump-inhibitors/

Torres, J., Mehandru, S., Colombel, J. and Peyrin-Biroulet, L. (2017). Crohn's disease. *Lancet* **389**(10080): 1741–1755.

Ungaro, R., Mehandru, S., Allen, P. et al. (2017). Ulcerative colitis. *Lancet* **389**(10080): 1756–1770.

Warren, J.L., Bacon, W., Harris, T. et al. (1994). The burden and outcomes associated with dehydration among US elderly, 1991. *American Journal of Public Health* **84**(8): 1265–1269.

World Health Organization. (2014). *The Selection and Use of Essential Medicines: Report of the WHO Expert Committee, 2013 (including the 18th WHO model list of essential medicines and the 4th WHO model list of essential medicines for children)* Geneva: World Health Organization.

Zarghami, M. and Rezapour, M. (2017). Loperamide dependency: a case report. *Addiction and Health* **9**(1): 59–63.

Multiple-choice questions

1. An example of a proton pump inhibitor (PPI) is:
   (a) Omeprezole
   (b) Ranitidine

(c) Simvastatin

(d) Gliclazide

2. Peptic ulcer is a term to describe an ulcer found in which areas of the body?

   (a) Stomach, oral cavity, oseophagus

   (b) Oesophagus, stomach, duodenum

   (c) Small intestine, stomach, duodenum

   (d) Anus, large intestine, oral cavity

3. Loperamide is an opioid medication, Paramedics should be aware that in extreme doses it can have severe adverse effects, including:

   (a) Sinus bradycardia

   (b) Prolonged PR

   (c) Wide QRS

   (d) All of the above

4. The most common type of antiemetic used to combat motion sickness is:

   (a) H1 receptor antagonists

   (b) Dopamine D2 antagonists

   (c) Serotonin (5-HT3) antagonists

   (d) H2 receptor antagonists

5. Below what age does metoclopramide become contraindicated in the JRCALC guidelines?

   (a) 18 months

   (b) 21 years

   (c) 18 years

   (d) 12 years

6. Which antacid would you use to treat loose stools?

   (a) Aluminum hydroxide

   (b) Magnesium hydroxide

   (c) Both

   (d) Neither

7. An example of a H1 receptor antagonist antiemetic is:

   (a) Chlorpromazine

   (b) Ondanestron

   (c) Metaclopramide

   (d) Cyclizine

8. Which of these is not a common cause of constipation?

   (a) Becoming less active

   (b) Stress, anxiety, depression

   (c) A new prescription of codeine

   (d) Eating oily foods

9. Chest pain that worsens when the patient lies down or bends over is generally associated with:

   (a) Gastric-related pain

   (b) Cardiac-related pain

   (c) Premenopause

   (d) All of the above

10. Which groups are at increased risk of dehydration secondary to diarrhoea?

    (a) Elderly patients

    (b) Young children

    (c) Certain ethnic minorities

    (d) All of the above

11. Which of these is *not* a common cause of absent bowel sounds?
    (a) Complete blockage of the bowels
    (b) Strangulation of the bowel
    (c) Peritonitis
    (d) Ulcerative colitis

12. Red flags for dehydration include:
    (a) Pyrexia and hypertension
    (b) Profound hypotension, oliguria/anuria
    (c) Weakness, confusion, tachycardia, profound hypotension, oliguria/anuria
    (d) None of the above

13. Risk factors for peptic ulcer include:
    (a) Long-term use of non-steroidal anti-inflammatory drugs
    (b) *Helicobacter pylori* infections
    (c) In rare circumstances, tumours
    (d) All of the above

14. Loperamide is likely to be prescribed to a patient who is complaining of:
    (a) Constipation
    (b) Nausea
    (c) GORD
    (d) None of the above

15. A peptic ulcer is:
    (a) Any ulcer in the stomach, duodenum or esophagus
    (b) Any ulcer in the stomach only
    (c) Any ulcer in the duodenum only
    (d) Any ulcer in the oesophagus only

Chapter 15

Medication and the nervous system

Geoffrey Bench, Alastair Dolan, Lena Solanki, Paul Doherty, Charlotte White, Ricky Lawrence and Emma Beadle

Aim

The aim of the chapter is to provide the reader with an introduction to pharmacology relating to common neurological disorders in the prehospital setting.

Learning outcomes

After reading this chapter the reader will be able to:

1. Explain the most common medications used in the management of Parkinson disease, epilepsy, dementia and strokes
2. Describe the mechanism and side-effects of the drugs used to treat common neurological conditions
3. Discuss the red flags you would consider in relation to medications used in neurological conditions
4. Discuss the treatment and management of patients with common neurological conditions, highlighting any red flags.

Introduction

This chapter will address conditions that affect the nervous system and the medication commonly prescribed for those conditions, and outline the drugs paramedics can administer. It is essential that the student paramedics and paramedics practise within the parameters of local policy and procedure, adhering at all times to their Code of Conduct.

Due to the number of conditions that affect the nervous system, the focus will be on the most common conditions that paramedics encounter in the prehospital setting. Some of the mental

Fundamentals of Pharmacology for Paramedics, First Edition. Edited by Ian Peate, Suzanne Evans, and Lisa Clegg.
© 2022 John Wiley & Sons Ltd. Published 2022 by John Wiley & Sons Ltd.

health conditions that affect the nervous system will be explored in Chapter 16. By the end of this chapter readers will have greater understanding of neurological conditions, how they are managed and the treatments available in everyday paramedic practice to ensure safe and effective care. The conditions included within this chapter are Parkinson disease, dementia, epilepsy and stroke.

The nervous system

The nervous system (NS) is a complex and sophisticated system. It acts as the master controller and communication system of the body (Marieb, 2004). It consists of both the central nervous system (CNS) and the peripheral nervous system (PNS). The CNS contains the brain and spinal cord whereas the PNS is made up of nerves and ganglia. Changes that occur inside and outside the body are detected by the NS and acted upon to control and co-ordinate vital aspects of bodily functions to maintain homeostasis. The NS helps us breathe, regulates blood pressure and heart rate, aids with digestion, allows us to eat, drink, gather new thoughts and skills, etc. The main functions of the NS overlap each other. By using millions of sensory receptors, it gathers information (sensory input), monitors changes that occur both inside and outside the body which in turn elicit a response (motor) by activating effector organs. This occurs by voluntary (involvement of thought) and involuntary control without conscious control (autonomic).

Parkinson disease and parkinsonism

262

Parkinson disease (PD) occurs in all ethnic groups and can be described as idiopathic or having no specific cause. PD has no definite cause but is thought to 'result from a genetically determined vulnerability to particular environmental factors' such as toxins, recreational drug abuse, head trauma and genetic influences (Jones, 2011).

Parkinson disease most commonly affects the elderly and is defined as a progressive neurological disorder of the basal ganglia. Parkinsonian patients show a substantially reduced concentration of dopamine in their basal ganglia; this is due to a continuing degeneration of the dopaminergic neurons of the substantia nigra located in the basal ganglia of the brain (Donizak and McCabe, 2017). The basal ganglia in patients without PD have an effect on voluntary motor control, procedural learning relating to routine behaviours such as eye movement, as well as emotional and cognitive functions.

The number of people diagnosed with PD worldwide is around 10 million; in the UK it is about 145 000 (www.parkinsons.org).

Figure 15.1 shows an image of the brain and the substantia nigra in Parkinson disease.

Although there are numerous causes of parkinsonism, for example cerebral ischaemia, stroke, viral encephalitis or other pathological damage, the most common cause is PD. PD can be characterised by slow initiation of movements, known as bradykinesia, muscle rigidity and tremors. Collectively, these symptoms are known as the 'parkinsonian triad'.

Patients start to show direct symptoms of parkinsonians when more than 80% of the dopaminergic neurons of the substantia nigra have degenerated (Dawson et al., 2002). The terms 'On' and 'Off' are often used by practitioners to describe the different stages of motor variants: the 'On' period where the patient's PD symptoms are under control and the 'Off' period when the symptoms are worsening due to medication ineffectiveness. 'PD is progressive with continued loss of dopaminergic neurons, which in turn leads to worsening of the clinical symptoms. Untreated PD eventually results in dementia and subsequent death' (Dawson et al., 2002).

People with PD may present with characteristic signs which include:

- speech impairments
- inability to perform skilled tasks
- a shuffling gait
- a blank 'mask-like facial expression (Dawson et al., 2002).

The neurotransmitter acetylcholine opposes the dopamine neurotransmitter involved in the co-ordination of motor responses. This is important as many of the therapies against the progression of PD and the loss of motor function are directed at addressing the imbalance between these neurotransmitters. Research suggests that a decline in dopamine levels would increase acetylcholine production and

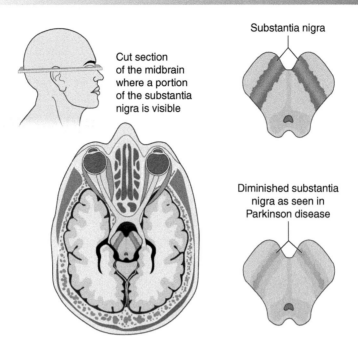

Substantia nigra

Cut section
of the midbrain
where a portion
of the substantia
nigra is visible

Diminished substantia
nigra as seen in
Parkinson disease

Figure 15.1   Parkinson disease and the substantia nigra.

these high levels of acetylcholine are the cause of uncontrolled, involuntary movements known as dyskinesia (Parkinson's News Today, 2019). Drugs taken for treatment of PD increase the amount of dopamine in the brain; they may act as a 'dopamine substitute by stimulating the parts of the brain where dopamine works or block the action of other factors that break down dopamine' (Parkinson's UK, 2019).

Parkinson drugs that paramedics may encounter in the prehospital setting are detailed in Table 15.1.

The potential harms and benefits of PD agents are shown in Table 15.2.

Table 15.1   Drugs used for Parkinson disease.

Drugs	Actions
Levodopa (co-beneldopa and co-careldopa)	Converts to dopamine in the brain
MAO-B inhibitors (rasagiline, selegiline, safinamide)	Enzymes that chemically break down the dopamine within the brain
Dopamine agonists (pramipexole, ropinirole)	Initiate actions of dopamine when levels are low
COMT inhibitors (entacepone, opicapone)	Enzymes that metabolise or degrade neurotransmitters (dopamine)
Amantadine	Increases dopamine release and blocks dopamine reuptake
Anticholinergics (procyclidine, trihexphenidyl)	Block the action of the neurotransmitter acetylcholine inhibiting nerve impulses responsible for involuntary muscle movements and bodily functions
Apomorphine	Dopamine agonist
Rotigotine skin patch (Neupro®)	Dopamine agonist administered through the skin

Source: Based on Inacio P. (2019). Imbalance in dopamine and acetylcholine levels may drive disease progression. https://parkinsonsnewstoday.com/

Table 15.2   Potential benefits and harms of dopamine agonists, levodopa and MAO-B inhibitors.

	Levodopa	Dopamine agonists	Monoamine oxidase B (MAO-B) inhibitors
Motor symptoms	More improvement in motor symptoms	Less improvement in motor symptoms	Less improvement in motor symptoms
Activities of daily living	More improvement in activities of daily living	Less improvement in activities of daily living	Less improvement in activities of daily living
Motor complications	More motor complications	Fewer motor complications	Fewer motor complications
Adverse events (excessive sleepiness, hallucinations and impulse control disorders)	Fewer specified adverse events	More specified adverse events	Fewer specified adverse events

Source: Based on Patricia Inacio PhD. 2019., Imbalance in Dopamine and Acetylcholine levels may drive disease progression, Parkinson's news today.

Episode of care

You are called to attend a 53-year-old male who has suddenly became lethargic and will not respond or does not want to respond to his normal daily living activities. His wife on scene states that he seems extremely fatigued and that this is unusual for him. She states that her husband was diagnosed with Parkinson disease about 2 years ago and that he takes levodopa (co-beneldopa) 100 mg four times a day. On further questioning, the patient's wife states that she had noticed a pungent smell of urine over the last day, when helping her husband dress. The patient has no other significant medical history.

Baseline observations

Pulse	Respiration rate	SpO$_2$	Temperature	Blood glucose	Blood pressure	GCS
85	18	98% on air	38.1°C	5.1mmol/L	105/70	14/15

What are your thoughts?

Underlying causes of lethargy in Parkinson patients can be due to the motor symptoms making the muscles tired but it is important to identify and treat illnesses that are not related to PD. It is important to interpret the baseline observations and take into account any new medications prescribed. Gaining a comprehensive history from a relative or carer, has this happened before? What was the treatment plan? What was the outcome?

What is your plan?

A comprehensive history will allow the clinician to make the correct decision for either transportation to the emergency department or referral to another healthcare practitioner.

Infections

Parkinson patients are prone to bladder infections due to the reduction of muscle control related to their illness and they have a difficult time passing urine. Ineffective emptying of the bladder acts as a breeding ground for bacteria. If the urinary tract infection is not treated, this could lead to a more systemic infection, i.e. sepsis. The patient needs referral to their GP for further investigations and antibiotics if indicated.

Dementia

The word 'dementia' describes over 200 different types of progressive neurological disorders that affect the brain.

As we go through life, the effects of ageing slowly start to affect our lives. We all suffer from memory problems to some degree as we get older. For some people, these early memory problems can indicate a medical condition such as dementia. It is a progressive disease that is irreversible with a decline of cognitive function, behavioural abilities, independent and social living.

Dementia patients can become tired and stressed, making them more anxious, which can lead to depression as well as physical illnesses.

There are a number of factors that can lead to the development of dementia.

- *Genetics:* a person's genetic history is known to have a role in the development of the disease though the effects may differ considerably.
- *Medical history:* people who experience conditions such as multiple sclerosis, Down syndrome, HIV, diabetes and metabolic syndrome are at higher risk of developing dementia.
- *General lifestyle:* sedentary lifestyles and excessive use of drugs or alcohol consumption can increase the risk of developing dementia.
- *Age:* getting older will increase the risk of developing dementia in combination with other conditions such as high blood pressure or those at risk from other diseases such as acute coronary syndrome and cerebrovascular accidents.

Due to an increase of the ageing population, those with dementia worldwide is estimated to be around 50 million, with nearly 10 million new cases each year.

Understanding of dementia and its cause is not clear but is improving, with research into the involvement of a nuclear protein called TDP-43 causing proteinopathy, where certain proteins become structurally abnormal, disrupting cell function. This is associated with hippocampal sclerosis and dementia, known as limbic-predominant age-related TDP-43 encephalopathy or LATE, predominantly found in those 80 and older. TDP-43 protein is also associated with the disease pathology of Alzheimer disease, found in up to 57% of Alzheimer disease patients (Boer et al., 2020).

265

Drugs used in dementia

There are many different types of drugs that may be used to treat the specific symptoms of dementia, such as antipsychotics, antianxiolytics and antidepressants (Table 15.3). The goal of treatment is to maintain current health. The most popular medications are cholinesterase inhibitors and memantine.

Cholinesterase inhibitors work by increasing acetylcholine, a chemical in the brain that aids in memory and judgement. It is believed that this may delay dementia-related symptoms and may even prevent it from worsening.

Table 15.3 Dementia drugs that paramedics may encounter in the prehospital setting.

Drugs	Actions
Donepzil	Inhibits the enzyme function of acetylcholinesterase which breaks down acetylcholine. This allows for higher concentrations of acetylcholine to facilitate communication between the synapses of nerve cells in the brain
Galantamine	Weak acetylcholinesterase inhibitor; binds to the choline binding site, thereby blocking the action of acetylcholinesterase and increasing availability of choline
Rivastigmine	Binds to acetylcholinesterase, making it inactive. This stops acetylcholinesterase from destroying choline, which helps towards increasing levels
Memantine	Not a cholinesterase inhibiter. Blocks the effects of glutamate, which is known to cause excessive stimulation in Alzheimer disease

Source: Based on Drugbank.com. www.alzheimers.org.uk/about-dementia/treatments/drugs/
how-do-drugs-alzheimers-disease-work

Cautions

Cholinesterase inhibitors are known to have significant interactions with a number of comorbidities, as shown in Table 15.4, and also side-effects, shown in Table 15.5.

Table 15.4   Interactions of cholinesterase inhibitors.

Cardiac	Respiratory	Gastrointestinal	Lymphatic	Neurological	Environmental
Coronary artery disease	Asthma	Peptic ulcers	Hepatic dysfunction	Seizures	Alcoholic cirrhosis
Bradycardia	Obstructive pulmonary disease		Thyroid	Epilepsy	
	Effects				
	Constriction of the bronchi	Increase gastric secretions and contractions	Cholinesterase is metabolised by the liver and can lead to hyperthyroidism	Can cause convulsions and tremors	Can cause convulsions and tremors

Source: Based on Drugs.com. (2020). Donepezil Side Effects. www.drugs.com/sfx/donepezil-side-effects.html

Table 15.5   Side-effects of cholinesterase inhibitors: minor, severe and rare.

	Donepezil	Galatamine	Rivastigmine	Memantine
Respiratory	Cough Dry mouth SOB Tachypnoea Wheezing	Dyspnoea SOB Tachypnoea		Dyspnoea
Cardiovascular	Arrhythmia BP Chest pain Dizziness Drowsiness Tachycardia	Arrhythmia Chest pain Dizziness Syncope Tachycardia	AV block Arrhythmia Dizziness Drowsiness HTN Syncope	Dizziness Drowsiness Embolism Heart failure HTN
Abdominal Genitourinary	Appetite loss Constipation Diarrhoea Melaena Nausea Polyuria Vomiting	Decreased urination Diarrhoea Dry mouth Dyspepsia	Abdominal pain Dehydration Diarrhoea Gastric ulcer Hepatitis Incontinence Nausea Pancreatitis UTI Vomiting	Constipation Vomiting
Integumentary	Bleeding Bruising Hives Itching Sweating	Reddening Sunken eyes Sweating	Skin reactions	Fungal infections
Musculoskeletal	Joint pain Muscle cramps Stiffness Swelling Tiredness Tremors Weakness Weight loss	Anorexia Fatigue Tremors Weight loss	Abnormal gait Fatigue Weight loss	Fatigue Impaired balance

(Continued)

Table 15.5 (Continued)

	Donepezil	**Galatamine**	**Rivastigmine**	**Memantine**
Neurological	Aggression Agitation Blurred vision Burning sensations Delusion Depression Headache Mood changes Nightmares Restlessness	Blurred vision Confusion	Anxiety Confusion Depression Hallucinations Headache Insomnia Nightmares Parkinsonism Seizure Tremor	Confusion Hallucinations Seizures

AV, atrioventricular; BP, blood pressure; HTN, hypertension; SOB, shortness of breath; UTI, urinary tract infection.

Epilepsy

Epilepsy is a neurological condition which is characterised by at least one of the following.

- Two or more unprovoked seizures occurring more than 24 hours apart.
- One unprovoked seizure and a probability of further seizures after two unprovoked seizures, occurring over the next 10 years.
- Diagnosis of an epilepsy syndrome (NICE, 2019).

Epilepsy and status epilepticus are connected to excessive activation of excitatory neurons or a reduction of inhibitory neurotransmission (Jones-Davis and MacDonald, 2003). Epilepsy is not an illness or disease, it is a controllable neurological condition managed with antiepileptic drugs (AEDs). Alternative management can be surgery, when optimal management cannot be achieved.

There are over 40 different presentations of seizures which include focal, focal aware, tonic, absence, myoclonic and tonic clonic. Seizures occur due to sudden, spontaneous uncontrolled depolarisation of neurons, as a result of excessive excitation or loss of normal inhibitory mechanisms. This depolarisation causes abnormal sensory or motor activity and possible unconsciousness.

In essence, the origin of seizures is a malfunction of the ion (sodium, potassium, calcium) channels. Neurotransmitters travel across synapses between neurons. They cross the synaptic cleft between neurons and attach to receptors on the adjoining neuron. Some neurotransmitters function to excite the joining neuron (e.g. glutamate) to send a subsequent electrical signal. The function of other neurotransmitters is to inhibit the joining neuron (e.g. GABA) and inhibit electrical impulses conducted down that neuron. These chemical and electrical pathways enable the neurons to function normally.

A fundamental principle of the pathophysiology of epilepsy is that seizures result from an imbalance in the normal excitatory and inhibitory mechanisms. The two main classes of neurons responsible for such properties are glutamatergic and GABAergic neurons.

The incidence of epilepsy is approximately 50 million worldwide (www.epilepsysociety.org). Epilepsy is a significant cause of mortality. People with epilepsy have a reduced life expectancy of 8 years compared to the rest of the population.

There are many underlying conditions which can lead to epilepsy, including brain damage during prenatal or perinatal care, head injuries, stroke, brain tumours, infections of the brain and certain genetic conditions. One in three people diagnosed with epilepsy may have a family member with the condition (NHS, 2020). In 50% of cases the cause of epilepsy is not identified (World Health Organization, 2018).

Seizures may be caused by a trigger such as stress, flashing lights (photosensitivity epilepsy), alcohol and lack of sleep. Many patients will describe an abnormal experience moments before the seizure presents, describing feelings of hallucinations/flashing lights, unusual smell or taste, numbness or tingling in limbs, déjà vu or feelings of sadness/joy. An epilepsy aura is a focal aware seizure and the patient will remain conscious and alert, remembering the experience (Epilepsy Society, n.d.). This is a pre-emptive warning that a greater seizure is likely to occur.

Table 15.6   Common AEDs seen in the prehospital setting.

Sodium valproate (Epilim®, Episenta®, Epival®)	Carbamazepine (Tegretol®)	Lamotrigine (Lamictal®)	Levetiracetam (Keppra®, Desitrend®)

Antiepileptic medication

Currently two-thirds of epilepsy patients are actively managing their condition with AEDs (Table 15.6). Healthcare professionals aim to manage the patient's seizures through optimal therapy, thus enhancing the health outcomes to maintain social, educational and employment activity which can be adversely affected through this chronic condition. Monotherapy is the optimal management for epilepsy patients, with sodium valproate described as an ideal therapy for generalised and unclassifiable epilepsy. The SANAD (Standard and New Antiepileptic Drugs) trial identified lamotrigine and/or carbamazepine as the optimum therapy for focal seizures (Marson et al., 2007).

Healthcare professionals managing epilepsy patients should tailor their treatment with an individualised plan, considering the prevalence of the seizures, manifestations, comedication and comorbidity. The lifestyle and preferences of the individual, family and carers should be discussed before prescribing an optimal AED management plan. This is due to the potential side-effects of the drugs; for example, sodium valproate must be avoided in females of child-bearing age and those who are pregnant in order to avoid birth defects in the baby (MHRA, 2018).

Depending on the presentation of the AED, they can be administered as tablet, capsules, liquid and syrups daily. Poor compliance with drug therapy can result in an increased likelihood of seizures, potentially leading to status epilepticus.

Psychogenic non-epileptic seizures (PNES) versus bilateral tonic clonic seizures (BTCS)

Convulsions in adults and children in the prehospital setting can be challenging to distinguish, leading to incorrect diagnosis of epilepsy (Table 15.7). Psychogenic non-epileptic seizures are a common cause of prolonged seizures and are often mistaken for status epilepticus, resulting in incorrect management and treatment. Administering emergency drug treatment such as diazepam can cause adverse side0effects such as respiratory depression, aspiration and death. Therefore, paramedics on scene should gain an accurate history from individuals, seeking an emergency care plan to aid decision making for the patient.

Thorough recording of the characteristics of the patient's seizure will aid in the diagnosis of a PNES. Doctors/specialists encourage the use of video recording of the seizure to aid in making a formal diagnosis retrospectively.

Emergency medication in the prehospital setting

Paramedics typically carry diazepam in their drug packs, either an ampule of 10 mg in an oil-in-water emulsion making up to 2 mL or a rectal tube containing 2.5 mg, 5 mg or 10 mg diazepam.

Current guidelines states diazepam should be administered to patients who have prolonged seizures (lasting 5 minutes or more) or a repeated convulsion (three or more in 60 minutes). The patient is currently convulsing which is not secondary to uncorrected hypoxia or hypoglycaemic episode (JRCLAC, 2021).

Diazepam will depress the actions of the CNS, causing a sedative effect. Caution should be exercised for patients who have consumed alcohol, are prescribed antidepressants and other CNS depressants due to an increased likelihood of side-effects. Diazepam in the emergency setting is typically a safe drug to administer but must be avoided if there is known hypersensitivity.

Administration of diazepam can cause respiratory depression, so be prepared to ventilate the patient using a bag-valve-mask and have this prepared before administration of the drug. Hypotension has also been noted in patients who have been rapidly removed from their location. Allow a 10-minute recovery period before extrication; if this is unachievable, keep the patient flat.

Buccal midazolam is a medication similar to diazepam and known epileptic patients, children will usually have an emergency tube of prefilled midazolam. If this medication is available, clinicians should prioritise administering it over intravenous diazepam due to the complexity of cannulation in children,

Table 15.7 Differentiating psychogenic non-epileptic seizures (PNES) from bilateral tonic clonic seizures (BTCS).

Signs that favour PNES	Signs that favour BTCS
During seizure	*During seizure*
Fluctuating intensity/location	Consistent, repeated, rhythmic myoclonic jerking
Brief pauses, tremor or slow flexion/extension movements	'Shock-like' movement
Arms and legs often not synchronised	Arms and legs mostly synchronised
Convulsion may move from one body area to another	Convulsions may spread from focal to generalised and clonic merging to clonic
May respond (e.g. speech, NPA insertion, etc.)	Unresponsive GCS 3 or 4 (grunting)
Tongue biting rare	Lateral tongue biting common
Eyes mostly shut	Eyes often open
Mouth often shut	Mouth often open
Pupils reacting	Pupils not reacting
May carry out purposeful movement	No purposeful movement
Normal SpO_2, no cyanosis	Low SpO_2 or cyanosis
May be prolonged (>3 min)	Typically short(<90 sec)
Pelvic thrusting common	Pelvic thrusting rare
Postictal	*Postictal*
Rapid end to convulsion	Gradual slowing down of seizure
Rapid recovery	Gradual recovery
Normal breathing	Noisy laboured breathing
History	*History*
Onset over 15 years	Onset under 10 years
Recurrent 'status epilepticus' (misdiagnosis)	Alcohol misuse
PTSD or psychological distress	Provoked seizures (e.g. brain injury)

GSC, Glasgow Coma Scale: NPA, nasopharyngeal airway; PTSD, post-traumatic stress disorder.
Source: Modified from JRCALC (2021).

administering en route to hospital. Buccal midazolam should only be administered if the clinician is confident in this skill; most caregivers on scene will have already administered a first dose of buccal midazolam. Clinicians can subsequently administer a second dose 10 minutes after the first dose.

Administering buccal midazolam

Patients who have been prescribed buccal midazolam will usually have an individualised treatment plan for an emergency situation (Figure 15.2). Clinicians should follow the epilepsy passport plan, utilising the prefilled syringe of midazolam, checking the dosage, date and quality. Prefilled syringes are 2.5 mg, 5 mg, 7.5 mg or 10 mg. Medication should be administered into the oral mucosa, aiming for the gums and providing gentle stimulation to ensure the medication is absorbed and not trickling into the airway.

Administering rectal diazepam

It may be appropriate for patients to receive rectal diazepam instead of intravenous (IV) diazepam due to inability to gain IV access. This will mostly be seen in paediatric and elderly patients. As previously noted, the rectal tubes will be in various dosages and it is imperative to check the clinical

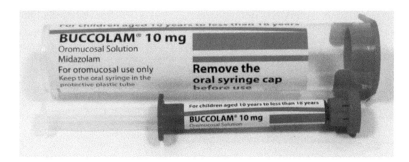

Figure 15.2   Emergency buccal midazolam presentation. Source: © Epilepsy Awareness Ltd.

Table 15.8   Adverse reactions associated with common antiepileptic drugs.

Drug	Adverse reactions
Carbamazepine	Rash, headache, ataxia, tremor, diplopia, hyponatraemia, hepatic failure
Gabapentin	Peripheral oedema, behaviour changes, acute pancreatitis, hepatitis, acute renal failure, Stevens–Johnson syndrome
Lamotrigine	Rash, headache, dizziness, ataxia, blurred vision, hepatic failure
Levetiracetam	Behavioural changes, headache, dizziness
Pregabalin	Dizziness, ataxia, confusion, renal failure, heart failure
Sodium valproate	Nausea, vomiting, hepatic and pancreatic failure

Source: Based on Brown, C. (2016). Pharmacological management of epilepsy. *Progress in Neurology and Psychiatry* **20**(2): 27–34c.

guidelines for drug dosage before administering the medication. Due to the route of medication, inform individuals on scene and maintain dignity where possible. The nozzle on the tube will have a marker indicating where to stop; general guidance is 2.5 cm for children and 4–5 cm for adults (JRCALC, 2021). When inserting the medication, keep a firm hold on the tube while removing, otherwise the medication will retract back into the nozzle.

Adverse reactions associated with common antiepileptic drugs are detailed in Table 15.8.

Strokes (including transient ischaemic attacks)

Over 13 million people suffer a stroke worldwide each year, of which 5.5 million die from the stroke (World Stroke Organization, 2020). The incidence of stroke and TIA increases with age; in one study more than 75% of events happened in people over the age of 65 (Rothwell et al., 2005). However, though strokes and TIAs are mostly associated with the elderly, anyone at any age can have a stroke; it is thought that around two out of 100 000 children worldwide are affected each year (betterhealth. vic.gov.au).

About 15% of strokes are haemorrhagic; 85% of haemorrhagic strokes are from intracranial aneurysms, 10% from a non-aneurysmal perimesencephalic haemorrhage and vascular abnormalities, including arteriovenous malformation, account for the other 5% (CKS, 2020; JRCALC, 2019). Haemorrhagic strokes are generally more severe and associated with higher fatality, with 1 in 10 patients dying before reaching hospital, and a higher fatality rate compared to ischaemic strokes within the first 3 months and beyond, intracranial haemorrhage being the more disabling and devastating (JRCALC, 2019). Though subarachnoid haemorrhage (SAH) is an intracranial bleed, the clinical presentation differs from other strokes and typically presents with a sudden onset of severe headache, with vomiting and no focal neurology signs (ISWP, 2016; JRCALC, 2019).

Definition of a stroke and a transient ischaemic attack

The World Health Organization (2002) defines a stroke as 'rapidly developing clinical signs of focal (or global) disturbance of cerebral function, lasting more than 24 hours'. This definition and the term 'stroke' cover a number of different pathologies causing lost neurological function and cerebral damage (Sacco et al., 2013).

The JRCALC (2019) identifies two types of stroke: those caused by ischaemia resulting in cerebral infarction and those caused by intracerebral haemorrhage. Ischaemic strokes account for 85% of strokes; they are caused by a thrombus (a complication from atherosclerosis), an embolus from a clot in the heart or larger artery (caused by atrial fibrillation or atherosclerosis) or fatty embolism from ruptured atherosclerotic plaque (CKS, 2020). This results in ischaemia of the distal tissue beyond the blockage; if blood flow is not restored then that tissue dies (Caroline, 2014).

Transient ischaemic attacks (TIA) have no formal WHO definition, though the generally used one is 'an acute loss of focal cerebral or ocular function with symptoms lasting less than 24 hours'. Tthere is also a recently suggested definition of 'an event lasting less than 1 hour without cerebral infarction on magnetic resonance imaging scan' (ISWP, 2016). The causes of TIAs are thought to be similar to those that cause ischaemic strokes, with reduced blood flow and perfusion of the cerebral and ocular tissue (JRCALC, 2019). The IWSP (2016) states that 'all suspected cerebrovascular events need to be investigated and treated urgently', as the risk from stroke in the first month after a TIA is very high and for up to a year after.

There are a number of risk factors associated with the development of strokes and TIAs (Table 15.9); some of these are modifiable, others are not (CKS, 2020).

Assessment of a stroke

The ISWP (2016) highlights the importance of public awareness in recognising the signs and symptoms of a stroke and of stroke prevention, using campaigns such as the FAST campaign in the UK. The ISWP (2016) notes that research suggests that one-off campaigns have little effect and repeated and continuous campaigns are better. However, there is a weak link between awareness and recommended behaviours, prompting the importance of the healthcare professional (HCP) as a source of healthcare education, as these campaigns have a higher impact on HCPs (ISWP, 2016).

There are a number of tools used in healthcare for the recognition of a stroke. The two recommended by NICE are FAST for prehospital and lay public use and the Recognition of Stroke in the Emergency room (ROSIER) for within the emergency department (ISWP, 2016; JRCALC, 2019; NICE, 2019; Rudd et al., 2016). ROSIER is a superior tool in the recognition of strokes within the emergency department, although a study by the London Ambulance Service found that it was not better than the FAST tool for prehospital recognition (JRCALC, 2019). The ISWP (2016) and JRCALC (2019) both recognised that the person may still be having a stroke and be FAST negative. The recommendation is that if there is any suspicion of stroke in the FAST-negative patient, the patient should still be treated for a stroke. JRCALC (2019) and NICE (2019) emphasize that a blood glucose level needs to be

Table 15.9   Risk factors associated with the development of strokes and TIAs.

Lifestyle	Established cardiovascular disease	Other
Poor diet	Hypertension	Age
Smoking	Atrial fibrillation	Gender[a]
Alcohol	Infective endocarditis	Hyperlipidaemia
Substance misuse	Valvular disease	Diabetes
Lack of exercise	Carotid artery disease	Sickle cell disease
	Congestive heart failure	Antiphospholipid disease
	Congenital or structural heart disease	Other hypercoagulation disorders
		Chronic kidney disease
		Obstructive sleep apnoea

[a] Although men are more likely to have a stroke at a younger age than women, women's risk is increased with current use of the contraceptive pill, migraines with aura, pre-eclampsia and in the immediate postpartum period. Source: CKS (2020).

assessed in any patient with a sudden onset of neurological symptoms as hypoglycaemia can mimic the signs and symptoms of a stroke.

It is recommended that all patients with suspected stroke be transferred to a specialist acute stroke unit after initial assessment (NICE, 2019). As TIAs and strokes initially present with the same signs and symptoms and for the prehospital clinician it is difficult to determine one from the other, conveying to a specialist acute stroke unit is recommended. However, there are different criteria depending on commissioning arrangements for transport to a hyperacute stroke unit (HASU) (JRCALC, 2019).

Treatment

Pharmacological treatment prehospital is limited in the treatment of a stroke and the emphasis is on recognition, management of life-threatening conditions and rapid transfer to an appropriate hospital (JRCALC, 2019).

The use of oxygen is only recommended if the patient is hypoxic, to achieve an oxygen saturation of >94% as per the JRCALC guidelines (JRCALC, 2019).

NICE (2019) states that hypoglycaemia needs to be excluded as a cause of neurological symptoms before a stroke or TIA can be confirmed. For the prehospital clinician, this means that any hypoglycaemia needs to be corrected before managing a suspected stroke (JRCALC, 2019). The current definition of hypoglycaemia for ambulance services is a blood glucose level of <4 mmol/L in the known diabetic patient and <3 mmol/L in the non-diabetic patient (JRCALC, 2019). Treatment for hypoglycaemia would depend on the level of consciousness and the patient's ability to swallow; the options available to the prehospital clinician include glucose 40% oral gel, glucagon or glucose 10% (JRCALC, 2019).

One of the most influential factors in the management of stroke and TIA patients is time, in particular the time from the onset of symptoms to hospital and then to brain scan (JRCALC, 2019; NICE, 2019).

Thrombolysis is indicated for those patients identified as having an ischaemic stroke within 4.5 hours from onset of symptoms (NICE, 2012, 2019). Thrombectomy with thrombolysis is indicated for those patients with an onset of symptoms within 6 hours and based on computed tomographic angiography (CTA) or magnetic resonance imaging (MRA) (NICE, 2019). Thrombectomy with or without thrombolysis is also considered for patients with an acute ischaemic stroke who were well up to 24 hours before, again depending on CTA and MRA imaging (NICE, 2019). The ISWP (2016) suggests imaging within 1 hour of arrival to hospital for those patients with a suspected stroke.

It is agreed that referral or transport to a specialist acute stroke unit for any patient suspected of a stroke or TIA, even when the onset of symptoms is outside the time scales mentioned above, is of great benefit. The single location of a multidisciplinary team for acute assessment and management, secondary preventive measures and rehabilitation for stroke patients, and preventive measures for those who have had a TIA, has been shown to improve patient outcomes for up to 1 year after the event (ISWP, 2016; JRCALC, 2019; NICE, 2019).

The recommendation within stroke units, once haemorrhagic stroke has been excluded and if presenting within the 4.5 hour window, is for thrombolysis using alteplase (for patients aged between 18 and 79 years old) (BNF, 2021; NICE, 2019). Alteplase comes under a group of drugs called fibrinolytic drugs used for thrombolytic therapy; paramedics may be familiar with tenecteplase which is used for the treatment of myocardial infarctions within some UK ambulance services (Galbraith et al., 2015; JRCALC, 2019). Alteplase is a plasminogen activator; plasminogen is a proenzyme in the blood which can be converted to the enzyme plasmin which breaks down fibrin in blood clots and other clotting factors present (Galbraith et al., 2015; NICE, 2012). Alteplase is used to accelerate this process in cases of acute ischaemic strokes, the aim being to restore blood flow and perfusion of the distal tissue (NICE, 2012).

The advantages of alteplase over other thrombolytics such as streptokinase is that it is clot specific, meaning it only activates the plasminogen within the clot; this results in fewer haemorrhagic episodes due to generalised plasminogen activation and the action of streptokinase (Galbraith et al., 2015). Alteplase does not stimulate the production of antibodies, like streptokinase, and can be used repeatedly with little fear of anaphylactic reaction (Galbraith et al., 2015). The main adverse effect is haemorrhagic events; other common side-effects of all fibrinolytics include nausea and vomiting, pulmonary oedema, fever, chills, hypotension, ecchymosis, pericarditis, angina, cardiogenic shock

272

and cardiac arrest (BNF, 2021). Though anaphylactic reaction is among the common side-effects the BNF indicates that this is due to hypersensitivity to gentamicin residue from the manufacturing process (BNF, 2021).

The initial dose of alteplase is 900 µg/kg (maximum dose 90 mg), 10% given as an intravenous injection bolus, the remainder as an intravenous infusion over 60 minutes.

Patients presenting with an acute ischaemic stroke should be started on an antiplatelet agent as soon as possible and certainly within 24 hours (NICE, 2019). NICE recommends starting people with suspected TIA on a daily dose of 300 mg aspirin (if not contraindicated). In the community, patients should be referred to a specialist unit for further assessment and preventive treatment. A protein pump inhibitor should also be offered, especially for those patients with a history of dyspepsia (NICE, 2019).

Aspirin has a number of actions and is part of a group of drugs known as salicylates, which have analgesic, antipyretic and anti-inflammatory actions; aspirin is the only drug in this group that has significant antiplatelet action (Galbraith et al., 2015). Aspirin inhibits the enzyme cyclo-oxygenaese which is needed in the synthesis of thromboxane. Thromboxane is released when platelets bind to collagen fibres to form a platelet plug as part of the clotting mechanism. Thromboxane inhibits adenylate cyclase, an enzyme which is used to make cyclic adenosine monophosphate (cAMP), which inhibits the adhesiveness of the platelets; any change in the concentration of cAMP has an effect on the adhesiveness and aggregation of platelets (Galbraith et al., 2015).

Dosage for acute ischaemic stroke is 300 mg aspirin (if not contraindicated) either orally or per rectum as soon as possible and within 24 hours of symptoms for 2 weeks or until long-term antico-agulant treatment is started (NICE, 2019).

Once acute treatment has started, emphasis shifts to the long-term and secondary preventive treatment, which should be started as soon as possible (ISWP, 2016). Long-term management starts with advising the patient about modifying risk factors around lifestyle, encouraging healthier eating habits, exercise, stop smoking advice and reducing alcohol intake (CKS, 2020). NICE (2019) and ISWP (2016) recommend that alongside lifestyle changes, a review of medication and the start of secondary preventive medication should take place to prevent further vascular events.

Episode of care

You receive a call to attend in the centre of town to a 30-year-old female patient. On arrival at the scene, you see a female patient in an agitated state being helped by friends and the police. The friends say that she started acting strangely about 2 hours ago. They say that they have been drinking for the last 4 hours and just thought that their friend was drunk but noticed about 30 minutes ago that her face looks dropped and that she seems unable to smile properly.

On examination, you notice that the patient appears frustrated and scared. She is unable to use appropriate words but appears to understand what you are saying and fully co-operates with your examination. You also notice that the left side of her face is dropped and she is only able to move the right side of her face.

Baseline observations

Resp rate	Pulse rate	Oxygen stats	Blood pressure	Blood glucose level	Temperature	GCS		
18 rpm	90 bpm	98%	127/90	2 mmol/L	36.7 °C	13		
						Eyes	Voice	Motor
						4	3	6

F.A.S.T. positive = Face dropped on left side, use of inappropriate words.

What are your thoughts?

It is important to establish a timeline of events so that the patient gets treatment quickly as the time window for thrombolysis is 4.5 hours. You should also be aware of any further deterioration and possible airway compromise and inadequate breathing. The patient is frustrated, possibly due to being unable to communicate. Establishing a method of communication will help with calming and reassuring the patient.

What is your plan?

A good history of events and timeline is important. Consider if there have been any previous episodes that may have led up to this event. Also a good past medical history, social and family history might highlight any risk factors. Drug history also highlights any risks; remember to ask about over-the-counter medications, contraception pills or devices, alternative therapies and any illicit drugs.

The key to the management of this patient is rapid recognition of symptoms and their cause. The correction of hypoglycaemia is an important step in excluding this as a cause of the symptoms; once corrected, then a stroke or TIA can be suspected. Rapid transport to an appropriate hospital is vital, preferably one with a hyperacute stroke unit to start initial treatment and further rehabilitation and support for ongoing care and treatment.

Considerations

The above symptoms could be due to the patient being drunk as she has been drinking for the last 4 hours. Be careful with this assumption as alcohol can hide symptoms of more serious pathology, so question further. Be aware of the confirmation bias present here as the patient has been drinking, is of a young age and female, and is having a hypoglycaemic event; each of these could lead to incorrect treatment of this patient. Careful observation of the patient's actions and behaviour is needed alongside a thorough history of events.

The patient also has hypoglycaemia and that can mimic the sign and symptoms of a stroke or TIA. Alcohol consumption can also cause hypoglycaemia. However, the patient is F.A.S.T. positive and understands what you are saying and is cooperating with your requests.

Conclusion

This chapter has covered four neurological conditions that paramedics encounter in the prehospital setting. It has addressed the common medications associated with those conditions, the pharmacodynamics, administration and side-effects. The nervous system is an extremely complex system and new conditions/disease are being discovered regularly so it is important for clinicians to maintain high standards of patient care.

References

Boer, E., Orie, V., Williams, T. et al. (2020). *TDP-43 proteinopathies: a new wave of neurodegenerative diseases.* https://jnnp.bmj.com/content/jnnp/92/1/86.full.pdf

British National Formulary (BNF). (2021). *Methylprednisolone.* London: British Medical Association and Royal Pharmaceutical Society.

Caroline, N. (2014). *Emergency Care in the Streets*, 7th edn. Burlington: Jones and Bartlett Learning.

Clinical Knowledge Summaries (CKS). (2020). *Stroke and TIA.* https://cks.nice.org.uk/topics/stroke-tia/

Dawson, J., Riede, P. and Taylor, M. (2002). *Crash Course: Pharmacology*, 2nd edn. London: Mosby.

Donizak, J. and McCabe, C. (2017). Pharmacology management of patients with Parkinsion's disease in the acute hospital setting: a review. *British Journal of Neuroscience Nursing* **13**(5): 220–225.

Epilepsy Society. (n.d.). *Epileptic seizures.* https://epilepsysociety.org.uk/about-epilepsy/epileptic-seizures

Galbraith, A., Bullock, S., Manias, E., Hunt, B. and Richards, A. (2015). *Fundamentals of Pharmacology: An Applied Approach for Nursing and Health.* London: Routledge.

Intercollegiate Stroke Working Party (ISWP). (2016). *National Clinical Stroke Guidelines*, 5th edn. London: Royal College of Physicians.

Joint Royal Colleges Ambulance Liaison Committee (JRCALC). (2021). *JRCALC Clinical Practice Guidelines, Convulsions in Adults, Psychogenic Non-Epileptic Seizures (PNES).* Bridgwater: Class Professional Publishing.

Jones, K. (2011). *Neurological Assessment. A Clinician's Guide.* Oxford: Churchill Livingstone.

Jones-Davis, D. and MacDonald, R. (2003). GABA receptor function and pharmacology in epilepsy and status epilepticus. *Current Opinion in Pharmacology* **3**(1): 12–18.

274

Marieb, E. (2004). *Human Anatomy and Physiology*, 6th edn. San Francisco: Pearson.

Marson, A.G., Appleton, R., Bake,r G.A. et al. (2007). A randomised controlled trial examining the longer-term outcomes of standard versus new antiepileptic drugs. The SANAD trial. *Health Technology Assessment* **11**(37): iii–iv, ix–x, 1–134.

Medicines and Healthcare products Regulatory Agency (MHRA). (2018) *Midazolam for Stopping Seizures*. www.medicinesforchildren.org.uk/midazolam-stopping-seizures

National Health Service (NHS). (2020). *Epilepsy*. www.nhs.uk/conditions/epilepsy/

National Institute for Health and Care Excellence (NICE). (2012). *Alteplase for treating acute ischaemic stroke*. www.nice.org.uk/guidance/ta264

National Institute for Health and Care Excellence (NICE). (2017). *Parkinson's disease in adults [NG71]*. www.nice.org.uk/guidance/ng71

National Institute for Health and Care Excellence (NICE). (2019). *Stroke and transient ischaemic attack in over 16s: diagnosis and initial management*. www.nice.org.uk/guidance/ng128

Parkinsons UK. (2019). *Homepage*. www.parkinsons.org.uk/

Parkinson's News Today. (2019). *Parkinson's Stages*. https://parkinsonsnewstoday.com/parkinsons-stages/

Rothwell, P.M., Giles, M., Flossmann, E. et al. (2005). A simple score (ABCD) to identify individuals at high early risk of stroke after transient ischaemic attack. *Lancet* **366**: 29–36.

Rudd, M., Buck, D., Ford, G.A. and Price, C.I. (2016). A systematic review of stroke recognition instruments in hospital and prehospital settings. *Emergency Medical Journal* **33**: 818–822.

Sacco, R.L., Kasner, S., Broderick, J. et al. (2013). An updated definition of stroke for the 21st century. *Stroke* **44**: 2064–2089.

World Health Organization. (2002). *The World Health Report 2002: Reducing Risks, Promoting Healthy Life*. Geneva: World Health Organization.

World Health Organization. (2018). *Epilepsy*. www.who.int/news-room/fact-sheets/detail/epilepsy

World Stroke Organization. (2020). www.world-stroke.org/

275

Further reading/resources

Diagnoses in the UK. www.dementiastatistics.org/statistics/diagnoses-in-the-uk/

- Understanding Dementia.www.dementiauk.org/understanding-dementia/what-is-dementia/?msclkid=709a c90120a41997c67aa9113d22e17e&utm_source=bing&utm_medium=cpc&utm_campaign=Dementia%20 Information%20%5BTier%203%5D&utm_term=define%20dementia&utm_content=Information%20-%20 Dementia%20Definition
- Drugbank.com. Galantamine. https://go.drugbank.com/drugs/DB00674
- Drugbank.com. Donepzil. https://go.drugbank.com/drugs/DB00674
- Drugbank.com. Rivastigmine. https://go.drugbank.com/drugs/DB00674
- Drugbank.com. Memantine. https://go.drugbank.com/drugs/DB00674
- www.alzheimers.org.uk/about-dementia/treatments/drugs/how-do-drugs-alzheimers-disease-work
- https://bnf.nice.org.uk/drug/galantamine.html
- https://bestpractice.bmj.com/topics/en-gb/319#:~:text=The%20aetiology%20is%20also%20often%20 multifactorial%2C%20with%20several,embolisation%2C%20thrombosis%2C%20lacunar%20 infarction%2C%20hypoxia%2C%20hypoglycaemia%2C%20or%20ischaemia.
- Gazettereview.com. Brain Atrophy in Advanced Alzheimer's Disease. https://gazettereview.com/wp-content/ uploads/2015/04/Alzheimers-Disease.jpg
- www.bing.com/images/search?view=detailV2&ccid=YyizLzhb&id=B33635825776BD77863584B8E38073620 DCAEB79&thid=OIP.YyizLzhbyQa8P6nKKToGBwHaEp&mediaurl=https%3A%2F%2Fwww.americanscientist. org%2Fsites%2Famericanscientist.org%2Ffiles%2F2018-106-3-152-perspective-2-figcap.jpg&exph=726&ex pw=1156&q=pictures+of+the+the+hippocampal&simid=608020700793274944&ck=B5F931BD5E2C41DF4 E9B2B9FF23B907C&selectedindex=124&form=IRPRST&ajaxhist=0&vt=0&sim=11
- www.drugs.com/mcd/dementia
- www.epilepsysociety.org
- www.health.harvard.edu/a_to_z/parkinsons-disease-a-to-z
- www.healthline.com/health/dementia-drugs-and-medication#effectiveness
- www.nationalmssociety.org
- www.Parkinsons.org.uk
- www.progressnp.com/article/pharmacological-management-epilepsy/
- www.mytutor.co.uk/answers/23361/A-Level/Biology/How-can-donepezil-improve-communication-between-nerve-cells/
- www.who.int>health topics>stroke-cerebrovascular accident

- www.epilepsy.org.uk/press/facts
- www.who.int/news-room/fact-sheets/detail/epilepsy
- https://cks.nice.org.uk/topics/epilepsy/
- www.rch.org.au/neurology/patient_information/antiepileptic_medications/
- www.gov.uk/guidance/valproate-use-by-women-and-girls
- www.sciencedirect.com/topics/neuroscience/hippocampal-sclerosis

Multiple-choice questions

1. Parkinson's disease is defined as:
   (a) A progressive neurological disorder of the basal ganglia
   (b) An organ-specific immune-mediated inflammatory condition that affects the central nervous system
   (c) A neurological condition characterised by two or more unprovoked seizures occurring more than 24 hours apart
   (d) Rapidly developing clinical signs of focal (or global) disturbance of cerebral function, lasting more than 24 hours.

2. Parkinsonian patients show reduced levels of:
   (a) Acetylcholine
   (b) Dopamine
   (c) Glutamate
   (d) Adrenaline

3. Drugs taken for treatment of Parkinson disease:
   (a) Increase the amount of dopamine in the brain
   (b) Decrease the amount of glutamate in the brain
   (c) Decrease the amount of dopamine in the brain
   (d) Increase the amount of adrenaline in the brain.

4. Cholinesterase inhibitors:
   (a) Help increase the amount of the neurotransmitter acetylcholine in the brain
   (b) Help decrease the amount of the neurotransmitter acetylcholine in the brain
   (c) There is little evidence that the neurotransmitter acetylcholine has any notifiable effect to the brain
   (d) Acetylcholine blocks the function of neurons.

5. The action of donepezil will allow for a higher concentration of:
   (a) Acetylcholinesterase
   (b) Acetylcholine
   (c) Cholinesterase
   (d) Glutamate.

6. Memantine:
   (a) Is a potentially disease modifying treatment because it is considered 'neuroprotective'
   (b) Is an 'N-methyl-D-aspartate (NMDA) receptor agonist
   (c) Can only help with Lewy body dementia
   (d) Is likely to be prescribed for patients with mild cognitive impairment.

7. One of the characteristics for diagnosing epilepsy is:
   (a) At least two unprovoked seizures occurring more than 24 h apart
   (b) Three unprovoked seizures occurring more than 48 h apart
   (c) Unknown pyrexia in an infant (2–5) years of age
   (d) An unexplained rash with pyrexia and seizure.

8. Which is an uncommon trigger of a seizure?
   (a) Flashing lights (photosensitivity)
   (b) Alcohol

   (c) Stress
   (d) Exercise
9. Sodium valproate is also known as:
   (a) Epilim
   (b) Episenta
   (c) Tegretol
   (d) Epival.
10. The WHO definition of stroke is:
   (a) 'Rapidly developing clinical signs of facial (or global) disturbance of cerebral function lasting more than 24 hours'
   (b) 'An acute loss of focal or ocular function with symptoms lasting less than 24 hours'
   (c) 'An event lasting more than 1 hour without cerebral infarction on magnetic resonance imaging scan'
   (d) All of the above.
11. Which is not an advantage of alteplase?
   (a) It is clot specific.
   (b) Fewer haemorrhagic episodes.
   (c) Can be used repeatedly.
   (d) No anaphylactic reaction.

12. The emphasis of prehospital treatment of an acute stroke is:
   (a) 300 mg of aspirin and high-flow oxygen to prevent further infarction of the brain tissue
   (b) High-flow oxygen to prevent further infarction of the brain tissue
   (c) Ensuring a good ROSIER assessment is done to confirm that this is a stroke
   (d) Recognition and management of life-threatening conditions and rapid transfer to an appropriate hospital.
13. Drugs used to control the symptoms of dementia can have adverse effects on which of the following?
   (a) Cardiac system
   (b) Respiratory system
   (c) Abdominal system
   (d) All of the above
14. Drugs used to control the symptoms of dementia are known as:
   (a) ACE inhibitors
   (b) Cholinesterase inhibitors
   (c) Proton pump inhibitors
   (d) Monoamine oxidase inhibitor.
15. Which is not a presentation of a prefilled syringe of midazolam in the prehospital setting?
   (a) 15 mg
   (b) 5 mg
   (c) 7.5 mg
   (d) 10 mg

Chapter 16

Medications used in mental health

Liam Rooney

Aim

This chapter provides the reader with an introduction to some of the common psychotropic medications used to treat mental health disorders (MHD).

Learning outcomes

After completing this chapter, the reader should be able to:

1. Expand knowledge and understanding on MHD you will encounter as a paramedic
2. Develop an understanding of the pharmacology related to the drugs used in MHD
3. Develop an understanding of the risks associated with medications used to treat MHD
4. Explore the role of the paramedic, to aid those in an emergency as a result of medication use.

Test your knowledge

1. Name some mental health disorders you may come across in the course of your duty
2. What are neurotransmitters?
3. How many classes of antidepressant drugs are there and can you name any?
4. What drug is recommended for use in the emergency treatment of ingested toxins/overdose?
5. Some drugs used to treat MHD were initially intended for unrelated conditions. Can you name any?

Introduction

There are many different MHDs, with different presentations. These include depression, anxiety disorders, bipolar disorder, schizophrenia and other psychoses, dementia, substance use disorders and developmental disorders such as autism. They are generally categorised by a combination of abnormal

Fundamentals of Pharmacology for Paramedics, First Edition. Edited by Ian Peate, Suzanne Evans, and Lisa Clegg.
© 2022 John Wiley & Sons Ltd. Published 2022 by John Wiley & Sons Ltd.

thoughts, perceptions, emotions, behaviour and relationships with others (World Health Organization (WHO), 2019b). COVID-19 has had a strong psychological impact on the global population, with some studies suggesting that levels of stress, depression, anxiety and the risk of post-traumatic stress disorder (PTSD) have increased due to fear of the disease, its consequences and lockdown measures (Passavanti et al., 2021).

There are effective treatments for MHD, many of which involve the use of psychotropic medications. Most of these medications act through neurotransmitters, having a direct effect on the brain and consequently behaviour. It is common practice for medications classified for a particular use or condition to be prescribed for treatment of a different condition; for example, valproate, an anticonvulsant, is prescribed for manic episodes associated with bipolar disorder. As discussed in Chapter 5, understanding the pharmacokinetics (what the body does with the medications) and pharmacodynamics (what the medication does to the body) of common psychotropic medications is key to identifying any issues a paramedic may encounter in the prehospital environment.

Neurotransmitters

The primary functions of the central nervous system (CNS) are to control and co-ordinate other body systems. Nerve pathways within the CNS connect areas of the brain that serve similar functions. Neurons in these pathways are linked together by synapses. These neurons release neurotransmitters, regulating transmission across these synapses, so nerve impulses are conducted along the nerve pathways to different areas of the brain, influencing the level of activity. While there are a significant number of neurotransmitters identified in the brain, key neurotransmitters that are relevant to this chapter are listed in Table 16.1.

Some MHDs are associated with abnormal changes in the amount of, or activity of, a specific neurotransmitter. Most medications used for MHDs act on the brain by affecting neurotransmitter concentrations and activity. When a neuron releases a neurotransmitter across a synapse, it binds to a receptor site on the dendrites of the adjoining neuron. Figure 16.1 illustrates this synapse process.

Neurotransmitters can be either excitatory or inhibitory. *Excitatory* neurotransmitters attach to the receptor of the adjoining neuron, generating action potentials along the nerve axon, stimulating that neuron to release more neurotransmitters, and so on, generating nerve impulses which transmit information along the nerve pathway. *Inhibitory* neurotransmitters impede the generation of these action potentials on the adjoining neuron due to the response of their inhibitory receptor action,

Table 16.1   Key neurotransmitters.

Neurotransmitter	Function
Acetylcholine	Powerful regulator of neuronal activity throughout the peripheral nervous system and CNS. Important in maintaining cognitive function. Damage to cholinergic neurons of the CNS associated with Alzheimer and Parkinson disease
Glutamate	The primary excitatory neurotransmitter in CNS with powerful excitatory effects
Gamma-aminobutyric acid (GABA)	A derivate of glutamate, primary inhibitory neurotransmitter, found only in the CNS. It controls many processes, including the brain's overall level of excitation
Dopamine	A monoamine neurotransmitter with several pathways (D_1–D_5). Involved in multiple functions, including motor control, reward and reinforcement, and motivation
Noradrenaline	A monoamine neurotransmitter, the primary neurotransmitter in the sympathetic nervous system, controls blood pressure, heart rate, liver function, among many other functions
Serotonin (5HT)	Another monoamine with numerous receptors, involved in functions such as sleep, memory, appetite, mood and other functions. Also produced in the GI tract in response to food
Histamine	Last of the major monoamines, plays a role in metabolism, temperature control, regulating various hormones, and controlling the sleep–wake cycle, among other functions

CNS, central nervous system; GI, gastrointestinal.

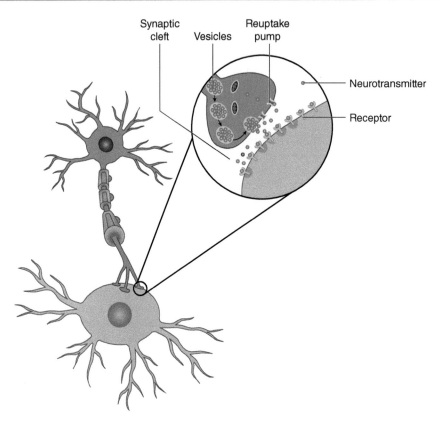

Figure 16.1   The synapse. Source: Queensland Brain Institute (2017).

reducing neural activity. Released neurotransmitters are inactivated and reabsorbed (reuptake) into their respective nerve endings. Whether a neurotransmitter is excitatory or inhibitory depends on the receptor to which it attaches (Hitner and Nagle, 2012).

Reflection

As a paramedic, you will attend a patient who has had a cerebrovascular accident, a stroke. Oxygen deprivation of the brain due to ischaemia causes a build-up of the neurotransmitter glutamate in the interstitial fluid of the CNS. Lack of oxygen causes the glutamate transporters to fail so glutamate accumulates in the interstitial space between the neurons and glia, overstimulating the neurons leading to cell death. This destruction of neurons through prolonged activation of excitatory synaptic transmission is called excitotoxicity (Tortora and Derrickson, 2011).

Antidepressants

Depression is a broad and diverse diagnosis. Severity of the disorder is determined by the number and severity of symptoms, as well as the degree of functional impairment (National Institute for Health and Care Excellence (NICE), 2009). It can substantially impair people's ability to function normally at work and school, and cope with daily life. At its most severe, depression can lead to suicide (WHO, 2019a). Drug treatments, such as antidepressants, are not recommended for use in people diagnosed with mild depression or with subthreshold depressive symptoms, but should be considered for those with moderate or severe depression, or those with persistent mild or subthreshold

Table 16.2   The stepped care model.

Focus of the intervention	Nature of the intervention
STEP 1: All known and suspected presentations of depression	Assessment, support, psychoeducation, active monitoring and referral for further assessment and interventions
STEP 2: Persistent subthreshold depressive symptoms; mild to moderate depression	Low-intensity psychosocial interventions, psychological interventions, medication and referral for further assessment and interventions
STEP 3: Persistent subthreshold depressive symptoms or mild to moderate depression with inadequate response to initial interventions; moderate and severe depression	Medication, high-intensity psychological interventions, combined treatments, collaborative care and referral for further assessment and interventions
STEP 4: Severe and complex depression; risk to life; severe self-neglect	Medication, high-intensity psychological interventions, electroconvulsive therapy, crisis service, combined treatments, multiprofessional and inpatient care

Source: Adapted from Depression in adults: recognition and management. Retrieved from: https://www.nice.org.uk/guidance/cg90 (2009).

symptoms who have not responded to psychosocial interventions such as psychotherapy or cognitive behaviour therapy (CBT) (NICE, 2009). Table 16.2 shows the stepped care approach.

Complex depression includes depression that shows an inadequate response to multiple treatments, is complicated by psychotic symptoms and/or is associated with significant psychiatric comorbidity or psychosocial factors. The class of drug prescribed will be based on the individual patient's requirements, taking into consideration the presence of concomitant disease, existing therapy, previous response to antidepressant therapy and suicide risk, as there is little difference in their efficacy (Joint Formulary Committee, 2021a).

Selective serotonin reuptake inhibitors

Selective serotonin reuptake inhibitors (SSRIs) are the most prescribed medication for the treatment of depression, first-line pharmacotherapy for depression and other MHDs due to their safety, efficacy and tolerability. Overdoses of SSRIs usually do not have serious consequences due to this increased safety profile and tolerability compared to other antidepressants (Chu and Wadhwa, 2020). Examples of SSRIs include citalopram, escitalopram, fluoxetine, paroxetine and sertraline. It is thought that depressive illnesses are attributed to a deficiency in the neurotransmitter serotonin (5HT). SSRIs decrease this deficiency by inhibiting reuptake of synaptic serotonin by the presynaptic neuron. This enables the serotonin to remain in the synapse for longer, which enables the neurotransmitter (serotonin) to repeatedly stimulate its postsynaptic receptors, thereby increasing serotonin activity.

There are more than 15 serotonin receptor subtypes and an SSRI may have more affinity or less affinity with a particular receptor subtype. They have little effect on other neurotransmitters, and have less impact on muscarinic, adrenergic, cholinergic and histaminergic receptors than other antidepressants, consequently leading to fewer side-effects. Common side-effects include insomnia, agitation, nausea, gastrointestinal (GI) upset and sexual dysfunction. Monitoring by the patient's doctor is imperative when beginning treatment with antidepressants, ensuring treatment response is adequate. SSRIs may take up to 6 weeks to achieve this adequate response (Hantsoo and Mathews, 2019).

Withdrawal or discontinuation syndrome may occur if SSRIs are abruptly stopped, doses are missed or reduced. These symptoms are usually mild and self-limiting but may be severe, particularly if the medication is stopped abruptly. Table 16.3 describes in detail the reported symptoms of withdrawal syndrome from SSRI discontinuation. Pharmacokinetics such as the half-life and metabolites produced by a particular SSRI may explain the potential for withdrawal syndrome if doses are missed. For example, all the SSRIs mentioned have a half-life of 24–36 hours, except for fluoxetine, whose half-life ranges from 4 to 16 days. SSRIs are metabolised by microsomal liver enzymes and excreted in the urine (McDermott, 2021).

Table 16.3   Symptoms of withdrawal syndrome

System involved	Symptoms
General	Flu-like symptoms, fatigue, weakness, tiredness, headache, tachycardia, dyspnoea
Balance	Gait instability, ataxia, dizziness, lightheadedness, vertigo
Sensory	Paraesthesias, electric shock sensations, myalgias, neuralgias, tinnitus, altered taste, pruritus
Visual	Visual changes, blurred vision
Neuromotor	Tremor, myoclonus, ataxia, muscle rigidity, jerkiness, muscle aches, facial numbness
Vasomotor	Sweating, flushing, chills
Sleep	Insomnia, vivid dreams, nightmares, hypersomnia, lethargy
Gastrointestinal	Nausea, vomiting, diarrhoea, anorexia, abdominal pain
Affective	Anxiety, agitation, tension, panic, depression, intensification of suicidal ideation, irritability, impulsiveness, aggression, anger, bouts of crying, mood swings, derealisation and depersonalisation
Psychotic	Visual and auditory hallucinations
Cognitive	Confusion, decreased concentration, amnesia
Sexual	Genital hypersensitivity, premature ejaculation

Source: Fava et al. (2015).

Tricyclic antidepressants (TCAs)

Tricyclic antidepressant medication predominantly blocks the reuptake of both serotonin and noradrenaline, although to different extents, also acting to antagonise alpha-cholinergic (alpha-1 and alpha-2), muscarinic and histamine receptors. Some are more selective for their serotonergic properties, such as clomipramine, or noradrenergic properties, such as imipramine. They can also be divided by their sedative properties. Amitriptyline, clomipramine, dosulepin and trimipramine are examples of sedative TCAs, while imipramine, lofepramine and nortriptyline are less sedative. Because of their varying degrees of antimuscarinic and anticholinergic side-effects, and a lower threshold for overdose, they are not typically used as first-line treatment for depression as they are usually less well tolerated in comparison to SSRIs (Joint Formulary Committee, 2021a).

The most common side-effects are dry mouth, constipation and dizziness. Blurred vision, urinary retention, confusion and tachycardia could be due to the blockade of cholinergic receptors. Blockade of adrenergic receptors may cause dizziness and orthostatic hypotension. Histamine blockade may lead to sedation, increased appetite, weight gain and confusion. TCAs should be used with caution in patients with pre-existing ischaemic heart disease as there is a possibility of cardiovascular complications (Moraczewski and Aedma, 2020). Some TCAs are now commonly used for the treatment of other conditions, such as neuropathic pain in adults and enuresis in children.

Due to the narrow therapeutic index of TCAs, intentional or unintentional overdose is possible. Prehospital activated charcoal may be used to absorb any ingested medication not absorbed by the gastrointestinal tract. TCA overdose may induce cardiotoxicity symptoms such as wide QRS complexes or even cardiac arrest. A medication paramedics may have access to, depending on their jurisdiction, to alleviate cardiotoxicity symptoms of TCA overdose is sodium bicarbonate, which can increase the pH of blood plasma, decreasing the concentration of active free TCA medication (Moraczewski and Aedma, 2020; PHECC, 2018).

Monoamine oxidase inhibitors

Monoamine oxidase inhibitors (MAOIs) are used less frequently than other antidepressants due to the dangers of dietary and drug interactions, side-effects and safety concerns. They are generally used when other treatment options have been unsuccessful.

Monoamine oxidase inhibitor medication blocks the monoamine oxidase enzyme. This enzyme breaks down different amine neurotransmitters in the brain, among them serotonin, dopamine, noradrenaline and tyramine. By inhibiting the breakdown of these neurotransmitters, their levels are increased, allowing them to continue their effect. Tyramine, one of the neurotransmitters inhibited by MAOIs, has a role in regulating blood pressure. Because of the accumulation of these amine neurotransmitters, the metabolism of some amine medications is also inhibited, potentially causing a hypertensive crisis. Common cough and decongestant medications are examples of these amine medications, as these contain pseudoephedrine, a sympathomimetic (Joint Formulary Committee, 2021a).

Some foods contain high levels of tyramine, such as:

- mature cheese
- salami
- pickled herring
- meat
- yeast extracts like Bovril°, Oxo° and Marmite°
- some beers, lagers and wine.

As food ages, levels of tyramine can increase, so over-ripe fruits and stale foods should also be avoided. Patients should be aware of these issues and are advised to eat fresh foods only. This danger of interaction persists for up to 2 weeks on discontinuation with MAOIs due to the washout period of these medications (Stavert, 2021).

Monoamine oxidase inhibitors have either a reversible or irreversible effect on neurotransmitters. Moclobemide is a reversible MAOI, phenelzine, tranylcypromine and isocarboxazid are irreversible. They should not be taken with any other antidepressants, especially SSRIs, due to the potential for serotonin syndrome, discussed below. Concomitant use of some analgesics, such as tramadol, may increase the risks of this potentially fatal syndrome. Common side-effects include dry mouth, constipation, nausea, dizziness, drowsiness, insomnia, blurred vision, tremor,and postural hypotension (Laban and Saadabadi, 2020).

Serotonin and noradrenaline reuptake inhibitors

Serotonin and noradrenaline reuptake inhibitors (SNRIs) inhibit the reuptake of serotonin and noradrenaline with varying levels of potency and affinity.Venlafaxine and duloxetine are examples of SNRIs, while reboxetine inhibits only noradrenaline with minimal effects on other neurotransmitters.

Venlafaxine is a relatively weak serotonin inhibitor and weaker noradrenaline inhibitor. It has a 30:1 serotonin:noradrenaline affinity ratio; as dose increases, noradrenaline binding increases. This gives this medication clear dose progression which can be beneficial in an individual's treatment. Therefore, at low doses, the side-effect profile is similar to SSRIs as it predominantly affects serotonin levels, insomnia, agitation, nausea, GI upset and sexual dysfunction. At higher doses it may cause hypertension, diaphoresis, tachycardia, tremors,and anxiety due to its noradrenergic effects (Sansone and Sansone, 2014).

Duloxetine also has a dominant serotonergic effect compared to its noradrenergic effect, but to a lesser degree than venlafaxine. It has a 10:1 affinity ratio, making it a more potent SNRI. It also demonstrates a weak dopamine reuptake. Common side-effects include dry mouth, nausea, headache, dizziness, constipation, insomnia and hypertension. It is also licensed for use in the treatment of diabetic neuropathy and urinary incontinence (Joint Formulary Committee, 2020a; Shelton, 2018).

Reboxetine is a potent noradrenaline reuptake inhibitor with a weak serotonergic effect and no effect on dopamine. Evidence suggest it is not an effective treatment for depressive disorders and it is linked to an increased incidence of adverse effects (Eyding et al., 2010). Side-effects include sexual dysfunction, insomnia, decreased appetite, anxiety, palpitations, paraesthesia, hypo/hypertension, skin reactions, nausea/vomiting and urinary disorders (Joint Formulary Committee, 2020c).

Serotonin syndrome

Serotonin syndrome is a relatively uncommon but potentially life-threatening consequence of too much serotonin in the synapses of the brain. It can occur due to overdose of SSRIs or more com-

Table 16.4 Symptoms of serotonin syndrome.

Altered mental status	Autonomic dysfunction	Neuromuscular abnormalities	Serious complications
Agitation	Tachycardia	Tremor	Rhabdomyolysis
Confusion	Hypertension	Clonus	Metabolic acidosis
Anxiety	Diaphoresis	Hyper-reflexia	Renal failure
Delirium	Diarrhoea	Muscle rigidity	Respiratory failure
Mania	Hyperthermia	Akathisia	Seizures
Coma	Mydriasis (dilated pupils)		Death
	Shivering		

Source: Modified from Zick et al. (2019).

monly, combining multiple medications that increase serotonin levels, such as MAOIs and SSRIs or SNRIs. Herbal remedies, for example St John's wort, and illicit drugs can contribute and must not be overlooked. Symptoms can range from mild to life-threatening, often categorised by changes in mental status, autonomic dysfunction and neuromuscular abnormalities. Onset can be rapid, developing after beginning treatment, increasing dosage or overdose. These symptoms are outlined in Table 16.4. Mild symptoms such as nervousness, nausea, diarrhoea, tremor and dilated pupils can progress to moderate symptoms such as increased reflexes, sweating, agitation, rhythmic muscle spasms and ocular clonus. Severe symptoms such as hyperthermia, delirium, rhabdomyolysis and sustained clonus or rigidity, usually bilaterally in the legs rather than arms, require emergency intervention in hospital (Chu and Wadhwa, 2020; Foong et al., 2018).

Other atypical antidepressants

Some drugs have unique pharmacological properties and do not easily fall into a particular class. Agomelatine is unique among antidepressants, in that it can regulate circadian rhythms due to melatonin receptor agonist properties. Mirtazapine is generally only used when other pharmacological interventions have been unsuccessful, and has sedative, antiemetic, antianxiolytic and appetite stimulant effects (Jilani et al., 2021). Vortioxetine has a unique mechanism of action with a distinct clinical profile, which has proven effective as an alternative therapy for patients with documented failure of other antidepressants (Chen et al., 2017).

Clinical consideration: activated charcoal

The administration of activated charcoal is recommended for the emergency prehospital treatment of acute oral poisoning and oral drug overdose with antidepressant medication (Joint Formulary Committee, 2021d; JRCALC, 2019). The toxic effect will depend primarily on the individual substance used. Activated charcoal has well-documented adsorptive properties and is effective in reducing the absorption of a wide range of toxicants, including drugs taken in overdose. When orally administered, it does not get absorbed within the GI lumen so any ingested toxins that have not been absorbed by the GI lumen will bind to the activated charcoal, reducing the systemic absorption of the toxic agent. It can also enhance the elimination of some compounds after they have been absorbed. Elimination is through faecal excretion (Silberman et al., 2020). Usual dose for >12 years is 50 g within 1 hour of ingestion, 25 g for <12 years. Presentation is usually granules or suspension in water, 50 g/250 mL. If vomiting occurs after dosing, it should be treated with an antiemetic drug (e.g. cyclizine or ondansetron), as vomiting may reduce the efficacy of charcoal treatment.

Reflection

Patients who have features of poisoning or who have taken poisons with delayed action should be transported to hospital, even if they appear well. Treatment depends on the substance or toxin taken. It is advisable to look for further information about the degree of risk or management required. Many countries have their own poisons information service to help practitioners with regard to management, and this should be the first port of call when dealing with poisoning/overdose.

Anxiolytics

Anxiety disorders affect more than 280 million worldwide, making them the most prevalent form of MHD. Anxiety disorders include generalised anxiety disorder (GAD), post-traumatic stress disorder (PTSD), obsessive compulsive disorder (OCD) and phobic, social and panic disorders (Ritchie and Roser, 2018). While symptoms and diagnostic criteria differ for each, collectively, the WHO notes that anxiety is characterised by apprehension or fear, sometimes accompanied by physical symptoms such as headaches, trembling, fidgeting, restlessness, diaphoresis, tachycardia, dyspnoea and epigastric discomfort (WHO, 2019a). The use of antipsychotic or anxiolytic medication initially is not advised as it may mask the true diagnosis. Supplementing antidepressants with anxiolytics may be necessary in patients with some psychotic symptoms (Joint Formulary Committee, 2021a).

Pregabalin

An anticonvulsant, this medication is also used for neuropathic pain and GAD. The mechanism of action of pregabalin is thought to be different from all other anxiolytics. Although similar in structure to the inhibitory neurotransmitter GABA, it has no significant effects at GABA receptors. It is not a glutamate antagonist nor does it inhibit the reuptake of serotonin. Instead, it binds to voltage-gated calcium channels, reducing the release of excitatory neurotransmitters such as glutamate. This reduction in postsynaptic neuron stimulation is thought to be responsible for its anxiolytic, anticonvulsant and analgesic effects (Baldwin and Ajel, 2007). Side-effects are numerous and include dizziness, drowsiness, confusion, impaired concentration, abnormal appetite leading to weight gain, GI upset and headache. Pregabalin is rapidly absorbed with a bioavailability of >90%, its half-life is 6.3 hours and it is eliminated primarily by renal excretion as unchanged drug (EMC, 2021b).

Pregabalin is a Class C controlled substance in some countries. There are concerns about potentially fatal risks when interacting with alcohol or other medications that may cause CNS depression, particularly opioids. A recent European review of pregabalin safety data has identified reports of severe respiratory depression in some patients, without concomitant opioid use, prompting an advisory issued by the Medicines and Healthcare products Regulatory Agency (MHRA) and Commission on Human Medicines (CHM), to consider adjustments in dosing for patients at higher risk of respiratory depression, including those with compromised respiratory function, those taking other CNS depressants and those over 65 years of age (Joint Formulary Committee, 2021e; MHRA, 2021).

Benzodiazepines

Benzodiazepines are indicted for short-term use only in severe anxiety. They are the most used anxiolytics and hypnotics, acting at benzodiazepine receptors which are associated with GABA receptors. As discussed earlier, GABA is the primary inhibitory neurotransmitter in the CNS, reducing the excitability of neurons; it produces a calming effect on the brain. Benzodiazepines increase the activity of GABA receptors, enhancing this calming effect (Griffin et al., 2013). Anxiolytic benzodiazepine treatment should be limited to the lowest possible dose for the shortest period. Dependence may become an issue, especially in patients with a history of alcohol or drug abuse and those with personality disorders.

Examples of drugs you are likely to encounter are diazepam, lorazepam and alprazolam (Joint Formulary Committee, 2021c). They are usually well absorbed in the GI tract; elimination depends on whether they are short or long acting. Short-acting benzodiazepines (alprazolam, lorazepam) have a median elimination half-life of 1–12 hours, long-acting benzodiazepines between 40 and 250 hours. For diazepam, a long-acting benzodiazepine, the elimination half-life increases by 1 hour for each year of age; for example, the elimination half-life in a 75-year-old would be 75 hours. Common side-effects for all benzodiazepines include drowsiness, lethargy and fatigue. Dizziness, inco-ordination, slurred speech, vision disturbances, mood swings and euphoria may be experienced at higher doses, as well as aggression and hostile behaviour (Griffin et al., 2013).

Benzodiazepine withdrawal syndrome can develop at any time up to 3 weeks after stopping a long-acting benzodiazepine, due to accumulation of the drug in the fatty tissues, but may occur within a day of stopping a short-acting one. Therefore, withdrawal should be gradual, as abrupt cessation may induce symptoms such as confusion, convulsion, toxic psychosis or a condition resembling delirium tremens (Joint Formulary Committee, 2021c).

Buspirone

Buspirone displays anxiolytic activity but lacks sedative, anticonvulsant and muscle relaxant activity. It is thought to act as an agonist of presynaptic and partial antagonist of postsynaptic $5HT_{1A}$ receptors. This initiates changes in 5HT neurotransmission, which is thought to benefit the treatment of anxiety. Relative to other anxiolytics, buspirone has low toxicity and potential for abuse and there is no associated risk of dependence or withdrawal due to lack of effects on the GABA receptors (Wilson and Tripp, 2021). It has little efficacy as an acute anxiolytic as response to treatment may take up to 2 weeks. Common side-effects include abdominal pain, chest pain, confusion, fatigue, paraesthaesias, nausea and vomiting (Joint Formulary Committee, 2021b). It is rapidly absorbed in the GI tract, with peak plasma levels noted at 60–90 minutes after oral administration, with equilibrium of plasma levels reached 2 days after repeated dosing (EMC, 2020).

Beta-blockers

Beta-blockers (e.g. propranolol) are sometimes used in the management of anxiety. Although they do not affect psychological symptoms of anxiety, worry, tension and fear, they do reduce autonomic symptoms, palpitations and tremors. Therefore, patients with predominantly somatic symptoms may be prescribed these to alleviate the onset of worry and fear (Joint Formulary Committee, 2021c). You can read more about beta-blockers in Chapter 10.

Hypnotics

Sleep disorders are common, and sometimes serious enough to interfere with normal physical, mental, social and emotional functioning. While non-pharmacological measures are deemed the appropriate first step in tackling insomnia, medication may or may not be used in conjunction with these measures. Long-term use of benzodiazepines and non-benzodiazepines, known as Z-drugs, have associated risks including falls, accidents, dependence and withdrawal symptoms, cognitive impairment and an increased risk of developing dementia and therefore should be avoided in the elderly. Recent studies have also raised similar safety concerns with melatonin, used in persons aged 55 years and older for the short-term treatment of insomnia (NICE, 2019).

Benzodiazepines

Although benzodiazepines are effective in the short term for improving sleep, adverse effects are common, including dizziness and drowsiness, sometimes lasting into the following day, potentially causing psychomotor impairment and affecting normal mental function. Nitrazepam and flurazepam are examples which have a prolonged action and may give rise to these effects. Temazepam, loprazolam and lormetazepam act for a shorter time and have little or no 'hangover effect'. If a patient is symptomatic for both daytime anxiety and insomnia, diazepam prescribed as a single night-time dose may be effective for both conditions (Barry, 2018; Joint Formulary Committee, 2021c).

Z-drugs

Zolpidem and zopiclone are non-benzodiazepine hypnotics, acting as benzodiazepine receptor agonists, enhancing GABA neuronal inhibition. Initially developed with the intention of overcoming some disadvantages of benzodiazepines, such as next-day sedation, dependence and withdrawal issues, no clear evidence of differences in effects between Z-drugs and short-acting benzodiazepines has been found (Barry, 2018). Zolpidem has a rapid absorption and onset of action; peak plasma levels can be achieved in as little as 30 minutes, with a short half-life of 2.4 hours (EMC, 2019b). Zopiclone is also absorbed rapidly, with a slightly longer onset of action, up to 2 hours before peak concentrations are reached, with a half-life of approximately 5 hours (EMC, 2016). Common side-effects include dry mouth, bitter taste, dizziness, fatigue, headache, nausea, vomiting and diarrhoea.

Pharmaceutical drugs used for non-medical purposes

Analgesics, anxiolytics and hypnotics are used by some people for non-medical purposes. These may be illegally sought or some, such as codeine, may be obtained without prescription.

287

Mood-stabilising medications

Bipolar disorder may consist of both manic and depressive periods separated by periods of normal mood, although those who only experience manic but not depressive periods are still classified as having this disorder (WHO, 2019b). Some studies have suggested that suicide rates among people with bipolar disorder may be up to 30 times higher than the general population. Indeed, an estimated 71% of those diagnosed have coexisting psychological and psychiatric conditions, such as anxiety, substance use disorders, personality disorders and attention deficit-hyperactivity disorder (ADHD).

Recommendations from NICE suggest an antipsychotic be offered when a person first develops manic episodes, such as haloperidol, olanzapine, quetiapine or risperidone. If these antipsychotics prove insufficient at their maximum licensed dosage, lithium may be considered. The anticonvulsant valproate may also be considered if lithium is not tolerated or unsuitable (NICE, 2020).

Lithium

Lithium has multiple pharmacodynamic effects and it has proved difficult to establish which ones are responsible for its mood-stabilising properties (Alda, 2015). Careful monitoring of patients taking lithium must take place due to its narrow therapeutic window. The difference between subtherapeutic, therapeutic and toxic dosage is small. Signs of lithium toxicity may include vomiting and diarrhoea, ataxia, muscle weakness, twitching, tremors and confusion. Convulsions, coma, hypotension, dehydration leading to electrolyte imbalance and possible renal failure may result from severe toxicity. Increasing fluid intake to increase urine output may be all that is required to eliminate excess drug from the system, otherwise gastric lavage may be considered if performed within 1 hour of ingestion (Joint Formulary Committee, 2021f). Non-steroidal anti-inflammatories (NSAIDs), such as ibuprofen, should be avoided, as these can increase the plasma concentrations of lithium (NICE, 2020).

Valproate

Sodium valproate is traditionally used as an antiepileptic drug but is also used in the long-term treatment of bipolar disorder. It is thought to increase GABA activity, but its exact effect on mood stabilisation is not well understood. It is contraindicated in women or girls of child-bearing age unless other treatments have proved ineffective or are not tolerated and a rigorous pregnancy prevention programme is followed by both prescriber and patient (EMA, 2018; NICE, 2020). Common side-effects include abnormal behaviour, weight gain, drowsiness, confusion, diarrhoea and urinary disorders. Overdose may present with CNS depression, coma, hypotension and circulatory collapse (EMC, 2021a).

Antipsychotics

A psychotic episode causes the person to lose some contact with reality. This may involve seeing, hearing or in some cases feeling, smelling or tasting things that do not exist outside their mind but feel very real to the person. A quite common hallucination is hearing voices. Hallucinations and delusions are recognised as positive psychotic symptoms. Negative psychotic symptoms include emotional apathy, social withdrawal and self-neglect. Psychotic disorders include schizophrenia, schizoaffective disorder and delusional disorder (Joint Formulary Committee, 2021f; NHS, 2019).

Antipsychotic medications are effective for treating positive psychotic symptoms but may be less effective for treating negative psychotic symptoms. Many patients will require life-long treatment as discontinuation has a high relapse rate (Stavert, 2021).

There are two distinct types of antipsychotic medications available: first- and second-generation drugs. First-generation antipsychotics (also known as 'typical') predominantly block only dopamine D_2 receptors, which may cause a range of undesirable side-effects, particularly acute extrapyramidal symptoms (EPS) and elevated prolactin hormone. Second-generation antipsychotics (also known as 'atypical') are more diverse and act on a range of receptors, dopamine, serotonin and others, so have more distinct clinical profiles. This leads to a lower risk of EPS, although the extent varies between drugs; however, they are associated with metabolic adverse effects, primarily weight gain and glucose intolerance (Joint Formulary Committee, 2021f). Examples of typical antipsychotics are chlorpromazine, flupentixol, haloperidol and trifluoperazine, atypical examples include amisulpride, olanzapine, quetiapine and risperidone. The plasma half-life of most antipsychotics is 15–30 hours, hepatic transformation accounting for their entire clearance. As well as oral preparations, medication can be administered as a depot injection, a formulation which releases gradually, permitting less frequent administration.The drug acts for 2–4 weeks but may produce acute side-effects.These treatments are reserved for those at risk of relapse who have difficulty adhering to oral medication regimens (Jones and Jones, 2016).

Antipsychotic-related side-effects

Extrapyramidal symptoms

One of the main disadvantages of antipsychotic medications, EPS include the conditions acute dystonia, akathisia, pseudo-parkinsonism and tardive dyskinesia, as a result of direct or indirect D_2 receptor blockade. Acute dystonias are involuntary movements, restlessness, muscle spasms, protruding tongue often accompanied by symptoms of Parkinson disease such as tremor, abnormal shuffling gait, dysarthric speech and dysphagia. Akathisia is defined as the inability to remain still.

Cardiovascular side-effects

The antagonism of alpha-1 adrenergic and alpha-1 adrenaline receptors leads to cardiovascular side-effects such as postural hypotension, tachycardia and arrhythmias. Postural hypotension can lead to syncope and fall-related injuries, especially in the elderly. Overall risk tends to be dose related but QT prolongation is of concern in patients who take doses exceeding the recommended maximum (Harris et al., 2009).

Endocrine side-effects

As dopamine inhibits prolactin release, blockade of dopamine pathways leads to a rise in prolactin levels causing hyperprolactinaemia. This condition may lead to symptoms such as sexual dysfunction, reduced bone density, menstrual disruption, breast enlargement and lactation; weight gain is a common side-effect.

Neuroleptic malignant syndrome

The rarest but most important adverse reaction, this syndrome is life-threatening if not recognised and treated. It may occur within 24 hours of initiating treatment, with 65% occurring within the first 7 days. Progression of symptoms is quite fast and reaches peak intensity within 72 hours. Neuroleptic malignant syndrome does not usually develop from overdose and happens even if medication is within therapeutic range. Symptoms include hyperthermia (>38°C) with profuse diaphoresis, altered level of consciousness, including delirium, stupor and coma, muscle rigidity with tremors, autonomic dysfunction with tachycardia, blood pressure changes, drooling and incontinence. Treatment requires immediate cessation of the antipsychotic, with most symptoms being self-limiting. In severe cases, supportive care is required, including fluid replacement, fever reduction and support of cardiac, respiratory and renal function, with mortality approximately 5% (Doran, 2013; Joint Formulary Committee, 2021f).

Other side-effects

Typical antipsychotics generally block D_2 receptors while atypical antipsychotics block a variety of receptors, particularly acetylcholine (muscarinic), histamine, noradrenaline and serotonin, which gives rise to a wide range of side-effects. Decreased libido and decreased arousal lead to sexual dysfunction through blockade of dopamine, muscarinic and alpha-1 receptors. Drowsiness and sedation are common but lessen through continued use; they are caused by the antihistamine activity of some antipsychotics. Blockade of muscarinic receptors may cause blurred vision, dry mouth and eyes, constipation and urinary retention (Ritter et al., 2018).

289

Clinical consideration: acute behavioural disturbance

Most acutely disturbed patients or those with a mental health emergency can be treated using reassurance and de-escalation techniques. It is a clinical emergency as the patient may suffer collapse or cardiac arrest with little or no warning. Physical restraint may be warranted. Sometimes sedation or rapid tranquillisation is required. Appropriately qualified clinicians may use medicines parenterally to calm the patient sufficiently for clinical care or transport to be initiated.

There are currently three medications used for prehospital rapid tranquillisation: benzodiazepines (lorazepam and midazolam), antipsychotics or a dissociative agent (ketamine). It is contraindicated in cases where the patient has decreased vital signs, alcohol-related altered level of consciousness or respiratory depression, or is hypoperfused. Oral lorazepam 2 mg is the recommended dose, with a repeated dose if necessary. More commonly, midazolam is required, which is given by either intramuscular (IM) injection or intranasal (IN) administration (see Skills in Practice feature) through an atomiser device, at a dose of 5 mg, with up to two repeated doses allowed to achieve effect. In paediatric patients, the dose is 0.1 mg/kg IN (repeat twice as required). Midazolam has an intense sedative and sleep-inducing effect. It also exerts an anxiolytic, anticonvulsant and a muscle relaxant effect. It has a short duration because of rapid metabolic transformation (EMC, 2019a). The aim of this procedure is to calm the patient without reducing their level of consciousness, but if the patient is already physiologically compromised, this may occur inadvertently. It is vital that resuscitative equipment is available and ready prior to administration.

Skills in practice: intranasal medication administration

The intranasal route of medication administration is a useful and reliable form of drug delivery. The nasal mucosa is well supplied by blood vessels, ensuring a rapid absorption, avoiding first-pass metabolism and enhancing drug bioavailability. It is achieved using a mucosal atomiser device (MAD), which attaches directly to a Luer-Lock syringe and atomises medication to a fine mist. Delivery of intranasal medication is painless, inexpensive and easy (Our Lady's Hospital for Sick Children, 2016). For volumes between 0.5 mL and 2.0 mL, drug absorption is optimised if both nostrils are used, half of the dose in each nostril. If volumes >2.0 mL are required, an alternative route of administration should be sought.

Equipment required:

- Luer-Lock syringe
- filter needle for drawing medication
- mucosal atomiser device (single-patient use)
- medication.

Figure 16.2 illustrates the procedure for using a MAD.

1. Wash/decontaminate hands.
2. Withdraw required dose of medication into syringe. An extra 0.1 mL should be drawn up to account for dead space in unprimed devices.
3. Connect the MAD to the Luer-Lock connector on the syringe.
4. Place the tip of the MAD snugly against the nostril, aiming slightly upward and outward.
5. Briskly compress the syringe plunger to deliver the medication.
6. Dispose of used equipment using local policy and procedure.
7. Wash/decontaminate hands.
8. Document actions.

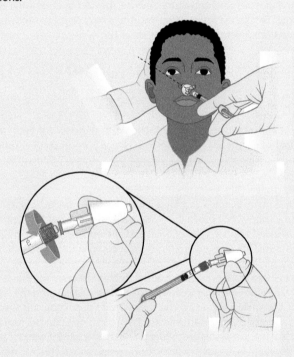

Figure 16.2 MAD nasal device procedure.

Episode of care TCA overdose

A 58-year-old female was attended by an emergency ambulance following a call by the patient's daughter who reported her Mum had taken an overdose. An advanced paramedic solo responder was also dispatched to assist ambulance crew. On arrival, the patient had an altered level of consciousness and was very distressed. It was quickly established that the patient had taken an overdose of amitriptyline 40 minutes earlier, prescribed to her husband for a chronic pain condition.

Treatment was initiated by paramedics; activated charcoal was indicated (it was less than 1 hour since ingestion), and the patient was alert enough to swallow the preparation.

Baseline vital signs were as follows.

- Pulse: 126 beats per minute
- Respiratory rate: 12 breaths per minute
- Oxygen saturation: 98% on room air
- Temperature: 37.6 °C
- Pupils: Dilated size 6, reactive
- Blood pressure: 110/66 mmHg
- GCS: 13

These findings are consistent with typical anticholinergic symptoms. Abnormal ECG findings were wide QRS complexes with prolonged PR and QT intervals. As the paramedics were preparing the patient for transport, she began seizing. Midazolam 5 mg was administered IN, while IV access was obtained. Respiratory support was initiated. Sodium bicarbonate 8.4% was indicated due to the anticholinergic poisoning and wide QRS arrhythmia. Dose required is 1 mEq (milliequivalent)/kg, maximum 50 mEq IV (50 mL) bolus, as per prehospital clinical guidelines. Seizure activity ceased, the patient was transferred to the ambulance and vital signs were repeated.

- Pulse: 54 beats per minute
- Respiratory rate: assisted ventilations with BVM and 100% oxygen
- Oxygen saturation: 99% on 100% oxygen
- Blood pressure: 86/54 mmHg
- GCS: 3
- Blood glucose: 4.8 mmol/L

Sodium chloride (NaCl) (0.9%) 250 mL infusion to address hypotension was started. Repeated ECG noted narrowing of QRS complex with reduced PR and QT interval. On arrival at the emergency department, the patient's level of consciousness had increased and she was maintaining her own airway with adequate respiratory effort (Clark et al., 2015).

Dementia

Dementia is characterised by progressive cognitive impairment. There may be memory loss, communication difficulties, changes in personality and spatial awareness issues. Alzheimer's is the most common type, accounting for 60–70% of total cases. Vascular, mixed dementia (Alzheimer and vascular), dementia with Lewy bodies, Huntington's disease and Creutzfeldt–Jakob disease are other less common types. Medication used for treatment of dementia aims to decelerate the progression of the disease as there is no cure at present. As discovered earlier, with Alzheimer's, damage to cholinergic neurons in the brain leads to a reduction of acetylcholine in the brain. For mild to moderate disease, medications that block the enzyme which breaks down the acetylcholine are used to prevent further loss of acetylcholine. These medications are called acetylcholinesterase (AChE) inhibitors. For moderate to severe disease, the glutamate inhibitor memantine is recommended (NICE, 2018).

Acetylcholinesterase inhibitors

The three AChE inhibitors recommended for the treatment of Alzheimer's are donepezil, galantamine and rivastigmine. The three drugs, although achieving the same therapeutic goal, are different from each other. Donepezil is a long-acting, selective, reversible AChE inhibitor. It has 100% oral bioavailability and a half-life of 70 hours, so once-daily dosage is sufficient. Higher dosage showed mild improvement in cognitive function but caused an increase in cholinergic side-effects. Galantamine is a selective, competitive, rapidly reversible AChE inhibitor. It is also a nicotinic agonist and enhances the nicotinic receptors in the presence of AChE. Twice-daily dosage is recommended as the plasma half-life is 7 hours. Rivastigmine is a powerful, slow, non-competitive, reversible AChE inhibitor. It has good absorption and an oral bioavailability of 40%, and twice-daily treatment is recommended; it is excreted through urine and has relatively few drug-to-drug interactions. It is also available in a transdermal patch.

Common side-effects of AChE inhibitors are GI upset, including nausea and vomiting, and diarrhoea. Headaches, dizziness, insomnia and psychiatric disturbances may also occur (Colović et al., 2013; Harris et al., 2009; Joint Formulary Committee, 2018).

Memantine

Memantine is a treatment option for those who have moderate Alzheimer disease and are not tolerant of AChE therapy, or those with severe disease. It may also be used as an adjunct to AChE inhibitors in moderate to severe disease on the recommendation of a specialist clinician. As discussed, overexposure to the excitatory neurotransmitter glutamate leads to neuronal death, excitotoxicity, due to ischaemia. A receptor involved in this process is the glutamate N-methyl-D-aspartate (NMDA) receptor. Memantine is a voltage-dependent, moderate-affinity, uncompetitive NMDA antagonist, blocking the effects of elevated levels of glutamate that may lead to neuronal dysfunction. This delays progression of symptoms (NICE, 2018). Side-effects include constipation, headaches, drowsiness and dizziness. Less common are confusion, hallucinations and fatigue.It has a 100% bioavailability, a half-life of 3–8 hours and is renally excreted.

Attention deficit-hyperactivity disorder

Paramedics attend patients of all ages so it is appropriate to include the most prevalent paediatric neurodevelopmental disorder, attention deficit-hyperactivity disorder (ADHD), and the medications used for it. It is a behavioural disorder characterised by hyperactivity, impulsiveness and inattention, which may lead to psychological, social, educational or occupational difficulties because of the functional impairment. While some may experience all symptoms, some patients are predominantly hyperactive and impulsive, while others are primarily inattentive. The two main categories of medication used in the treatment of ADHD are stimulants and non-stimulants.

Stimulants

Methylphenidate or lisdexamfetamine are recommended as first-line treatment for ADHD. Dexamfetamine is also a consideration if the patient has a beneficial response to lisdexamfetamine but cannot tolerate its longer duration of effect. Lisdexamfetamine and dexamfetamine are amphetamines; these are slow-release formulations, delivering more stable concentrations of drug, below that required to produce euphoria, and therefore with a reduced potential for abuse (Ritter et al., 2018). The primary pharmacological effects of stimulants are related to increased central dopamine and noradrenaline activity in certain regions of the brain. Common side-effects of stimulants include aggression, alopecia, arrhythmias, abdominal pain, dry mouth, cough, movement disorders, muscle cramps, nausea, palpitations and vomiting. Overdose of amphetamines causes wakefulness, excessive activity, paranoia, hallucinations and hypertension, followed by exhaustion, convulsions, hyperthermia and coma.The early stages of overdose are managed by benzodiazepines, temperature control and anticonvulsants, and respiratory support may be required (Joint Formulary Committee, 2021d).

Non-stimulants

Non-stimulant medication such as atomoxetine or guanfacine may be prescribed by a specialist if stimulant medication has not achieved the desired benefit, is not suitable, not tolerated or ineffective, or there is a coexisting condition which precludes stimulant therapy.

Atomoxetine is a selective noradrenaline reuptake inhibitor, achieving its therapeutic effects by increasing the concentrations of synaptic noradrenaline in the CNS, without directly affecting the serotonin or dopamine transporters (EMC, 2021c). Common side-effects include headache, abdominal pain, decreased appetite, nausea, vomiting and somnolence. Severe adverse effects are uncommon, with mostly mild or moderate effects reported (Garnock-Jones and Keating, 2009).

Guanfacine is a selective alpha-2 adrenergic receptor agonist, enhancing noradrenaline neurotransmission, producing a beneficial effect on cognitive function and improvement in attention and working memory (Huss et al., 2015). Common side-effects include anxiety, decreased appetite, arrhythmias, drowsiness, dizziness, GI upset and skin reactions. Somnolence and sedation may occur during initial treatment or on dose increase. Discontinuation or dose reduction is recommended if symptoms are clinically significant or persistent. Overdose symptoms may include initial hypertension, bradycardia, lethargy, respiratory depression and hypotension (Joint Formulary Committee, 2020b).

As discussed, paramedics should contact their local poison information centre for further advice in all cases of overdose with medications.

Conclusion

There are many different MHDs with many different presentations, many different medications used to treat them, and many different side-effects and adverse events that are possible. This chapter has provided the reader with insight into these disorders and the classes of medications encountered in a practice setting. Understanding how these medications work will give you an insight into how they may be affecting the patient or how they may interact with other medication.

Find out more about these conditions

The following are a list of conditions associated with mental health disorders. Take some time and write notes about each of the conditions. Think about the medications that may be used in order to treat these conditions and be specific about the pharmacokinetics and pharmacodynamics. Remember to include aspects of patient care. If you are making notes about people you have offered care and support to, you must ensure that you have adhered to the rules of confidentiality.

The condition	Your notes
Depression	
Bipolar disorder	
Schizophrenia and other psychoses	
Anxiety disorders	
Dementia and Alzheimer disease	

Glossary

Akathisia	A movement disorder that makes it hard for a person to stay still; causes an urge to move that the person cannot control.
Anticonvulsant	A category of drugs treating seizures.
Antiemetic	Category of drugs preventing nausea.
Autonomic	Part of the peripheral nervous system responsible for involuntary bodily functions.
Cardiotoxicity	Injury to the heart muscle.
Circadian rhythm	Wake–sleep cycle.
Clonus	Involuntary muscular contractions and relaxations.
Cognitive behavioural therapy	A talking therapy that can help manage problems by changing the way the person thinks and behaves.
Concomitant	Occurring or existing at the same time.
Delirium tremens	Condition characterised by rapid onset of confusion, shaking, shivering, irregular heart rate and sweating.
Diaphoresis	Sweating.
Dyspnoea	Difficulty breathing.
Dystonia	Uncontrollable and sometimes painful muscle spasms.
Efficacy	The ability to produce the desired or effective result.
Electroconvulsive therapy	Small electric currents passed through the brain, intentionally triggering a brief seizure.
Enuresis	Bedwetting.
Excitotoxicity	Injury to neurons caused by release of excitatory neurotransmitter.
Gastric lavage	Gastric suction or stomach washout.
Melatonin	Naturally occurring hormone produced by the pineal gland in the brain.
Neuropathic	Nerve origin.
Neurotransmitters	Chemical messengers transmitting a signal from a neuron across the synapse to a target cell.
Paraesthesia	A sensation, such as tingling or numbness.
Primary insomnia	Difficulty in initiating or maintaining sleep, early waking or non-restorative, poor-quality sleep.

Psychiatric comorbidity	The coexistence of two or more psychiatric disorders.
Psychosocial	The effect of social factors on thoughts and behaviours.
Psychotherapy	Treatment to change behaviours and overcome psychological issues.
Psychotropic	Medications that have effects on psychological function.
Rhabdomyolysis	Death of muscle tissue and release of toxins into the bloodstream.
Somnolence	Drowsiness, sleepiness.
St John's wort	A flowering plant, believed to have some benefits in depression treatment.
Sympathomimetic	Physiological effects characteristic of the sympathetic nervous system by promoting the stimulation of sympathetic nerves.
Therapeutic index	A ratio comparing the blood concentration at which a drug causes a therapeutic effect to the amount that causes toxicity.
Washout	Time taken for concentrations of drugs to be eliminated.

References

Alda, M. (2015). Lithium in the treatment of bipolar disorder: pharmacology and pharmacogenetics. *Molecular Psychiatry* **20**(6): 661–670.

Baldwin, D. and Ajel, K. (2007). Role of pregabalin in the treatment of generalized anxiety disorder. *Neuropsychiatric Disease and Treatment* **3**(2): 185–191.

Barry, M. (2018). *Guidance on appropriate prescribing of benzodiazepines and z-drugs (BZRA) in the treatment of anxiety and insomnia.* www.hse.ie/eng/about/who/cspd/ncps/medicines-management/bzra-for-anxiety-insomnia/bzraguidancemmpfeb18.pdf

Chen, G., Højer, A., Areberg, J. and Nomikos, G. (2017). Vortioxetine: clinical pharmacokinetics and drug interactions. *Clinical Pharmacokinetics* **57**(6): 673–686.

Chu, A. and Wadhwa, R. (2020). *Selective Serotonin Reuptake Inhibitors.* www.ncbi.nlm.nih.gov/books/NBK554406/

Clark, S., Catt, J. and Caffery, T. (2015). *Rapid diagnosis and treatment of severe tricyclic antidepressant toxicity.* www.ncbi.nlm.nih.gov/pmc/articles/PMC4612524/

Colović, M.B., Krstić, D.Z., Lazarević-Pašti, T.D., Bondžić, A.M. and Vasić, V.M. (2013). Acetylcholinesterase inhibitors: pharmacology and toxicology. *Current Neuropharmacology* **11**(3): 315–335.

Doran, C. (2013). *Prescribing Mental Health Medication.* Abingdon: Routledge Taylor & Francis Group, 350–359.

Electronic Medicines Compendium (EMC). (2016). *Zopiclone 7.5mg Tablets – Summary of Product Characteristics.* www.medicines.org.uk/emc/product/5894/smpc#gref

Electronic Medicines Compendium (EMC). (2019a). *Midazolam 5mg in 1ml Injection – Summary of Product Characteristics.* www.medicines.org.uk/emc/medicine/23636

Electronic Medicines Compendium (EMC). (2019b). *Zolpidem 10 mg Film-Coated Tablets – Summary of Product Characteristics.* www.medicines.org.uk/emc/product/8188/smpc

Electronic Medicines Compendium (EMC). (2020). *Buspirone 5mg Tablets – Summary of Product Characteristics.* www.medicines.org.uk/emc/product/5736/smpc

Electronic Medicines Compendium (EMC). (2021a). *Depakote 250mg Tablets – Summary of Product Characteristics.* www.medicines.org.uk/emc/product/6102/smpc

Electronic Medicines Compendium (EMC). (2021b). *Pregabalin 150 mg Capsules, Hard - Summary of Product Characteristics.* www.medicines.org.uk/emc/product/7132/smpc

Electronic Medicines Compendium (EMC). (2021c). *Strattera 10mg Hard Capsules – Summary of Product Characteristics.* www.medicines.org.uk/emc/product/5531/smpc

European Medicines Agency (EMA). (2018). *Valproate and related substances.* www.ema.europa.eu/en/medicines/human/referrals/valproate-related-substances-0

Eyding, D., Lelgemann, M., Grouven, U. et al. (2010). Reboxetine for acute treatment of major depression: systematic review and meta-analysis of published and unpublished placebo and selective serotonin reuptake inhibitor-controlled trials. *BMJ* **341**(1): c4737–c4737.

Fava, G., Gatti, A., Belaise, C., Guidi, J. and Offidani, E. (2015). Withdrawal symptoms after selective serotonin reuptake inhibitor discontinuation: a systematic review. *Psychotherapy and Psychosomatics* **84**(2): 72–81.

Foong, A., Grindrod, K., Patel, T. and Kellar, J. (2018). Demystifying serotonin syndrome (or serotonin toxicity). *Canadian Family Physician* **64**: 720–727.

Garnock-Jones, K. and Keating, G. (2009). Atomoxetine. *Pediatric Drugs* **11**(3): 203–226.

Griffin, C.E. 3rd, Kaye, A.M., Bueno, F.R. and Kaye, A.D. (2013). Benzodiazepine pharmacology and central nervous system-mediated effects. *Ochsner Journal* **13**(2): 214–223.

Hantsoo, L. and Mathews, S. (2019). Pharmacological treatment of depressive disorders. In: *APA Handbook of Psychopharmacology* (eds S.M. Evans and K.M. Carpenter). Washington, DC: American Psychological Association, pp.141–164.

Harris, N., Baker, J. and Gray, R. (2009). *Medication Management in Mental Health*. Oxford: Wiley-Blackwell.

Hitner, H. and Nagle, B. (2012). *Pharmacology*, 6th edn. New York: McGraw-Hill.

Huss, M., Chen, W. and Ludolph, A. (2015). Guanfacine extended release: a new pharmacological treatment option in Europe. *Clinical Drug Investigation* **36**(1): 1–25.

Jilani, T., Gibbons, J., Faizy, R. and Saadabadi, A. (2021). *Mirtazapine*. www.ncbi.nlm.nih.gov/books/NBK519059

Joint Formulary Committee. (2018). *British National Formulary (BNF): Dementia*. London: British Medical Journal (BMJ) and Pharmaceutical Press.

Joint Formulary Committee. (2020a). *British National Formulary (BNF): Duloxetine*. London: British Medical Journal (BMJ) and Pharmaceutical Press.

Joint Formulary Committee. (2020b). *British National Formulary (BNF): Guanfacine*. London: British Medical Journal (BMJ) and Pharmaceutical Press.

Joint Formulary Committee. (2020c). *British National Formulary (BNF): Reboxetine*. London: British Medical Journal (BMJ) and Pharmaceutical Press.

Joint Formulary Committee. (2021a). *British National Formulary (BNF): Antidepressant Drugs*. London: British Medical Journal (BMJ) and Pharmaceutical Press.

Joint Formulary Committee. (2021b). *British National Formulary (BNF): Buspirone Hydrochloride*. London: British Medical Journal (BMJ) and Pharmaceutical Press.

Joint Formulary Committee. (2021c). *British National Formulary (BNF): Hypnotics and Anxiolytics*.London: British Medical Journal (BMJ) and Pharmaceutical Press.

Joint Formulary Committee. (2021d). *British National Formulary (BNF): Poisoning, Emergency Treatment*. London: British Medical Journal (BMJ) and Pharmaceutical Press.

Joint Formulary Committee. (2021e). *British National Formulary (BNF): Pregabalin*. London: British Medical Journal (BMJ) and Pharmaceutical Press.

Joint Formulary Committee. (2021f). *British National Formulary (BNF): Psychoses and Related Disorders*. London: British Medical Journal (BMJ) and Pharmaceutical Press.

Joint Royal Colleges Ambulance Liaison Committee (JRCALC). (2019). *JRCALC Clinical Guidelines*. Bridgwater: Class Publishing Ltd.

Jones, A. and Jones, M. (2016). Reviewing depot injection efficacy in the treatment of schizophrenia. *Nursing Standard* **30**(33): 50-60.

Laban, T. and Saadabadi, A. (2020). *Monoamine Oxidase Inhibitors (MAOI)*. www.ncbi.nlm.nih.gov/books/NBK539848/

McDermott, C. (2021). *MIMS Ireland - Depression Supplement* 2021. www.mims.ie

Medicines and Healthcare products Regulatory Agency (MHRA). (2021). *Pregabalin (Lyrica): reports of severe respiratory depression*. www.gov.uk/drug-safety-update/pregabalin-lyrica-reports-of-severe-respiratory-depression

Moraczewski, J. and Aedma, K. (2020). *Tricyclic Antidepressants*. www.ncbi.nlm.nih.gov/books/NBK557791/

NHS. (2019). *Psychosis*. www.nhs.uk/mental-health/conditions/psychosis/overview/

National Institute for Health and Care Excellence (NICE). (2009). *Depression in adults: recognition and management*. www.nice.org.uk/guidance/cg90

National Institute for Health and Care Excellence (NICE). (2018). *Recommendations. Dementia: assessment, management and support for people living with dementia and their carers*. www.nice.org.uk/guidance/ng97/chapter/Recommendations#pharmacological-interventions-for-dementia

National Institute for Health and Care Excellence (NICE). (2019). *Attention deficit hyperactivity disorder: diagnosis and management*. www.nice.org.uk/guidance/ng87

National Institute for Health and Care Excellence (NICE). (2020). *Bipolar disorder: assessment and management*. www.nice.org.uk/guidance/cg185

Our Lady's Hospital for Sick Children. (2016). *Guideline on the delivery of intranasal medication using mad (mucosal atomiser device)*. www.olchc.ie/Healthcare-Professionals/Nursing-Practice-Guidelines/Intranasal-Medication-using-Muscosal-Atomiser-Device-MAD-Oct-2016.pdf

Passavanti, M., Argentieri, A., Barbieri, D. et al. (2021). The psychological impact of COVID-19 and restrictive measures in the world. *Journal of Affective Disorders* **283**: 36–51.

Prehospital Emergency Care Council (PHECC). (2018). *Medication Formulary – Sodium Bicarbonate injection BP*, p.161. www.phecit.ie/Custom/BSIDocumentSelector/Pages/DocumentViewer.aspx?id=oGsVrspmiT0dOhDFFXZvIz0q5GYO7igwzB6buxHEgeDBS9BbdRZpZNKt9Y89hp%252bGEhGQslpxcyrk4LlD4mqoKVIIS8fTY5J4n9kis07L5AerdqOnkw1wT420D1B2squ1oo9F9c25TpBl%252b3U%252baqdDiVOmcN6k1CYjcsscD%252fi1%252fxamYjGwM82FlrSynKr9Vrt%252b

Queensland Ambulance Service. (2020). *Clinical Practice Procedures. Drug Administration/Intranasal*. www.ambulance.qld.gov.au/docs/clinical/cpp/CPP_Intranasal.pdf

295

Queensland Brain Institute. (2017). *Neurotransmitters*. https://qbi.uq.edu.au/brain/brain-physiology/what-are-neurotransmitters

Ritchie, H. and Roser, M. (2018). *Mental Health*. https://ourworldindata.org/mental-health#anxiety-disorders

Ritter, J., Rang, H., Dale, M. et al. (2018). *Rang and Dale's Pharmacology*, 9th edn. Philadelphia: Elsevier, pp.598–600.

Sansone, L. and Sansone, R. (2014). *Serotonin Norepinephrine Reuptake Inhibitors: A Pharmacological Comparison*. www.ncbi.nlm.nih.gov/pmc/articles/PMC4008300/

Shelton R.C. (2018). Serotonin and norepinephrine reuptake inhibitors. In: *Antidepressants* (eds M. Macaluso and S. Preskorn). Cham: Springer.

Silberman, J., Galuska, M. and Taylor, A. (2020). *Activated Charcoal*. www.ncbi.nlm.nih.gov/books/NBK482294/

Stavert, L. (2021). Medications used in mental health. In: *Fundamentals in Pharmacology for Nursing and Healthcare Students* (eds I. Peate and B. Hill). Chichester: John Wiley & Sons Ltd.

Tortora, G. and Derrickson, B. (2011). *Principles of Anatomy and Physiology* 13th edn. Chichester: John Wiley & Sons Ltd.

World Health Organization (WHO). (2019a). *ICD-10 Version:2019 Chapter 5 Mental and Behavioural Disorders*. https://icd.who.int/browse10/2019/en#/V

World Health Organization (WHO). (2019b). *Mental disorders*. www.who.int/news-room/fact-sheets/detail/mental-disorders

Wilson, T. and Tripp, J. (2021). *Buspirone*. www.ncbi.nlm.nih.gov/books/NBK531477

Zick, J., Rettey, S., Cunningham, E. and Thomas, C. (2019). Serotonin syndrome: how to keep your patients safe. *Current Psychiatry* **18**(7): 38–42.

Further reading

Guidance on appropriate prescribing of benzodiazepines and z-drugs (BZRA) in the treatment of anxiety and insomnia. www.hse.ie/eng/about/who/cspd/ncps/medicines-management/bzra-for-anxiety-insomnia/bzraguidancemmpfeb18.pdf

Harris, N., Baker, J. and Gray, R. (2009). *Medications Management in Mental Health*. Chichester: Wiley-Blackwell.

McKnight, S.E. (2020). *De-Escalating Violence in Healthcare*. Indianapolis: Sigma Theta Tau International Honor Society of Nursing.

Spencer, S., Johnson, P. and Smith, I. (2018). *De-escalation techniques for managing non-psychosis induced aggression in adults*. https://doi.org/10.1002/14651858.CD012034.pub2

Resources

- A–Z glossary of street drug names: www.taltofeank.com
- Mind, a UK-based charity dedicated to information and support for all mental health-related issues: www.mind.org.uk

Multiple-choice questions

1. What is the name of the group of medicines used to treat mental health disorders?
   (a) Analgesics
   (b) Antiemetics
   (c) Psychotropics
   (d) Anticholinergics
2. Which of these is not classified as a mental health disorder?
   (a) Depression
   (b) Bipolar disorder
   (c) Autism
   (d) Epilepsy
3. Neurotransmitters can be described as being either:
   (a) Positive or negative
   (b) Excitatory or inhibitory

(c) Acting or non-acting

(d) Agonist or antagonist.

4. Which neurotransmitter is important for maintaining cognitive function?
   (a) Acetylcholine
   (b) GABA
   (c) Noradrenaline
   (d) Serotonin (5HT)

5. The destruction of neurons through prolonged activation of excitatory synaptic transmission is called:
   (a) Cardiotoxicity
   (b) Neurotoxicity
   (c) Hepatotoxicity
   (d) Excitotoxicity.

6. Current evidence suggests the first-line pharmacotherapy for depression and other MHD due to their safety, efficacy, tolerability is:
   (a) Selective serotonin reuptake inhibitors (SSRIs)
   (b) Tricyclic antidepressants (TCAs)
   (c) Serotonin and noradrenaline reuptake inhibitors (SNRIs)
   (d) Antipsychotics.

7. What is another common use for tricyclic antidepressants?
   (a) Anticonvulsant for seizures
   (b) Insomnia and other sleep disorders
   (c) Anxiety
   (d) Neuropathic pain in adults

8. Suicidal behaviour is associated with MHD; which disorder is more strongly linked to suicidal behaviours than others?
   (a) Alzheimer disease
   (b) Generalised anxiety disorder
   (c) Bipolar disorder
   (d) Attention deficit-hyperactivity disorder

9. With more than 280 million affected worldwide, the most prevalent form of MHD is:
   (a) Substance abuse disorders
   (b) Anxiety disorders
   (c) Psychotic disorders
   (d) Dementia.

10. The most used drugs in the anxiolytic and hypnotic class of drugs are:
    (a) Selective serotonin reuptake inhibitors (SSRIs)
    (b) Pregabalin
    (c) Benzodiazepines
    (d) Beta-blockers.

11. Melatonin can be described as:
    (a) A non-benzodiazepine hypnotic
    (b) A naturally occurring hormone
    (c) A naturally occurring element
    (d) A histamine receptor antagonist.

12. The conditions acute dystonia, akathisia, pseudo-parkinsonism and tardive dyskinesia are collectively known as what?
    (a) Extrapyramidal symptoms
    (b) Serotonin syndrome
    (c) Neuroleptic malignant syndrome
    (d) Delirium tremens

13. First-generation 'typical' antipsychotics generally block which receptors?
    (a) α_1 adrenergic receptors
    (b) $5HT_{1A}$ receptors
    (c) D_2 receptors
    (d) H_1 receptors
14. Acetylcholinesterase inhibitors are used for which condition?
    (a) Creutzfeldt–Jakob disease
    (b) Schizophrenia
    (c) Hyponatraemia
    (d) Alzheimer disease
15. The primary pharmacological effects of which stimulants used to treat ADHD are related to increased activity in certain regions of the brain?
    (a) Dopamine and adrenaline
    (b) Dopamine and noradrenaline
    (c) Dopamine and serotonin
    (d) Dopamine and GABA

Chapter 17

Immunisations

Michael Fanner

Aim

The aim of this chapter is to develop essential public health knowledge of infectious diseases and immunisations for paramedic practice, including fundamental epidemiological, pharmacological, social and clinical considerations of immunisations in paramedic consultations.

Learning outcomes

After completing this chapter, the reader will be able to:

1. Understand the fundamental epidemiological concepts and theories in preventing infectious diseases
2. Be familiar with vaccine design to underpin clinical practice knowledge
3. Appreciate public concerns in the acceptability and uptake of immunisations
4. Identify the role of the paramedic in health promotion and immunisation administration.

Test your knowledge

1. What are the key epidemiological concepts to consider in the prevention of infectious diseases?
2. What makes immunisations different from other medicines?
3. What routine immunisations are given in childhood?
4. Why is it important to appreciate public concerns surrounding immunisations?
5. What health promotion information and advice would you give to a patient prior to consenting for immunisation?

Introduction

Immunisations are one of the greatest global developments of modern medicine and after the provision of clean water and sanitation, with 26 separate diseases prevented by vaccination, the British Society for Immunology (2020) estimates that 2–3 million lives are saved each year. The universal offer of a diverse range of immunisations can provide significant protection from infectious diseases, with some immunisations offering up to 97% protection, for example after two doses of the measles, mumps and rubella (MMR) immunisation (Centers for Disease Control and Prevention, 2021). So, the simple construction one may form from this evidence is that if immunisations are clinically

Fundamentals of Pharmacology for Paramedics, First Edition. Edited by Ian Peate, Suzanne Evans, and Lisa Clegg.
© 2022 John Wiley & Sons Ltd. Published 2022 by John Wiley & Sons Ltd.

effective and economically sound at saving lives, why do individuals, communities and populations still become majorly affected by infectious diseases? This chapter will explore some of the reasons behind this.

At the time of writing this chapter, the first UK anniversary of the novel coronavirus and SARS-CoV-19 pandemic had arrived, so the timeliness of this chapter reinforces the importance of stressing public health messages and interventions surrounding infectious diseases in all clinical practice. Before Covid-19 in the UK, public perceptions of infectious diseases were perhaps less obvious than in developing nations with more visible detriment of infectious diseases. With first-hand witnessing of Covid-19, this perception has changed with unprecedented, emergency reprioritisation of health services, the social significance of government pandemic rules and the national rollout of new vaccines (Fanner and Maxwell 2021).

The public health knowledge of infectious diseases including immunisations requires a greater understanding than viewing health via an episodic care lens; a traditional, defining feature of paramedic care, historically a distinguishing characteristic from other professions. With the increasing numbers of paramedics now working in non-ambulance settings such as primary and urgent care, a more central role in preventing infectious diseases arises and the likelihood for directly administering immunisations with the associated health promotion is inevitable. This should not, however, detract from the importance of paramedics working in emergency settings embracing essential public health knowledge, whereby health promotion opportunities for immunisations may arise, such as Health Education England's Making Every Contact Count behaviour change approach.

As a general observation, all paramedics are likely to meet patients who have a varied interaction and experience with the NHS, so each paramedic–patient clinical interaction is vital to include exploration of immunisation history with associated health promotion, including if presenting medical complaints are related to vaccinatable infectious diseases. Paramedics may also be called to emergency situations due to suspected anaphylaxis in vaccination settings.

This chapter will explore the epidemiological concepts and theories in relation to infectious diseases, the pharmacology of immunisations, the public concerns about immunisations and the emerging role of the paramedic in immunisations.

Being mindful of clinical terminology

The terms 'immunisations, inoculations and vaccinations' are often used interchangeably or synonymously yet each is defined differently.

- *Inoculation*: the process of 'introducing' a pathogen into a human to stimulate an antibody production.
- *Vaccination*: the process of receiving a vaccine.
- *Immunisation*: the process that results in an acquired immune response to receiving a vaccine.

Stern and Markel (2005) advise that the preferred term is immunisation, as this is inclusive of an immunological agent (vaccination or inoculation) resulting in the development of an adequate immune response and immunity. Avoid terms such as 'shot', 'dose', 'bout', 'hit', 'jab' or 'injection' to solely define an immunisation.

Understanding the fundamental epidemiological concepts and theories in preventing infectious diseases

Infectious diseases and their resultant immunopathogenic mechanisms are some of the main aetiologies behind mass mortality throughout human history. The immunopathogenic mechanisms, or immunopathogenesis, can be defined as the development of disease with involvement of the immune system response. Infectious pathogens can exist as bacteria, fungi, parasites or viruses and are responsible for deadly diseases such as *Mycobacterium tuberculosis* (3300 years ago), coronaviruses including severe acute respiratory syndrome (SARS) 1 and 2 (2003 and 2019 respectively) and Middle East respiratory syndrome (MERS) (2013).

Essential ways of examining infectious diseases

Infectious diseases are communicable diseases and, unlike non-communicable diseases such as diabetes mellitus or asthma, can spread through communities and populations, regionally, nationally and internationally, as endemics, epidemics and pandemics. The spread of infectious disease can occur via different modes of transmission, including human-to-human contact and animal-to-human contact. Infectious disease spread can occur through ingestion, inhalation, skin penetration and mucosal membrane penetration and be transmitted horizontally or vertically (Balakrishnan and Bhanu Rekha, 2018). Horizontal transmission refers to spread across individuals within the same generation and vertical transmission refers to spread from individuals from one generation to the next. Sutherst (2004) points out that, through holistic assessment of ever-moving societal vulnerabilities to infectious diseases in the world, the infectivity status and transmission opportunities also change. Societal vulnerabilities can include urbanisation with poverty or wealth, climate variability, climate change, changes to land use, changes in human migration and changes in cultural practices (Sutherst 2004), thus illuminating the importance of the social determinants of health.

Sutherst (2004) identifies that adopting conceptual frameworks such as the disease triangle to consider the ecology and epidemiology of infectious diseases is important to evaluate the risks and opportunities for transmission. In order to conceptualise this, the disease triangle, or epidemiological triad (Celentano and Szklo, 2019), provides a visualised way of examining the varying factors of infectious disease status and transmissibility in any given situation.

The three main components of the disease triangle represent the complexity that can occur during infectious disease spread (including viral shed): a host (a human or animal, usually), a pathogen and the environment (such as living conditions or public transport). Each component has an interactional relationship with the other two components that is mediated by the degree of exposure and sensitivity which determines the likelihood of transmission through what is known as a vector (such as overcrowding, poor hand washing practices, poor ventilation or poor cleaning practices) (Figure 17.1). This framework enables a variety of ways for examining aetiological factors and

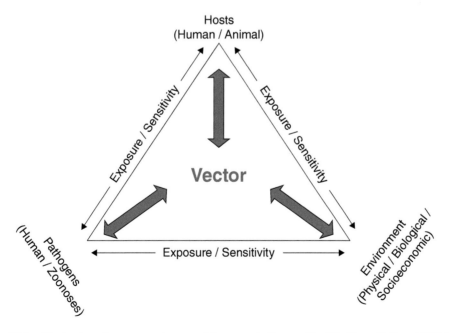

Figure 17.1   The host–pathogen–environment framework. Source: Modified from Sutherst (2004).

ecological drivers that facilitate the increase or decrease of infectious disease spread. With the presence and optimal uptake of a vaccine, the host can be near guaranteed protection from serious pathogenesis even if a vector allows for increased sensitivity and exposure to pathogens in physical, biological or socioeconomic environments. With optimal uptake, immunisation strategy has eradicated infectious diseases such as smallpox (Fenner et al., 1988). However, during pandemics of novel or non-vaccinatable infectious diseases, immunisation strategy or vaccines in development alone should not be relied upon to prevent spread, for example, human immunodeficiency virus 1 (Pitisuttithum and Marovich, 2020) and malaria (Frimpong et al., 2019).

The aforementioned discussion draws attention to immunisations, which should be appreciated from both epidemiological and social determinant perspectives in order to achieve optimal uptake and effect on individuals, communities and populations, such as herd immunity.

Herd immunity is an important immunisation goal, which is not as easily achieved when solely considered as a pandemic strategy by which naturally acquired immunity is established through the natural spread of infectious diseases. Herd immunity is defined as the minimal level of community protection, through immunisation uptake, for individuals susceptible to infectious agents from their proximity to and the presence of individuals with acquired immunity (whether through infection or immunisation) (McNaughton, 2020). McNaughton (2020) argues that herd immunity is better defined as a 'fire line', borrowed from the strategies employed to tackle wildfire by disrupting viral spread. McNaughton suggests that as with fire lines, where the width has to be determined according to the wildfire's behaviour, fuel and weather conditions (e.g. high winds), herd immunity efforts have to focus on those individuals who are more likely to be infected and those who are likely to be exposed in order to 'smother' viral spread. Herd immunity requires constant vigilance as the level of community protection can rapidly decrease with the birth of an estimated 140 million immunologically naive infants and the death of 60 million people, worldwide, every year.

Reflection: essential infectious diseases knowledge

The public health role of the paramedic is perhaps not an obvious feature of day-to-day clinical practice. Reflect upon why it is necessary for paramedics to understand essential knowledge on infectious disease as part of their professional development.

Becoming familiar with vaccine design to underpin clinical practice knowledge

All vaccines must go through large rigorous clinical trials before they can be fully approved for use by governmental regulatory bodies responsible for publicly available medicines, such as the Medicine and Healthcare products Regulatory Authority (UK). Clinical trial methodology ultimately tests for medicinal safety, quality and effectiveness, but these processes can take time and be costly. Unlike other drug groups, immunisations are not scientifically studied or understood through the traditional concepts of pharmacology, i.e. pharmacodynamics and pharmacokinetics, but instead are studied through the concepts of biotechnology and toxicity.

Vaccine design

Vaccines are pharmacologically designed to prevent or interfere with immunopathogenesis within the body by lessening the pathogen's effect through 'working with' the body's immune systems. The vaccine's 'work' prompts the body to initiate the innate immunity and activate antigen-presenting cells to attack one or more antigens (surface proteins) on an infectious pathogen by killing or preventing further replication through disablement (Pasquale et al., 2015; PHE, 2021). Immunisations do not provide an immediate therapeutic effect to patients, but simply put, provide enough immunologically active material of a particular pathogen to allow the body to produce a 'learned' immune response to prevent serious complication and, ultimately, death. The learning the immune system must undergo can take from a number of days to several weeks to be immunologically alert and prepared to target future pathogens. Therefore, the biotechnological engineering of vaccines aims to ultimately create immunisations to behave like infections (or threats) or interact with the immune system to develop a response and resultant internal development of what is known as immunological memory (Nicholson, 2016).

Josefsberg and Buckland (2012) observe that the evolution of vaccines is correlational to the advancement of vaccine production methods; methods that evolve as scientific understanding of immunogenic biology improves. Modern human vaccine development requires significant basic science knowledge of a target infectious disease, including the natural trajectory, aetiology, epidemiology and pathogenesis, in order to identify the right immune response to be effective across immunologically heterogeneous populations (Zepp, 2010). The development of vaccines can take many years, if not decades, to be rolled out but in a global crisis, this development can be expedited through political commitment.

The 2013–2016 Ebola outbreak in West Africa caused more than 11 000 deaths and cost the economy billions of dollars but despite nearly a decade of vaccine development, a vaccine was not available until after a year of the epidemic (British Society for Immunology, 2020). This vaccine dilemma can also be observed with the current SARS-CoV-2 pandemic, whereby it took just over a year for the first available vaccines to be rolled out after the first cases of the novel coronavirus in late 2019 in China.

The European Medicines Agency (EMA) (2005) advises that pharmacokinetic studies are generally not necessary for vaccine trials as the kinetic properties of antigens within vaccines do not provide beneficial information for dosing determinations. The EMA does advise that such studies may be relevant if vaccines contain new adjuvants or excipients. Adjuvants, such as mineral salts, emulsions and aluminium, are substances added to stimulate amplified inflammatory and immune responses with highly purified antigens that are incapable of such effect (Pasquale et al., 2015); however, not all vaccines include adjuvants (Josefsberg and Buckland 2012). Vaccines with adjuvants can result in more frequent and noticeable local reactions, such as a sore arm (Kool et al., 2008).

Table 17.1 illustrates the six main classifications of vaccines.

Vaccine failure

No vaccines can provide 100% protection from infectious diseases and a small number of vaccinated individuals can end up becoming infected. There are two types of failure: primary and secondary. Primary failure is defined as when an individual fails to make an immunological response to a vaccine, whereas secondary failure is when an individual initially immunologically responds to a vaccine, but their protection fades over time (PHE, 2021).

Appreciating public concerns in the acceptability and uptake of immunisations

Immunisations present rather different challenges by which the intended effect is not only to achieve optimal health for individual patients, but more so for the health of the community. Being given a medicine prophylactically may seem unnecessary or even controversial to some, which can create public concern about immunisation programmes. Immunisations have many benefits on an individual level, such as preventing serious disease manifestation or hospitalisation, but the true and optimal effect of immunisation requires much wider uptake at the population level.

Immunisations can be understood through four different categories of offer in the clinical setting: routine, event-specific, occupational and travel. The majority of routine immunisations are offered during childhood and then periodically throughout adulthood. The uptake of childhood immunisations in UK, for example, is considered to be very good but since 2014 there has been a slow decline, with the uptake of completed courses at around 90%, whilst the goal is a sustained 95% (Bedford, 2020). Immunisation offers are continuously monitored according to infectious

Table 17.1 Classifications of vaccine biotechnology.

Classification of vaccine	Biotechnology of vaccine	Vaccine example
Whole pathogen vaccines	Use of whole disease-causing pathogen to produce a similar effect as seen in natural infection. Potentially dangerous to individuals due to risk of disease spread and death. This is the oldest method of vaccine biotechnology and has since been replaced by more modern vaccines	Edward Jenner's cowpox vaccine in 1797
Live attenuated vaccines	Contains whole bacteria or viruses that are genetically modified to 'weaken' or attenuate in order to create an immune response but not cause pathogenesis. This type of vaccine biotechnology has a strong and lasting immune response and is considered the best current vaccine. Caution should be raised with their use in individuals with immune system problems through medication or underlying illness due to an increased likelihood of pathogenesis	• Rotavirus vaccine • MMR vaccine • Nasal flu vaccine • Shingles vaccine • Chickenpox vaccine • BCG vaccine against TB • Yellow fever vaccine • Oral typhoid vaccine (not the injected vaccine)
Inactivated vaccines	Inactivated vaccines are similar to live attenuated vaccines but contain killed or altered whole bacteria or viruses, so they do not replicate. This type of vaccine biotechnology tends not to have as strong or lasting immune response but is suitable for individuals with immune system problems through medication or underlying illness due to an increased likelihood of pathogenesis	• Inactivated polio Vaccine • Japanese encephalitis vaccine • Hepatitis A vaccine • Influenza vaccine • Rabies vaccine
Subunit vaccines 1. Recombinant protein vaccines 2. Toxoid vaccines 3. Conjugate vaccines	Subunit vaccines do not contain any whole bacteria or viruses, but instead typically contain one or more specific surface proteins/antigens from the pathogen, sometimes referred to as acellular. This type of vaccine biotechnology allows the immune system to focus its attention on a small number of antigen targets. Subunit vaccines tend not to have as strong or lasting immune response as live attenuated vaccines so may require further booster doses. Often developed with adjuvants	
	Recombinant protein vaccines are made using bacterial or yeast cells to manufacture a vaccine. A small piece of DNA is taken from a bacterium or virus and inserted into manufacturing cells	• Hepatitis B vaccine • HPV vaccine • MenB vaccine
	Toxoid vaccines are made of inactivated toxins (poisonous proteins) released by some bacteria. The immune system responds in the same way to these toxins as to other surface antigens of the bacteria. This type of vaccine biotechnology has a strong and lasting immune response.	• Diphtheria vaccine • Tetanus vaccine • Pertussis vaccine
	Conjugate vaccines are joined with polysaccharides (complex sugars on the surface of bacteria) rather than proteins. Often conjugate vaccines are attached to diphtheria or tetanus toxoid protein to generate a stronger immune response to the polysaccharide	• Hib vaccine • MenC vaccine (in the Hib/MenC vaccine) • PCV (children's pneumococcal vaccine) • MenACWY vaccine

(Continued)

304

Table 17.1   (Continued)

Classification of vaccine	Biotechnology of vaccine	Vaccine example
Virus-like particles vaccines Outer membrane vesicles vaccines	Virus-like particles vaccines are naturally occurring or synthesised individual expressions of viral structural proteins and are non-infectious because they contain no viral genetic material	• Hepatitis B vaccine • HPV vaccine
	Outer membrane vesicles vaccines are relatively new type of vaccine biotechnology; they are a bleb of bacterial outer cell membrane that is non-infectious but stimulates an immune response	• MenB vaccine (meningococcal B vaccine)
Nucleic acid vaccines 1. RNA vaccines 2. DNA vaccines	Nucleic acid vaccines are a significantly promising vaccine biotechnology. Rather than providing a protein antigen of a pathogen, they provide genetic instructions of the antigen to the cells in the body and in turn the cells produce the antigen to stimulate an immune response	
	RNA vaccines use messenger RNA (mRNA) inside a lipid membrane. The lipid membrane protects the mRNA when it enters the body and helps the mRNA get into cells. Once inside the cell, the cell translates the mRNA into an antigen protein to then produce an immune response. The mRNA is then broken down and eliminated from the body	• Pfizer BioNTech and Moderna Covid-19 vaccines
	DNA vaccines are more stable than mRNA vaccines and do not need the same initial protection. DNA vaccines are typically administered with a technique called electroporation. This uses low-level electronic waves to allow the body's cells to take up the DNA vaccine. DNA must be translated to mRNA within the cell nucleus before it can subsequently be translated to protein antigens which stimulate an immune response	• No licensed DNA vaccines
Viral vectored vaccines • Replicating • Non-replicating	Viral vectored vaccines use harmless viruses to deliver the genetic code of target vaccine antigens to cells of the body, so that they can produce protein antigens to stimulate an immune response. Viral vectored vaccines are significantly cheaper to produce in most cases compared to nucleic acid vaccines and many subunit vaccines. This is a newer type of vaccine biotechnology	
	Replicating viral vectored vaccines retain the ability to make new viral particles alongside delivering the vaccine antigen. This type of vaccine biotechnology has the advantage of a replicating virus that can provide a continuous source of vaccine antigen over an extended period of time compared to non-replicating vaccines, and so is likely to produce a stronger immune response	• Ervebo (rVSV-ZEBOV) Ebola vaccine
	Non-replicating viral vectored vaccines do not retain the ability to make new viral particles during the process of delivering the vaccine antigen to the cell through removing key viral genes. This has the advantage that the vaccine cannot cause disease, and adverse events associated with viral vectored replication are reduced. However, vaccine antigen can only be produced as long as the initial vaccine remains in infected cells (a few days). This means the immune response is generally weaker than with replicating viral vectors and booster doses are likely to be required	• Oxford-AstraZeneca Covid-19 vaccine

Source: Adapted from Types of Vaccines (Vaccine Knowledge Project, Oxford Vaccine Group, University of Oxford): https://vk.ovg.ox.ac.uk/vk/types-of-vaccine

disease threat by governmental health departments or independent advisory expert committees on immunisations; for example, in the UK, the Joint Committee on Vaccination and Immunisation provides recommendations on immunisations, vaccine safety and national immunisation schedules to the government (Table 17.2). Routine immunisations are offered and are accessible to patients with general practitioner (GP) registrations, so paramedics should be mindful of patients

Table 17.2   UK immunisation schedule (PHE 2019b).

Minimum age according to vaccine licence	Diseases protected against	Vaccine given	Administration site
8 weeks old	Diphtheria, tetanus, pertussis (DTap), polio (IPV), *Haemophilus influenzae* type b (Hib), hepatitis b (HepB)	DTap/IPV/Hib/HepB	Thigh
	Meningococcal group B (MenB)	Men B	Thigh
	Rotavirus	Rotavirus	By mouth
12 weeks old	DTap, IPV, Hib, HepB	DTap/IPV/Hib/HepB	Thigh
	Pneumococcal (13 serotypes)	Pneumococcal conjugate vaccine (PCV13)	Thigh
	Rotavirus	Rotavirus	By mouth
16 weeks old	DTap, IPV, Hib, HepB	DTap/IPV/Hib/HepB	Thigh
	MenB	MenB	Thigh
1 year old (or after the child's first birthday)	Hib and meningococcal group C (MenC)	Hib/MenC	Upper arm/thigh
	Pneumococcal (13 serotypes)	PCV13	Upper arm/thigh
	Measles, mumps and rubella (MMR) (German measles)	MMR	Upper arm/thigh
	MenB	MenB booster	Thigh
Eligible paediatric age groups	Influenza (each year from September)	Live attenuated influenza vaccine	Both nostrils
	DTap and IPV	DTap/IPV	Upper arm
	MMR	MMR (check the first dose given)	Upper arm
3 years 4 months old or soon after	DTap and IPV	DTap/IPV	Upper arm
	MMR	MMR (check the first dose given)	Upper arm
Boys and girls aged 12–13 years	Cancers caused by human papillomavirus (HPV) types 16 and 18 (and genital warts caused by types 6 and 11)	HPV (two doses 6–24 months apart)	Upper arm
14 years old (school year 9)	Tetanus, diphtheria and IPV	Td/IPV (check MMR status)	Upper arm
	Meningococcal groups ACWY disease	MenACWY	Upper arm
65 years old	Pneumococcal (23 serotypes)	Pneumococcal polysaccharide vaccine (PPV)	Upper arm
65 years of age and older	Influenza (each year from September)	Inactivated influenza vaccine	Upper arm
70 years old	Shingles	Shingles	Upper arm

Source: Modified from PHE (2019b).

who are not registered. Adults with incomplete childhood immunisations can catch up at any point in their lives via their GP.

In addition to routine immunisations, patients may be eligible for event-specific immunisations due to 'dirty' injuries with the risk of tetanus infection. The tetanus vaccine is required if a patient is unvaccinated or more than 10 years have passed since their last tetanus vaccine. There is a high likelihood of paramedics seeing this type of clinical presentation in urgent and emergency care situations.

Vaccine acceptability

Due to the prophylactic nature of immunisations, the acceptability and uptake can be ethically complex and contextual for a variety of reasons (Bedford, 2020). Vaccine hesitancy can be defined as the 'delay in acceptance or refusal of vaccines despite availability of vaccine services' (Bedford, 2020, p. 302). Bedford (2020) has highlighted a non-exhaustive number of reasons for vaccine hesitancy.

- Complacency (do not perceive need for vaccine).
- Inconvenience (lack of accessibility to vaccines).
- Confidence (do not trust the vaccine or provider).
- Influence of the internet, social media and significant individuals or groups including family, friends and anti-vaccine (anti-vaxxer) movements.
- Patient-held beliefs about western medicine and anti-vaccine conspiracies.
- Patient attitudes towards vaccine safety and threat of infectious diseases.

Many western countries do not have mandatory vaccine policies so paramedics should only seek to promote essential evidence-based information to patients with 'anti-vax' views to avoid disrespect. If a paramedic is concerned about the safeguarding of a patient's welfare due to the patient's/parent's/carer's attitudes about vaccines, they should refer the patient through safeguarding procedures in line with their employer's policy.

Paramedics should be mindful of new or re-emerging pandemics which can arise as a direct result of insufficient immunisation uptake, or indeed infectious diseases without a vaccine. For example, the measles vaccine has been available from the NHS since 1968, but in 2019 the WHO withdrew the UK's 'measles-free' status due to an increase in cases, even after the UK had initially eliminated measles in 2017 (PHE, 2019a). Paramedics should be cognisant of the prevention of seasonal infectious diseases such as influenza or community-acquired bacterial pneumonias and 'normalise' such immunisations through reminding patients of their eligibility.

Clinical consideration: key points when assessing patients with vaccine hesitancy

Patients with mental capacity must make an autonomous and informed decision before consenting to receive medical care or intervention. Patients who are not sure if they want to be immunised should not be forced to receive one. Patients should be advised on the latest evidence base on immunisations as a way of providing the patient with the essential information required to make an informed decision. If a patient appears hesitant, with their permission you may wish to consider the following in your consultations.

1. Explain your profession's commitment to person-centred, evidence-based practice through empathic communication to establish rapport and trust.
2. Check what information the patient already has regarding the vaccine(s) as well as vaccinations in general.
3. Ask where the patient has received such information, including credible and unfounded sources of information.

4. Explain to the patient the vaccine(s) you wish to administer, including its indications, contraindications, potential side-effects, potential adverse reactions and the likely immunity cover as well as the concept of herd immunity/fire lines.
5. Listen and respond carefully to questions from the patient.
6. Remind the patient that they may wish to come back at another time once they have thought about the decision to vaccinate, unless it is an event-specific vaccination such as tetanus.
7. Patients who lack mental capacity should be referred to their GP. There is no such event as an 'emergency immunisation'.

Reflection: Immunisation information and advice opportunities

In your current clinical practice, reflect upon previous opportunities you have had where immunisation information and advice could have been useful.

Recognising the role of the paramedic in health promotion and immunisation administration

The nature of paramedic–patient relationships is rapidly changing, with an increasing number of paramedics working in clinical settings beyond emergency ambulances, such as primary care. Peate (2015) advises that as paramedics begin to widen their scope of practice, patient safety must remain the priority. The international literature suggests that paramedics can improve system performance and patient outcomes in primary care, but more research is required to explain exactly how (Bigham et al., 2013; Eaton et al., 2020). In light of the little research on paramedics' clinical practice surrounding immunisation, the three previous learning outcomes bring together a solid knowledge base on immunisations to begin to confirm the role of the paramedic, including conceptualising how infectious diseases spread, vaccine biotechnology and awareness of more sensitive issues associated with public concerns surrounding immunisations.

Reflection: the role of the paramedic

How can paramedics contribute to immunisation uptake through health promotion in prehospital care settings?

Immunisations as prescription-only medicines

In the UK, immunisations are legally defined as prescription-only medicine, with the sale, supply, administration and prescribing of medicines controlled by three key laws: Medicines Act 1968, Misuse of Drugs Regulations 2001 and Human Medicines Regulations 2012. Paramedics who have demonstrable clinical knowledge and competence and are independent prescribers can prescribe immunisations, but non-prescribing paramedics must follow a 'written instruction' by a doctor, dentist or non-medical prescriber through a prescription, patient group or patient-specific direction. Patient-specific directions are written instructions, produced after an individual clinical assessment, given and signed by a prescriber for another professional (note: not non-registered ambulance staff or healthcare assistants) to supply or administer medicines to a named patient (HCPC, 2021) (Figure 17.2). Patient group directions (PGD) are written instructions that are given and signed by a prescriber for a specific group of patients (with eligibility criteria) that enable the supply or administration by named professionals. PGDs are the most common form of written instruction with immunisations (HCPC, 2021) (Figure 17.3). The detailed information that should be present in a PGD can be found via the MHRA website: www.gov.uk/government/publications/patient-group-directions-pgds/patient-group-directions-who-can-use-them.

Embedding immunisation history taking in clinical assessment

Paramedics work towards a systems-based assessment in clinical practice, which provides the ideal framework to embed immunisation history taking. Prior to consenting and administering an immunisation or exploring immunisation options with patients, paramedics should also make sure they obtain an immunisation history. Patients may be poor historians with regard to their immunisation history so detailed clinical assessment, with specific questioning for each type of immunisation,

---

Patient Specific Direction (PSD)

Name of Patient   _Richard Brown _____

DOB   ____01/02/1960_____

Address   __2 Froom Cottages_____

                            ___Hertfordshire_____

                            ___HA10 9JU _____

I authorise for the above-named patient to receive the following vaccination:

Name of Vaccination:	BNT162b2 Pfizer-BioNTech Covid-19 vaccine
Dose	30µg in 0.3mL
Frequency	Twice. Second dose 10–12 weeks after first dose.
Site of injection/method of administration	IM deltoid region of the upper arm

and that this can be administrated by the Health Care Professional who is suitably qualified to do so and is employed by this general practice

Signed A Doctor_____

Print Name_____Alice Doctor_____

Position/role_____General Practitioner_____

Date _____20/10/2021 _____

Expiry date of this PSD_____31/12/2021 _____

Figure 17.2   Example of a patient-specific direction in general practice.

To see the complete NHS England PGD for the BNT162b2 Pfizer-BioNTech COVID-19 vaccine, please visit: https://www.england.nhs.uk/coronavirus/wp-content/uploads/sites/52/2020/12/C1219-Patient-Group-Direction-for-COVID-19-mRNA-vaccine-BNT162b2-Pfizer-BioNTech.pdf

To be completed by a Primary Care Paramedic upon administration of the vaccine

Name of Vaccine administered	BNT162b2 Pfizer-BioNTech COVID-19 vaccine
Batch Number	12345678
Expiry Date	08/05/2022
Dose	30µg in 0.3mL
Site of injection/method of administration	IM right deltoid
Date vaccine administered	29/10/2021
Contraindications to the vaccine	None known.
Notes	Patient informed of immunisation, its indications, contraindications, potential side effects, potential adverse reactions, the likely resultant immunity and to continue to follow COVID-19 rules including social distancing / face mask wearing. Patient also reminded about the requirement for a second dose in 10–12 weeks to complete immunisation course. Patient is on warfarin but has not taken this medication in the last 6 hours. Patient gave informed verbal consent.

Signed   _A. Paramedic_____

Print Name__ Adam Paramedic _____

Qualifications_____RP_____

Date   _____29/10/2021_____

Figure 17.3 Example of a patient group direction. Source: Based on Public Health England. (2021). Patient Group Direction for COVID-19 mRNA vaccine BNT162b2 (Pfizer/BioNTech).

should be undertaken, including accessing the patient's records and asking whether a patient may have a personally held immunisations record such as the Personal Child Health Record (or 'red book') or an 'Immunisation Record' from other countries.

Public Health England (2016) provides an algorithm for individuals with uncertain or incomplete immunisation status. The algorithm is underpinned by four general principles.

1. Unless there is a documented or reliable verbal vaccine history, individuals should be assumed to be unimmunised and a full course of immunisations planned.
2. Individuals coming to the UK part way through their immunisation schedule should be transferred onto the UK schedule and immunised as appropriate for age.
3. If the primary course has been started but not completed, resume the course – no need to repeat doses or restart course.
4. Plan catch-up immunisation schedule with minimum number of visits and within a minimum possible timescale – aim to protect individual in shortest time possible.

Not all patients can receive immunisations due to contraindications. It is, however, important to note that even if patients may feel they are contraindicated, this could be due to self-reported side-effects of previous immunisations rather than true contraindications, hypersensitivities or adverse reactions, so careful questioning is required with accurate documentation.

Public Health England (2017) stipulates seven specific situations where vaccination should be avoided.

- History of confirmed anaphylactic reaction to a previous vaccine dose.
- History of confirmed anaphylactic reaction to a component of the vaccine.
- Patients with primary or acquired immunodeficiency (1) or on current or recent immunosuppressive or immunosuppressive biological therapy (IBT) (2) as well as those in contact with them (3).
- Infants born to a mother who received IBT during pregnancy.
- Pregnant women.

Patients with egg allergies should be offered alternative egg-free/very low ovalbumin vaccines if possible.

Clinical consideration: consent

The Health and Care Professions Council advises registered practitioners of their duty to gain consent from patients before beginning an assessment or intervention and explicitly states that accountability for ensuring a legally competent consent always lies with the practitioner, not the patient.

Failure to ascertain informed consent can lead to both professional and legal action against the registered practitioner. Immunisation administration requires a qualified practitioner to give patient the necessary relevant and easy-to-follow information about the immunisation, the indications, the contra-dictions, potential side-effects, potential adverse reactions and the procedure itself as well as providing the opportunity for asking questions prior to consenting. This information may need to be provided in a variety of formats (e.g. verbal, written, Braille) to ensure equity of need. Qualified practitioners should fully explain the benefits and risks of immunisation, situating immunisations within wider concepts such as infectious diseases transmission and herd immunity to demonstrate community benefit.

Qualified practitioners should not pressure a patient in any way to receive a vaccine and use health promotion approaches, such as education or empowerment, to ascertain vaccine acceptability. Qualified practitioners should explain how the immunisation administration will be documented, in line with data protection legislation and Caldicott guidance.

The nature of consent, as understood within UK legislation, means that consent is only valid at the time it is given and is dependent on the offered information that is deemed necessary to make a reasonable decision. Consent is often subject to case law which can make universal changes to the way practitioners facilitate consent; for more information, please visit: www.gov.uk/government/publications/reference-guide-to-consent-for-examination-or-treatment-second-edition

Clinical consideration: anaphylaxis

Medicines should not be given to patients without the provision of emergency life-saving medications/equipment to be used in the event of anaphylaxis. The Resuscitation Council UK and Public Health England (2020) have produced guidance entitled 'Management of Anaphylaxis in the Vaccination Setting' although they advise that anaphylaxis is rare, with less than one anaphylaxis episode per million vaccine doses in the UK. The onset of anaphylaxis usually occurs within the first 15 minutes but can occur later. The classic features of anaphylaxis can include:

- itchy skin rash/urticaria (wheals) or swelling (angio-oedema), e.g. lips, face
- airway/breathing problems such as airway swelling, hoarse voice, stridor, shortness of breath, bronchospasms or persistent cough, tiring with effort of breathing, hypoxic confusion, cyanosis and respiratory arrest
- tachycardia and hypotension
- a sense of 'impending doom', loss of consciousness with no improvement once supine or head down position.

If anaphylaxis is recognised, urgent ambulance support should be requested (or different in acute hospital settings) and an anaphylaxis pack should be accessed immediately. Adrenaline (1:1000) should be administered as soon as possible to older children and adults (500 µg dose) and repeated if the above clinical features persist. Patients should be continuously monitored and remain lying supine until an ambulance or extra help arrives as death can occur if a patient stands, walks or sits up too suddenly. An automated external defibrillator should be available in case of cardiac arrest.

All suspected vaccine-induced adverse reactions should be reported via the MHRA's Yellow Card scheme and any patient with suspected anaphylaxis should be referred to their local allergy clinic.

For the full RCUK and PHE (2020) guidance, please visit: www.resus.org.uk/about-us/news-and-events/rcuk-publishes-anaphylaxis-guidance-vaccination-settings

Skills in practice: vaccination care

Paramedics must ensure they practise accountably within their scope of practice when administering immunisations, as defined by the Health and Care Professions Council, their employer's policies and professional indemnity insurance cover.

Before vaccine administration
- Check the clinical setting's policies and protocols for vaccine administration.
- Ensure vaccines have been stored correctly under cold chain conditions (see the Green Book for more information).
- Ensure vaccines are correctly labelled and are in their original packaging.
- Ensure vaccines are within their expiry date.
- Wash hands and wear protective personal equipment as required and follow universal precautions.
- Ensure the correct equipment for drawing the vaccine is available, including sterile syringes, needles and a sharps bin.
- Draw the vaccine only when it is ready to be administered to the patient. Note that only single-use needles must be used for drawing up and discarded after each use. When drawing vaccine from a vial, keep the vial on a firm surface and push the needle down into the vial to minimise needle stick injury.
- Once a vial has been opened, the following information should be documented on the vial itself.

- Date and time of the reconstitution (if required) or first opened.
- Initials of the health professional who opened the vial/reconstituted the vaccine.
- Date and time the vaccine must be used within.
- Stored correctly once opened but not in use.

Vaccine administration
- Introduce yourself and your role to the patient.
- Check patient details on the appointment/clinical system through asking patients questions to establish positive identifiers.
- Undertake a clinical assessment to ensure the appropriateness of the patient to receive the vaccine including all information as outlined in the Clinical consideration: consent box (page 311) to ensure informed consent.
- Wash/gel hands again.
- Ensure the reconstituted vaccine or vaccine is drawn to the correct dose as per the PSD or PGD and is administered according to the correct route: intramuscular, oral, nasal or intradermal. The majority of vaccines are administered intramuscularly in the deltoid area of the upper arm or the anterolateral aspect of the thigh (see Figures 17.4 and 17.5).
- Ensure that a sharps bin is next to you, so you do not have to travel to dispose of a needle.
- No vaccine should be administered into the same site as a previous vaccine within 7 days in order to be certain of avoiding adverse reactions.
- Skin preparation is not required if the skin looks visibly clean. If necessary, use water and soap to clean the skin and ensure it is dry before administration.
- If a patient is to have more than one vaccine via injection at the same time, a different limb should be used for administration for the subsequent vaccines. If only one limb is available, each vaccine should be administered approximately 25 mm apart.
- Intramuscular injections should be given with the needle at a 90° angle to the skin, with the skin held taut by using a finger and thumb technique to make a 'u' or 'n' shape with the non-injecting hand. The needle should be carefully inserted into the skin, being sure not to over- or underpenetrate. If bone is felt on needle insertion, the vaccinator should gently pull the needle back a few millimetres and begin to inject the vaccine. No aspiration of the injection is required to check correct positioning.
- Depending on the vaccine, the needle should remain in place for 10 seconds after pushing the syringe plunger to ensure no underdosing.
- Gently remove the needle from the patient and place straight into a sharps bin.
- Check the injection site for signs of bleeding, using a small piece of cotton wool if necessary. Use a small plaster to cover the injection site if the patient is not allergic to plasters.

Postvaccine care
- Continuously observe the patient for any adverse reactions for up to 15 minutes.
- Ensure the patient is comfortable.
- Ensure all patient documentation is completed including:
  - the vaccine name, batch number, expiry date
  - dose administered
  - administration site
  - date given
  - name and signature of the vaccinator.

313

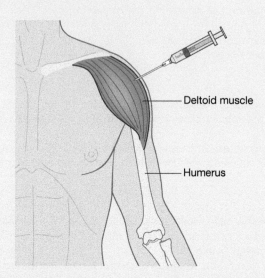

Figure 17.4   Location of the deltoid muscle. Source: Peate and Wild (2018).

314

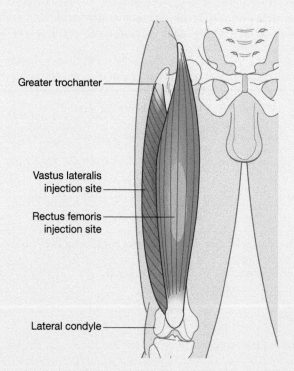

Figure 17.5   Location of the rectus femoris and vastus lateralis muscles of the thigh. Source: Peate and Wild (2018).

Episode of care

Mr Brooks calls 999 following an accident in his garden. He suffered a laceration to his left index finger whilst attempting to make cuttings from one of his roses with a very old pruning knife; he had originally felt faint but has since recovered.

Mr Brooks is seen at his home by Hannah Hanbury, an advanced paramedic practitioner in urgent care, solo working in a rapid response vehicle. Mr Brooks has been gardening all day and has visibly soiled hands. He is a 68-year-old man and has a firmly set 'doctor knows best' attitude to his engagement with healthcare yet also believes that a 'bit of dirt won't hurt you'. Mr Brooks has no significant medical history and is a retired builder. He lives with his wife in a small village, 15 miles from the nearest health facility.

Hannah decides that Mr Brooks does not need to attend hospital. She assesses, cleans and sutures Mr Brooks' hand and advises him to keep the dressing dry for the next 5 days and to go to the practice nurse at his general practice for review. Hannah asks Mr Brooks when he last received the tetanus vaccine. Mr Brooks informs her that he last had an injection when he was a child but knows that he had no 'childhood disease shots' due to his parents believing 'a bit of dirt is good for everyone'. Hannah advises Mr Brooks that due to his reported immunisation history, he would be recommended for the tetanus vaccine. Hannah recommends this vaccine due to the risk of tetanus infection caused by a bacterium called *Clostridium tetani* and the potential entrance of spores of the tetanus bacteria from the garden soil into his wound. Hannah also advises Mr Brooks of the relevant information about the tetanus vaccine including the contraindications, potential side-effects and potential adverse reactions.

Hannah advises Mr Brooks to attend the local Minor Injuries Unit (MIU) today to receive the tetanus vaccine and to inform his GP afterwards so his health records are up to date. On the Patient Report Form, Hannah documents Mr Brooks' injury through the ABCDE model and objectively states the advice she gave him regarding the tetanus vaccine with onward signposting to the MIU on discharge.

Conclusion

This chapter has provided an essential overview of the pharmacology of immunisations, and also presents wider, important disciplinary considerations in relation to the basic epidemiology of infectious diseases and public concerns about immunisations. Immunisations are integral medicines to public health and with the increasing numbers of paramedics now working within primary and urgent care settings, immunisation knowledge is more important than ever before. Without immunisations, many of the infectious diseases that we do not so often hear about would result in increased mortality and morbidity in our populations. This chapter should be read in conjunction with the continuously updated online Green Book, which provides all the latest guidance on vaccines and vaccination procedures and vaccinatable infectious diseases in the UK: www.gov.uk/government/collections/immunisation-against-infectious-disease-the-green-book.

The following infectious diseases are a list of conditions that can be prevented or reduced in pathogenic seriousness by immunisations. Take some time and write notes about each of the conditions. Think about the types of immunisations that are used to prevent each, including their biotechnological approaches. Remember to include aspects of patient care. If you are making notes about people you have offered care and support to, you must ensure that you have adhered to the rules of confidentiality.

The condition	Your notes
Influenza infection	
Tuberculous infection	
Severe acute respiratory syndrome coronavirus 2 infection	
Pneumococcal chest infection	
Tetanus infection	

References

Balakrishnan, S. and Bhanu Rekha, V. (2018). Herd immunity: an epidemiological concept to eradicate infectious diseases. *Journal of Entomology and Zoology Studies* **6**(2): 2731–2738.

Bedford, H. (2020). Immunisation: ethics, effectiveness, organisation. In: *Community Public Health Policy and Practice. A Sourcebook*, 3rd edn (eds S. Cowley and K. Whittaker). St Louis: Elsevier.

Bigham. B.L., Kennedy, S.M., Drennan, I. and Morrison, L.J. (2013). Expanding paramedic scope of practice in the community: a systematic review of the literature. *Prehospital Emergency Care* **17**: 361–372.

British Society for Immunology. (2020). *Protecting the world. Celebrating 200 years of UK vaccine research*. www.immunology.org/sites/default/files/BSI_Celebrate_vaccines_report_2020_FINAL.pdf

Celentano, D.D. and Szklo, M. (2019). *Gordis Epidemiology*, 6th edn. North York: Elsevier.

Centers for Disease Control and Prevention. (2021). *Measles, Mumps and Rubella (MMR) Vaccination: What Everyone Should Know*. www.cdc.gov/vaccines/vpd/mmr/public/index.html#:~:text=One%20dose%20of%20MMR%20vaccine%20is%2093%25%20effective%20against%20measles,(weakened)%20live%20virus%20vaccine

Eaton, G., Wong, G., Williams, V., Roberts, N. and Mahtani, K.R. (2020). Contribution of paramedics in primary and urgent care: a systematic review. *British Journal of General Practice* **70**(695): e421–e426.

European Medicines Agency (EMA). (2005). *Note for Guidance on the Clinical Evaluation of Vaccines*. www.ema.europa.eu/en/documents/scientific-guideline/note-guidance-clinical-evaluation-vaccines_en.pdf

Fanner, M. and Maxwell, E. (2021). Children with Long Covid: Co-producing a specialist community public health nursing response. *Journal of Health Visiting* **9**(10): 418–424.

Fenner, F., Henderson, D.A., Arita, I. Ježek, Z. and Ladnyi, I.D. (1988). *Smallpox and Its Eradication*. Geneva: World Health Organization.

Frimpong, A., Kusi, K.A., Ofori, M.F. and Ndifon, W. (2018). Novel strategies for malaria vaccine design. *Frontiers in Immunology* **9**: 1–14.

Health and Care Professions Council (HCPC). (2021). *Medicine entitlements*. www.hcpc-uk.org/about-us/what-we-do/medicine-entitlements/#:~:text=A%20paramedic%20may%20administer%20certain,administer%20medicines%20under%20this%20exemption.&text=Medicines-,A%20list%20of%20medicines%20included%20in%20this,available%20on%20the%20MHRA%20website

Josefsberg, J.O. and Buckland, B. (2012). Vaccine process technology. *Biotechnology and Bioengineering* **109**: 1443–1460.

Kool, M., Pétrilli, V., De Smedt, T. et al. (2008). Cutting edge: alum adjuvant stimulates inflammatory dendritic cells through activation of the NALP3 inflammasome. *Journal of Immunology* **181**: 3755–3759.

McNaughton, C.D. (2020). Herd immunity: knowns, unknowns challenges and strategies. *American Journal of Health Promotion* **34**(6): 692–694.

Nicholson, L.B. (2016). The immune system. *Essays in Biochemistry* **60**: 275–301.

Pasquale, A.D., Preiss, S., Da Silva, F.T. and Garçon, N. (2015). Vaccine adjuvants: from 1920 to 2015 and beyond. *Vaccines* **3**(2): 320–343.

Peate, I. (2015). Scope of practice: considering how the role of the paramedic continues to change. *Journal of Paramedic Practice* **7**(7): 330–331.

Peate, I. and Wild, K. (2018). *Nursing Practice: Knowledge and Care*, 2nd edn. Chichester: John Wiley & Sons Ltd.

Pittisuttithum, P. and Marovich, M.A. (2020). Prophylactic HIV vaccine: vaccine regimens in clinical trials and potential challenges. *Expert Review of Vaccines* **19**(2): 133–142.

Public Health England (PHE). (2016). *Individuals with uncertain or incomplete immunisation status*. https://assets.publishing.service.gov.uk/government/uploads/system/uploads/attachment_data/file/836241/Algorithm_immunisation_status_07_October_2019.pdf

Public Health England (PHE). (2017). *Contradictions and special considerations. Chapter 6. The Green Book*. https://assets.publishing.service.gov.uk/government/uploads/system/uploads/attachment_data/file/655225/Greenbook_chapter_6.pdf

Public Health England (PHE). (2019a). *Measles in England. Public health matters blog*. https://publichealthmatters.blog.gov.uk/2019/08/19/measles-in-england/

Public Health England (PHE). (2019b). *UK Immunisation Schedule. Chapter 11. The Green Book*. www.gov.uk/government/publications/immunisation-schedule-the-green-book-chapter-11

Public Health England (PHE). (2021). *Immunity and How Vaccines Work. Chapter 1. The Green Book*. https://assets.publishing.service.gov.uk/government/uploads/system/uploads/attachment_data/file/949797/Greenbook_chapter_1_Jan21.pdf

Resuscitation Council UK and Public Health England. (2020). *Management of Anaphylaxis in the Vaccination Setting*. www.resus.org.uk/about-us/news-and-events/rcuk-publishes-anaphylaxis-guidance-vaccination-settings

Stern, A.M. and Markel, H. (2005). The history of vaccines and immunizations: familiar patterns, new challenges. *Health Affairs* **24**(3): 611–621.

Sutherst, R.W. (2004). Global change and human vulnerability to vector-borne diseases. *Clinical Microbiology Reviews* **17**: 136–173.

Zepp, F. (2010). Principles of vaccine design – lessons from nature. *Vaccine* **28**(Suppl 3): C14–C24.

Further reading

Vickers, P.S. (2016). The immune system. In: *Fundamentals of Anatomy and Physiology for Nursing and Healthcare Students* (eds I. Peate and M. Nair). Chichester: John Wiley & Sons Ltd.

Multiple-choice questions

1. What is an infectious disease?
   - (a) A communicable disease that spreads through communities and populations, regionally, nationally and internationally
   - (b) Any disease that is perceived to be infectious by the public
   - (c) A non-communicable disease that spreads through communities and populations, regionally, nationally and internationally
   - (d) Any disease that has symptoms of vomiting and diarrhoea
2. How is the horizontal transmission of infectious diseases defined?
   - (a) The spread of pathogens from individuals from one generation to the next
   - (b) The societal vulnerabilities of infectious diseases
   - (c) The spread of pathogens across individuals within the same generation
   - (d) The spread of infectious diseases that can be foreseen on the horizon
3. Why are social determinants of health important to consider in infectious diseases spread?
   - (a) Because social determinants can directly impact on how infectious diseases are spread/controlled
   - (b) Because people living in poverty are more likely to be in contact with infectious diseases
   - (c) Because there is an evidence-based relationship between social determinants and infectious diseases
   - (d) All of the above
4. What can dramatically speed up vaccine development?
   - (a) Political commitment
   - (b) Social media discourse
   - (c) A vocal paramedic on social media
   - (d) A vocal medical doctor on social media
5. How are vaccines broadly designed?
   - (a) Through attention to biotechnology and toxicity
   - (b) Through attention to pharmacokinetic studies
   - (c) Through attention to vaccine acceptability with middle-class individuals
   - (d) Through attention to how much vaccines cost
6. How many main classifications of vaccines are there?
   - (a) 1
   - (b) 3
   - (c) 6
   - (d) 12
7. How many routine vaccines is an infant given by the time they reach 6 months old?
   - (a) 4
   - (b) 8
   - (c) 6
   - (d) 2
8. What is vaccine hesitancy?
   - (a) Delay in acceptance or refusal of vaccines despite availability of vaccine services
   - (b) Feeling nervous while receiving a vaccine

(c) A patient who believes in vaccines but does not attend their appointment

(d) A patient being indecisive about which arm they would like to receive the vaccine

9. What is the best approach to dealing with 'anti-vaxxers'?

(a) Tell them they are wrong and vaccinate them through force

(b) Provide evidence-based information about vaccines in an objective, neutral approach with their permission

(c) Pretend the vaccine is another non-vaccine medication and vaccinate them

(d) Provide them with your opinions about vaccines with their permission

10. What is a patient group direction?

(a) A written and signed instruction by a prescriber, produced after an individual clinical assessment, given by another professional

(b) A written and signed instruction by a prescriber for a specific group of patients with eligibility criteria, given by another professional

(c) A verbal drug recommendation by a prescriber for a specific patient

(d) A public sign directing patients to a group therapy session

11. How many general principles underpin Public Health England's (2016) algorithm for individuals with uncertain or incomplete immunisation status?

(a) 2

(b) 6

(c) 4

(d) 5

12. What would be considered the minimum necessary, relevant and easy-to-follow information alongside the immunisation a patient/client should be given in order to reach an informed understanding prior to consent?

(a) The indications and adverse effects

(b) The indications, contraindications andpotential adverse reactions

(c) The indications, contraindications, potential side-effects, potential adverse reactions and an opportunity to ask questions

(d) The indications, contraindications, adverse effects and effects of social media on immunisations

13. Why do paramedics need to know about immunisations?

(a) Increasing numbers of paramedics are now working in non-ambulance settings such as primary and urgent care

(b) In case presenting medical complaints are related to vaccinatable infectious diseases

(c) To provide opportunistic health promotion on immunisations through Making Every Contact Count

(d) All of the above

14. What is the suggested prevalence of anaphylaxis in UK vaccination settings?

(a) Less than nine anaphylaxes per million vaccine doses

(b) Less than five anaphylaxes per million vaccine doses

(c) Less than 24 anaphylaxes per million vaccine doses

(d) Less than one anaphylaxis per million vaccine doses

15. What is the name of the book that provides the latest information on vaccines and vaccination procedures, for vaccine-preventable infectious diseases in the UK?

(a) The Government Vaccine Book

(b) The Green Book

(c) The Blue Book

(d) The Vaccination Book

Normal Values

There are a variety of techniques that those who analyze blood use in the laboratory to identify the various components. These techniques can differ from laboratory to laboratory, it is essential that when assessment of blood results is undertaken, referral to the local laboratory's normal values is made. Variation occurs across the UK, Europe, and globally.

Haematology
Full blood count
Haemoglobin (males) 130–180 g/l
Haemoglobin (females) 115–165 g/l
Haematocrit (males) 0.40–0.52
Haematocrit (females) 0.36–0.47
MCV 80–96 fl
MCH 28–32 pg
MCHC 32–35 g/dl
White cell count $(4–11) \times 10^9$ l

White cell differential
Neutrophils $1.5–7 \times 10^9$ l
Lymphocytes $1.5–4 \times 10^9$ l
Monocytes $0–0.8 \times 10^9$ l
Eosinophils $0.04–0.4 \times 10^9$ l
Basophils $0–0.1 \times 10^9$ l
Platelet count $150–400 \times 10^9$ l
Reticulocyte count $(25–85) \times 10^9$ l or 0.5–2.4%

Erythrocyte sedimentation rate
Westergren
Under 50 years:
   Males 0–15 mm/1st hour
   Females 0–20 mm/1st hour
Over 50 years:
   Males 0–20 mm/1st hour
   Females 0–30 mm/1st hour

Plasma viscosity 1.50–1.72 mPa s[1] (at 25 °C)

Coagulation screen
Prothrombin time 11.5–15.5 seconds
International normalized ratio < 1.4
Activated partial thromboplastin time 30–40 seconds
Fibrinogen 1.8–5.4 g/l
Bleeding time 3–8 minutes

Coagulation factors
Factors II, V, VII, VIII, IX, X, XI, XII 50–150 IU/dl

Fundamentals of Pharmacology for Paramedics, First Edition. Edited by Ian Peate, Suzanne Evans, and Lisa Clegg.
© 2022 John Wiley & Sons Ltd. Published 2022 by John Wiley & Sons Ltd.

Factor V Leiden Present or not
Von Willebrand factor 45–150 IU/dl
Von Willebrand factor antigen 50–150 IU/dl
Protein C 80–135 IU/dl
Protein S 80–120 IU/dl
Antithrombin III 80–120 IU/dl
Activated protein C resistance 2.12–4.0
Fibrin degradation products <100 mg/l
D-dimer screen <0.5 mg/l

Hematinics
Serum iron 12–30 μmol/l
Serum iron-binding capacity 45–75 μmol/l
Serum ferritin 15–300 μg/l
Serum transferrin 2.0–4.0 g/l
Serum B_{12} 160–760 ng/l
Serum folate 2.0–11.0 μg/l
Red cell folate 160–640 μg/l
Serum haptoglobin 0.13–1.63 g/l

Haemoglobin electrophoresis
Haemoglobin A > 95%
Haemoglobin A2 2–3%
Haemoglobin F < 2%

Chemistry
Serum sodium 137–144 mmol/l
Serum potassium 3.5–4.9 mmol/l
Serum chloride 95–107 mmol/l
Serum bicarbonate 20–28 mmol/l
Anion gap 12–16 mmol/l
Serum urea 2.5–7.5 mmol/l
Serum creatinine 60–110 μmol/l
Serum corrected calcium 2.2–2.6 mmol/l
Serum phosphate 0.8–1.4 mmol/l
Serum total protein 61–76 g/l
Serum albumin 37–49 g/l
Serum total bilirubin 1–22 μmol/l
Serum conjugated bilirubin 0–3.4 μmol/l
Serum alanine aminotransferase 5–35 U/l
Serum aspartate aminotransferase 1–31 U/l
Serum alkaline phosphatase 45–105 U/l (over 14 years)
Serum gamma glutamyl transferase 4–35 U/l (<50 U/l in males)
Serum lactate dehydrogenase 10–250 U/l
Serum creatine kinase (males) 24–195 U/l
Serum creatine kinase (females) 24–170 U/l
Creatine kinase MB fraction <5%
Serum troponin I 0–0.4 μg/l
Serum troponin T 0–0.1 μg/l
Serum copper 12–26 μmol/l
Serum caeruloplasmin 200–350 mg/l
Serum aluminum 0–10 μg/l
Serum magnesium 0.75–1.05 mmol/l
Serum zinc 6–25 μmol/l
Serum urate (males) 0.23–0.46 mmol/l
Serum urate (females) 0.19–0.36 mmol/l
Plasma lactate 0.6–1.8 mmol/l

Plasma ammonia 12–55 μmol/l
Serum angiotensin-converting enzyme 25–82 U/l
Fasting plasma glucose 3.0–6.0 mmol/L
Haemoglobin A1 C 3.8–6.4%
Fructosamine <285 μmo/l
Serum amylase 60–180 U/l
Plasma osmolality 278–305 mosmol/kg

Lipids and lipoproteins
Target levels will vary depending on the patient's overall cardiovascular risk assessment
Serum cholesterol <5.2 mmol/l
Serum LDL cholesterol <3.36 mmol/l
Serum HDL cholesterol >1.55 mmol/l
Fasting serum triglyceride 0.45–1.69 mmol/l

Blood gases (breathing air at sea level)
Blood H^+ 35–45 nmol/l
pH 7.36–7.44
PaO_2 11.3–12.6 kPa
$PaCO_2$ 4.7–6.0 kPa
Base excess ±2 mmol/l

Carboxyhaemoglobin
Non-smoker <2%
Smoker 3–15%

Immunology/rheumatology
Complement C3 65–190 mg/dl
Complement C4 15–50 mg/dl
Total hemolytic (CH50) 150–250 U/l
Serum C-reactive protein <10 mg/l

Serum immunoglobulins
IgG 6.0–13.0 g/l
IgA 0.8–3.0 g/l
IgM 0.4–2.5 g/l
IgE <120 kU/l
Serum β_2-microglobulin <3 mg/l

Cerebrospinal fluid
Opening pressure 50–180 mmH$_2$O
Total protein 0.15–0.45 g/l
Albumin 0.066–0.442 g/l
Chloride 116–122 mmol/l
Glucose 3.3–4.4 mmol/l
Lactate 1–2 mmol/l
Cell count ≤5 mL^{-1}

Differential
Lymphocytes 60–70%
Monocytes 30–50%
Neutrophils None
IgG/ALB ≤0.26
IgG index ≤0.88

Urine
Albumin/creatinine ratio (untimed specimen) <3.5 mg/mmol (males)
<2.5 mg/mmol (females)
Glomerular filtration rate 70–140 mL/min

Total protein <0.2 g/24 hours
Albumin <30 mg/24 hours
Calcium 2.5–7.5 mmol/24 hours
Urobilinogen 1.7–5.9 µmol/24 hours
Coproporphyrin <300 nmol/24 hours
Uroporphyrin 6–24 nmol/24 hours
δ-Aminolevulinate 8–53 µmol/24 hours
5-Hydroxyindoleacetic acid 10–47 µmol/24 hours
Osmolality 350–1000 mosmol/kg

Faeces
Nitrogen 70–140 mmol/24 hours
Urobilinogen 50–500 µmol/24 hours
Fat (on normal diet) <7 g/24 hours

Answers

Chapter 1 Introduction to pharmacology

1. (d); **2.** (c); **3.** (b); **4.** (c); **5.** (b); **6.** (b); **7.** (d); **8.** (a); **9.** (c); **10.** (b); **11.** (c); **12.** (a); **13.** (d); **14.** (c); **15.** (c)

Chapter 2 How to use pharmaceutical and prescribing reference guides

1. (a); **2.** (a); **3.** (c); **4.** (c); **5.** (a); **6.** (b); **7.** (a); **8.** (a); **9.** (c); **10.** (d)

Chapter 3 Legal and Ethical Issues.

1. (b); **2.** (c); **3.** (c); **4.** (a); **5.** (d); **6.** (d); **7.** (a); **8.** (c); **9.** (c); **10.** (a); **11.** (d); **12.** (d); **13.** (d); **14.** (d); **15.** (d)

Chapter 4 Medicines management and the role of the Paramedic

1. (a); **2.** (c); **3.** (c); **4.** (b); **5.** (b); **6.** (a); **7.** (a); **8.** (b); **9.** (c); **10.** (b); **11.** (b); **12.** (a); **13.** (c); **14.** (a); **15.** (b)

Chapter 5 Pharmacodynamics and Pharmacokinetics

1. (a); **2.** (d); **3.** (c); **4.** (b); **5.** (a); **6.** (d); **7.** (b); **8.** (d); **9.** (a); **10.** (a); **11.** (c); **12.** (a); **13.** (a); **14.** (c); **15.** (a)

Chapter 6 Drug Formulations

1. (b); **2.** (b); **3.** (d); **4.** (b); **5.** (d); **6.** (c); **7.** (d); **8.** (c); **9.** (a); **10.** (c); **11.** (d); **12.** (c); **13.** (a); **14.** (c); **15.** (a)

Chapter 7 Adverse Drug Reactions

1. (a); **2.** (c); **3.** (b); **4.** (c); **5.** (a); **6.** (b); **7.** (a); **8.** (d); **9.** (d); **10.** (a); **11.** (a); **12.** (a); **13.** (c); **14.** (c); **15.** (d)

Chapter 8 Analgesics

1. (a); **2.** (d); **3.** (b); **4.** (d); **5.** (d); **6.** (d); **7.** (b); **8.** (d); **9.** (b); **10.** (b); **11.** (b); **12.** (d); **13.** (c); **14.** (a); **15.** (d)

Chapter 9 Antibacterials

1. (b); **2.** (d); **3.** (b); **4.** (c); **5.** (a); **6.** (d); **7.** (d); **8.** (d); **9.** (a); **10.** (a); **11.** (a); **12.** (b); **13.** (d); **14.** (d); **15.** (b); **16.** (c)

Fundamentals of Pharmacology for Paramedics, First Edition. Edited by Ian Peate, Suzanne Evans, and Lisa Clegg.
© 2022 John Wiley & Sons Ltd. Published 2022 by John Wiley & Sons Ltd.

Chapter 10 Medications used in the cardiovascular system

1. (c); **2.** (b); **3.** (a); **4.** (b); **5.** (b); **6.** (c); **7.** (d); **8.** (b); **9.** (c); **10.** (a); **11.** (a); **12.** (a); **13.** (c); **14.** (c); **15.** (d)

Chapter 11 Medications used in the renal system

1. (c); **2.** (a); **3.** (a); **4.** (d); **5.** (c); **6.** (b); **7.** (d); **8.** (c); **9.** (a); **10.** (c); **11.** (d); **12.** (b); **13.** (a); **14.** (a); **15.** (b)

Chapter 12 Medications and diabetes mellitus

1. (a); **2.** (d); **3.** (a); **4.** (b); **5.** (c); **6.** (b); **7.** (c); **8.** (a); **9.** (a); **10.** (b); **11.** (a)

Chapter 13 Medications used in the respiratory system

1. (b); **2.** (a); **3.** (b); **4.** (d); **5.** (a); **6.** (b); **7.** (a); **8.** (b); **9.** (c); **10.** (d); **11.** (b); **12.** (d); **13.** (b); **14.** (c); **15.** (c)

Chapter 14 Medications used in the gastrointestinal system

1. (a); **2.** (b); **3.** (d); **4.** (a); **5.** (c); **6.** (b); **7.** (d); **8.** (d); **9.** (a); **10.** (d); **11.** (d); **12.** (c); **13.** (d); **14.** (d); **15.** (a)

Chapter 15 Medication and the Nervous System

1. (a); **2.** (b); **3.** (a); **4.** (a); **5.** (b); **6.** (a); **7.** (a); **8.** (d); **9.** (c); **10.** (a); **11.** (d); **12.** (d); **13.** (d); **14.** (b); **15.** (a)

Chapter 16 Medications used in Mental Health

1. (c); **2.** (d); **3.** (b); **4.** (a); **5.** (d); **6.** (a); **7.** (d); **8.** (c); **9.** (b); **10.** (c); **11.** (b); **12.** (a); **13.** (c); **14.** (d); **15.** (b)

Chapter 17 Immunisations

1. (a); **2.** (c); **3.** (d); **4.** (a); **5.** (a); **6.** (c); **7.** (b); **8.** (a); **9.** (b); **10.** (b); **11.** (c); **12.** (c); **13.** (d); **14.** (d); **15.** (b)

Index

Fundamentals of Pharmacology for Paramedics, First Edition. Edited by Ian Peate, Suzanne Evans, and Lisa Clegg.
© 2022 John Wiley & Sons Ltd. Published 2022 by John Wiley & Sons Ltd.